Chinese

with Comm

MW00453288

Chinese Herbs

with Common Foods

Recipes for Health and Healing

Henry C. Lu, Ph.D.

Principal of the International College of Traditional Chinese Medicine, Vancouver, Canada

KODANSHA INTERNATIONAL

Tokyo • New York • London

This book is presented as an aid to understanding the theories and practices underlying the use of traditional Chinese herbs and is not intended to replace medical consultation and treatment. Please consult a doctor or other appropriate health professional for any problems you may be having. Neither the author nor publisher may be found liable for any adverse effects or consequences resulting from the use of any of the advice or preparations in this book.

Distributed in the United States by Kodansha America, Inc., 114 Fifth Avenue, New York, N.Y. 10011, and in the United Kingdom and continental Europe by Kodansha Europe Ltd., 95 Aldwych, London WC2B 4JF. Published by Kodansha International Ltd., 17-14 Otowa 1-chome, Bunkyo-ku, Tokyo 112-8652, and Kodansha America, Inc.

Copyright © 1997 by Kodansha International Ltd.
All rights reserved. Printed in Japan.
First edition, 1997
97 98 99 10 9 8 7 6 5 4 3 2 1
ISBN 4-7700-2074-0

Library of Congress Cataloging-in-Publication Data

A catalog record for this book is available from the Library of Congress

Contents

Preface

Foods and herbs are similar and also different. They are similar because they all have properties and actions; they are different because foods taste good, are relatively mild in action, and can be consumed every day, while herbs have an unpleasant taste, are fairly drastic in action, and cannot be consumed for a prolonged period of time.

In daily life, we eat foods to maintain good health. We become sick if we keep eating unbalanced foods. For example, if we continue to consume pungent foods excessively and for a lengthy period, we may perspire too much and develop eye disease; if we continue to consume sweet foods, we may accumulate an excessive quantity of water in the body. When we do get sick, we may eat balanced foods to cure ourselves, which is called a food cure. Since foods are relatively mild in action, consumption of foods alone may not be sufficient to cure disease; we may need to consume herbs to reinforce the effects of foods, which is why the Chinese have developed a system of "cooking with herbs for health." This system has been in existence in China from time immemorial, most probably dating back to many centuries before Christ.

If foods are relatively mild in action, and for that reason insufficient to cure disease in many cases, why don't we simply consume herbs as a cure? In point of fact, the Chinese have been consuming herbs for twenty or thirty centuries, which is how the system of Chinese herbology developed. But herbs are herbs. They don't taste good; we don't want to eat them if we can avoid it. In other words, foods taste good, but they are not strong enough to cure disease; herbs are strong enough to cure disease, but they don't taste good. It would be nice to enjoy the delicious taste of foods and benefit from the strong effects of herbs simultaneously when we are sick. It was to fulfill this common human desire that the Chinese developed a system of cooking with herbs for health. When we cook herbs with foods to eat at meals, they are used only in small amounts in comparison to other ingredients, so that we don't even know that we are consuming them—their unpleasant taste is masked by the delicious flavor of foods.

Chinese medicine is fundamentally different from Western medicine in its approach to disease. In the latter, all individuals with the same ailment are treated similarly. Ten people with hypertension are treated with the same drugs to cure it. In Chinese medicine, however, individuals suffering a disease like hypertension may be treated quite differently according to the type or syndrome of hypertension.

This book contains many hundreds of foods and herbs with pertinent information on each of them, including their properties, classes, actions, and indications. Diseases are classified into types to be treated differently. Foods and herbs are recommended for each type of disease according to Chinese experience, followed by sample recipes to cure it. You can use the foods and herbs listed under each type of disease to create your own recipes to cure your conditions. For this reason, this book is recommended not only for those who want to overcome illness and stay in good health, but also for the creative and curious who are interested in discovering the Chinese system of curative cooking with herbs.

PART I

PROPERTIES, ACTIONS, AND COOKING OF FOODS AND HERBS

CHAPTER 1 Terminology and Basic Theory of Chinese Medicine

Each discipline makes use of a substantial number of special terms, and Chinese medicine is no exception. Most terms will be unfamiliar to a layman; in fact, many of them cannot be easily translated using layman's language. Therefore, before you begin to read this book, it may prove helpful to understand the special terminology used and what it means in Chinese medicine, as well as the basic theory behind Chinese medicine. The basic intent of this book, however, is not merely to teach you the theory of Chinese medicine, but more importantly to enable you to identify your physical condition and problems and to cook herbs and foods for good health.

There are four important terms used in Chinese medicine which should be distinguished from each other.

Disease

A disease in Western medicine is also called a disease in Chinese medicine. Some of the diseases you will encounter in this book are: fascioliasis (infection of the body caused by a liver fluke), ecthyma (an infection of the skin marked by shallow lesions), erysipelas (acute febrile disease with localized inflammation of skin), dysphagia (difficulty in swallowing), chyluria (presence of chyle in the urine), hemiplegia (paralysis of one side of the body), hepatic ascites (accumulation of fluid in the liver), hydatid disease (the disease produced by the tapeworm), parotitis (inflammation of the parotid gland), pulmonary gangrene (death of tissue in the lungs), otitis media (inflammation of the middle ear), scrofula (tuberculosis of the lymph nodes), secretagogue (an agent that stimulates secreting organs), schistosomiasis (a parasitic disease caused by an infestation of blood flukes of schistosoma), stomatitis (inflammation of the mouth), tinea (any fungal skin disease), and tracheitis (an inflammation of the trachea).

Symptom

A symptom refers to an abnormal change in the body and its functions. Some of the symptoms you will encounter in this book are: abdominal pain, headache, diarrhea, hiccups, dizziness, constipation, stomachache, blood in urine, diminished urination, nosebleed, and shortage of milk in nursing mothers. In Western medicine, a symptom indicates disease. For example, pains over the lower right ribs or a little lower are a symptom which indicates the possibility of a disease of the gallbladder.

Sign

In Western medicine, signs are often considered "objective symptoms," such as shaking of the head and vomiting, but in Chinese medicine, signs refer to a manifestation of a particular syndrome, such as poor appetite, indigestion, and skinniness, all of which point to a stomach condition. Symptoms and signs may not always be distinguishable, because they may overlap in some cases. Furthermore, a sign need not be a symptom in that it may rule out the existence of a syndrome. For example, "no bad breath," "normal bowel movement," "no pain or swelling in the gums" are not symptoms at all but signs; in the presence of such signs, it is reasonable to suppose that the patient is not afflicted with the syndrome called hot stomach. The Chinese also use some peculiar words to describe a sign. One of them is "turbid" (or "muddy"). This word is often used to describe the look of urine that is not clear, just like turbid water, and is also used to describe the look of sputum that is not clear or watery.

Indeed, signs form the very foundation of diagnosis in Chinese medicine. Chinese physicians are very particular about signs, because only signs will tell them what syndrome is involved and enable them to suggest the appropriate treatment. For example, a doctor of Chinese medicine will not only ask the patient about urination in general, but in great detail. How frequently a patient passes urine, the quantity of urine discharged during urination, how difficult it is to discharge urine, any occurrence of drops in urine, the color of urine—whether it is reddish, yellowish, clear, turbid—all of these are important. When a patient has a nosebleed, the doctor will want to know about the color of the blood, whether it looks very dark or light red, fresh looking or old looking, whether there are blood clots, and the timing of bleeding.

Syndrome

A syndrome may be described as "a specific combination of disease and symptoms" in layman's terms. It refers to a fundamental condition of the body to be corrected by treatment, indicated by a group of symptoms and signs. There are a total of over three hundred common syndromes in Chinese medicine. For example, "stomach fire" is one of the six syndromes responsible for hyperthyroidism. It is indicated by a group of symptoms and signs including chronic thirst for cold drinks, a bitter taste in the mouth, bleeding and painful gums, toothache, sore throat, headache, nosebleed, constipation, and stomachache with burning sensations. For a patient with hyperthyroidism, overactive thyroid is the chief complaint to be dealt with, but the treatment should be aimed at correcting stomach fire, which is responsible for hyperthyroidism. However, six syndromes are possibly responsible for hyperthyroidism, so how does the doctor of Chinese medicine know which syndrome to treat? The doctor will have to go through six different groups of signs and symptoms to determine which syndrome is involved, and treat that particular syndrome accordingly.

Thus, in Chinese medicine, a doctor will treat syndromes, not diseases or symptoms or signs; for that reason, the objective of diagnosis is to establish the syndrome involved in each clinical case and treat it accordingly. Signs are the most crucial factor in identifying the syndrome, so much so that signs are spelled out in great detail. The following are a few examples:

Sputum may be divided into yellowish and sticky sputum, called hot sputum because it is due to heat or "hot syndrome"; white and clear sputum, called cold sputum because it is due to cold; or thin and green sputum, called wind sputum because it is due to wind. There are about ten different types of sputum caused by ten different syndromes.

Again, there are different types of thirst. Under normal circumstances, when a person is thirsty, he or she will want to drink water—the more thirst, the more water. But this may not be the case when one is sick. Thirst as a sign may be further divided into thirst with a desire to drink cold water, which is due to internal heat; thirst with a desire to drink hot water, which is due to spleen deficiency; thirst with no desire to drink water, which is due to damp heat; thirst at night, which is due to yin deficiency with abundant fire. There are about a dozen types of thirst caused by different syndromes.

If in reading through the signs for a given syndrome, you come across signs that you do not comprehend, chances are you have never experienced such signs. Also, you may come across some odd signs such as "too lazy to talk" (which is a Chinese phrase to describe someone who does not want to waste energy in talking) and "love of sighing" (which is a Chinese phrase to describe someone who sighs frequently).

The terminology and basic theory of Chinese medicine may be divided into the following four broad categories: climatic pathogens, classifications of symptoms, energy and body fluids, and internal organs.

Six Climatic Pathogens That Cause Disease

What causes disease? In Western medicine, germs and viruses are the primary culprits, but in Chinese medicine, there are six climatic pathogens considered as the primary causes of disease: wind, cold, heat and summer heat, dampness, dryness, and fire. When a climatic pathogen causes a disease or symptom, it becomes the syndrome responsible for that disease or symptom. As an example, when wind causes arthritis, the wind syndrome is responsible for the arthritis.

Wind

How does wind cause disease? Wind is a natural phenomenon in the atmosphere. It is air in motion, and we need it to maintain good health. When we feel hot, for example, we obviously need wind to cool our body; we leave our windows open in hot summer, because we need fresh air that will be brought in by the wind. Therefore, as natural climatic energy, wind is essential to human health. But wind can be a good or bad influence on our health, depending on the circumstances. When wind causes an imbalance, it becomes harmful to the human body, and is regarded as a hostile climatic energy to be avoided.

How do we know that a specific disease is caused by wind? Chinese physicians in the past have analyzed the nature of wind very carefully, and have found a few distinct characteristics.

First, wind tends to move upward and stay high; when wind causes disease, it often attacks the upper region of the human body to cause such symptoms as headache, sore throat, or cough—common symptoms in a bad cold. Second, wind moves fast and constantly changes. When a person is under attack by wind, it causes symptoms that move from one place to another, undergoing rapid change. For example, a type of rheumatism characterized by pain that wanders from one part of the body to another is caused by wind.

Wind syndrome (1)

There are quite a number of signs for this syndrome. To treat the wind syndrome, it is necessary to disperse or stop wind. Diseases and symptoms treated under this syndrome include arthritis, rheumatoid arthritis, and eczema.

Wind cold syndrome (2)

Wind cold refers to wind and cold attacking the body simultaneously. Common signs are lack of perspiration, cough, diarrhea, aversion to cold and wind, loss of voice, pain in the joints, and stuffed nose. To treat this syndrome, it is necessary to disperse wind and remove cold from the body. Diseases and symptoms caused by wind include amenorrhea (absent period), common cold and flu, cough, and dysmenorrhea (period pain).

Wind heat/wind hot syndrome (3)

Wind heat refers to wind and heat attacking the body simultaneously. Common signs are cough, headache, dizziness, aversion to wind and heat, thirst, toothache, and yellow urine. Diseases and symptoms treated under this syndrome include common cold and flu, cough, and ringing in the ears and deafness.

Wind warm superficial syndrome (4)

In this syndrome, the wind attacks the superficial region of the body (not the internal organs, which are in the deep region) to cause warm symptoms such as fever. Common signs are cough, fever, aversion to wind, headache, and thirst. For effective treatment, it is necessary to induce perspiration with pungent and cool herbs. Pneumonia is disease to be treated under this syndrome.

Cold

Cold is the dominant climatic energy in winter. There are three ways in which cold may attack the body. First of all, it may attack only the superficial region of the body, causing aversion to cold, fever without perspiration, headache with stiff neck, pain in the body, cough and asthma, pain in the bones, severe pain in a fixed region, and/or difficulty in moving the affected parts.

Second, cold may attack the deep region to cause pale complexion, fatigue, cold sensations particularly in the limbs which may be relieved by heat, discharge of watery stools or diarrhea in the early morning, abdominal pain, and/or puffiness in the lower limbs.

Third, cold may penetrate the body to attack the internal region directly, causing shivering with cold, numbness of the four limbs, spasmodic cold pain, slow and feeble breathing, cold air coming from the mouth and nose, and skin turning a purplish hue.

Cold syndrome (5)

Common signs of the cold syndrome are presented in the above description of cold. To treat this syndrome, it is necessary to expel cold from the body. Diseases and symptoms treated under this syndrome include arteriosclerosis (hardening of blood vessels), arthritis and rheumatoid arthritis, gallstones, and hiccups.

Heat, Summer Heat

Heat and summer heat are the dominant climatic energies in summer, but heat can occur in all seasons, while summer heat refers to heat in the summer only. When the body is under the attack of heat or summer heat, a person will experience high fever, thirst, and profuse perspiration. Summer heat is most harmful to body fluids because it sucks moisture and water from the body, which explains why the patient will experience extreme thirst, fatigue due to lack of body fluids, dry mouth and lips, constipation due to intestinal dryness, and scanty urine due to the shortage of water in the body.

Heat/hot syndrome (6)

To treat the hot syndrome, it is necessary to clear heat from the body. Diseases and symptoms treated under this syndrome include arthritis, rheumatoid arthritis, common acne, gallstones, and hiccups.

Summer heat syndrome (7)

To treat the summer heat syndrome, it is necessary to clear summer heat from the body. The common cold and flu are the symptoms to be treated under the summer heat syndrome.

Dampness

Dampness is the dominant climatic energy in late summer. Early summer rains make the ground very damp, and as summer progresses and the weather begins to cool, moisture on the ground fails to dry as quickly as in early and midsummer. Someone who walks in the rain, sleeps on the damp ground, lives in a damp environment, or wears wet clothes or swims a lot becomes an easy target for dampness, and may develop blisters on the skin and experience retention of water with puffiness and watery stools.

Dampness tends to flow into the joints like water to cause "damp arthritis" and "damp rheumatism," in which the patient often experiences an increase in symptoms when humidity is high. Dampness is heavy and moves slowly, which is why diseases caused by dampness take longer to heal. In this respect, dampness is the opposite of wind, which moves fast. When dampness causes pain, as in damp rheumatism and damp arthritis, the pain always stays in the same spot. As time goes on, swelling will occur due to an accumulation of dampness in the affected region. When dampness causes headaches, the person feels dull pain in the head and becomes sleepy, as if the head were wrapped up in a wet towel.

Dampness is heavy, with a tendency to move downward and attack the lower part of the body, causing swelling of the lower limbs. Dampness and heat often work together as a formidable team to cause discharge of yellowish urine, frequent but difficult urination, vaginal discharge with an offensive smell, and/or thirst but no desire to drink.

Summer heat and dampness may team up to attack the body in summer, causing congested chest, nausea with a desire to vomit, poor appetite, high fever, mental depression, and/or red complexion. During the summer when a patient feels thirsty but has no desire to drink, a physician of Chinese medicine may conclude the patient is suffering an attack of summer heat and dampness. This may occur in seasons other than summer due to a combination of dampness and heat (other than summer heat), in which case it is customarily called "damp heat" or "superficial damp heat" instead of "summer heat and dampness."

Why do summer heat and dampness team up to attack the body? This is not only because summer heat is the dominant climatic energy in summer, but also because there is high humidity in summer, and on top of that, people tend to consume more water and beverages in summer, thus becoming easy targets of dampness.

Dampness syndrome (8)

Diseases and symptoms treated under this syndrome include arthritis, rheumatoid arthritis, and cirrhosis.

Summer heat and dampness syndrome (9)

To treat the summer heat and dampness syndrome, it is necessary to simultaneously clear summer heat and eliminate dampness from the body. Gastroenteritis is a disease to be treated under this syndrome.

Damp heat (superficial damp heat) syndrome (10)
Damp heat refers to dampness and heat attacking the superficial region of the body. Common signs are excessive perspiration, diarrhea, thirst with no desire to drink, excessive vaginal discharge, and reddish, scanty urine. To treat damp heat, it is necessary to clear heat and eliminate dampness from the body simultaneously. Diseases and symptoms treated under this syndrome include diarrhea, diminished urination, dysentery, hepatitis, high cholesterol, seminal emission and premature ejaculation, blood in urine, cirrhosis (a chronic disease of the liver characterized by useless scar tissue), hemorrhoids (piles), and prostatitis (inflammation of the prostate gland).

Cold dampness syndrome (11)
Cold dampness means the body is under attack by cold and dampness simultaneously. Common signs are lack of perspiration, diarrhea, cold sensations, cough, headache, and pain in the joints. Diseases and symptoms treated under this syndrome include: diarrhea, dysmenorrhea (period pain), gastroenteritis (inflammation of the stomach and intestinal tract), irritable bowels, premenstrual syndrome (PMS or premenstrual tension), and vomiting.

Dryness

Dryness is the dominant climatic energy in autumn when there is low humidity in the atmosphere, which is why in autumn people are more likely to develop dry cough, sore throat with dryness, dry skin, dry nasal passages, thirst, scanty urine, and constipation with dry stools. Dryness can harm the lungs more easily than other organs. Unlike other pathogenic energies that attack the body through the skin and muscles, dryness attacks the body through the nose and the mouth, and for that reason renders the lungs most susceptible to an attack of dryness among the internal organs. Since dryness likes to attack the lungs, smoking is particularly harmful in making the lungs even drier.

When dryness originates from the internal conditions of the body itself, it is called internal dryness, mostly associated with an excessive consumption of alcohol and spices. The common symptoms arising from internal dryness are excessive perspiration, vomiting, chronic diarrhea, excessive bleeding, and chronic other ailments, all of which take a heavy toll in body fluids. In addition, internal dryness causes dry skin, dry, damaged hair, night sweats, unusual hunger, constipation with dry stools, discharge of scanty urine, poor vision, dry throat with cracked lips, and sleeplessness.

Fire

Fire is one of the odd terms in Chinese medicine that puzzles many a Western reader. The human body needs fire to maintain normal body temperature, just like a room needs heat to be warm; hence, fire is essential to human health and is called friendly fire. Fire as a hostile energy originates from the other five climatic energies and emotions. The Chinese use such phrases as "anger transforming into fire," "wind transforming into fire," or "dryness transforming into fire" to mean that "anger (or wind or dryness) produces heat, which transforms into fire, causing harm to the body."

When internal heat transforms into fire, it causes cracked lips, extreme thirst, insomnia, backache, cough, and asthma. The nature of fire is to burn upward and spread quickly. In severe cases, it may cause high fever, severe headache, coma, vomiting of blood, and/or discharge of blood from the mouth. In addition, fire opens up the pores all over the body, leading to profuse perspiration. Together with bleeding, vomiting, and diarrhea, there is a heavy toll in body fluids. Similarly, fire's extreme heat necessarily speeds up the rate of metabolism so that the body consumes more energy than usual, reducing the quantity left in the body.

When extreme heat turns into fire, it may produce toxic effects, called "toxic fire," which can "burn up" each and every part of the body to cause infections and inflammation, including infection of the eyes, throat, kidneys (nephritis), and urinary system, and inflammation of the lungs (pneumonia), boils, and carbuncles.

Deficiency fire syndrome (12)

Deficiency fire refers to an attack of fire on a person when the person is in a state of yin deficiency. Common signs are dry throat, hot sensations in the body, low-grade fever, ringing in the ears, insomnia, and toothache. Diseases and symptoms treated under this syndrome include hyperthyroidism (a condition caused by excessive secretion in the thyroid gland), impotence in men, pulmonary tuberculosis, and seminal emission or premature ejaculation.

Hot fire syndrome (13)

Hot fire means fire attacking the body to cause hot symptoms. Common signs are bleeding gums, bad breath, mouth cankers, and discharge of yellowish urine. To treat this syndrome, it is necessary to eliminate fire with cold herbs. Eczema is a disease treated under this syndrome.

Eight Principal Classifications of Symptoms

The eight principal classifications of symptoms are: yin, yang, superficial, deep, cold, hot, deficient, and excessive. Thus, a symptom may be either yin or yang, superficial or deep, cold or hot, deficient or excessive. This is why in Chinese medicine, we often use the terms "yin symptoms," "yang symptoms," "cold symptoms," "hot symptoms," "superficial symptoms," "deep symptoms," "deficient symptoms," and "excessive symptoms."

Yin vs. Yang Symptoms

Yin and yang symptoms represent two opposing forces or qualities in a relationship. All concepts and phenomena in the universe can be classified into yin and yang. For example, in terms of objects, the sun is yang and the moon is yin, heaven is yang and earth is yin, fire is yang and water is yin; in terms of movements, motion is yang and being at rest is yin. A chronic symptom is yin and an acute symptom is yang. Yin and yang are often used to denote energy. Yang energy is warm and travels on the body's surface to defend the body and keep it warm; yin energy travels inside the body to keep the body moist. All internal organs have both yin energy and yang energy. For example, yang energy of the lungs keeps the lungs warm and active while yin energy of the lungs keeps the lungs moist and stable.

Superficial vs. Deep Symptoms

Superficial and deep refer to the region in which a symptom occurs; in general, a symptom of the skin and muscles is a superficial one, a symptom involving internal organs is a deep one. A superficial symptom is most frequently observed at an early stage. It is normally caused by the six climatic energies mentioned earlier. On the other hand, a deep symptom is most frequently observed at its interim or later stage. Pain in the joints is a superficial symptom, because it does not involve any particular internal organ, but pain in the heart is a deep one, because of the deep region where the heart lies.

Cold vs. Hot Symptoms

A cold symptom is caused by cold climatic energy and is intensifed by the presence of coldness. A hot symptom is caused by hot climatic energy and is intensified by the presence of heat. However, a hot symptom is not identical with high body temperature as in a fever, because high body temperature is merely one possible aspect of a hot symptom (not all cases of hot symptoms display a high body temperature). And, of course, a patient may not have a hot symptom even though there is a fever.

Dry heat syndrome (14)

Dry heat means the body is under attack by dryness and heat simultaneously. Common signs are constipation, dry cough, and thirst. To treat this syndrome, it is necessary to moisten the internal region and clear heat from the body. Cough is a common symptom treated under this syndrome.

Excessive heat syndrome (15)

Excessive heat refers to an attack by heat while the body is not in deficiency. Common signs are pain in the throat, menstrual pain, high fever, thirst with craving for cold drinks, and constipation. To treat this syndrome, it is necessary to clear heat from the body. Abdominal pain is a common symptom treated under this syndrome.

Toxic-heat-penetrating-into-the-deep-region syndrome (16)

This syndrome refers to heat penetration into the deep region, affecting internal organs, the large intestine in particular. Common signs are abdominal pain, severe headache, diarrhea, and constipation. To treat this syndrome, it is necessary to clear heat from the internal region with cold herbs. Dysentery is a disease treated under this syndrome.

Internal heat syndrome (17)

Internal heat refers to an accumulation of heat in the internal region. Common signs are cold limbs, hot sensations in the palms of the hands or soles of the feet, and yellowish urine. To treat this syndrome, it is necessary to clear heat from the internal region with cold herbs. Amenorrhea (absent period) is treated under this syndrome.

Deficient vs. Excessive Symptoms

In general, a deficient symptom refers to one arising from a weak condition of the body, whereas an excessive symptom refers to one caused by climatic factors. A chronic symptom is a deficient symptom, because it most likely involves a weak physical condition. A new and acute symptom is an excessive symptom, because it is most likely due to an attack by climatic factors. The following are syndromes associated with deficient or excessive symptoms.

Deficiency of yin and yang syndrome (18)

This syndrome means both yin and yang are deficient. Common signs are cold sensations in the body, cold limbs, fatigue, speaking in a low or feeble voice, dizziness, palpitation, and excessive perspiration. To treat this syndrome, it is necessary to tone yin and yang. Diseases and symptoms treated under this syndrome include coronary heart disease (a condition caused by decreased flow of blood to the heart muscles), dizziness, and prostatitis (inflammation of the prostate gland).

Deficient yin with excessive yang syndrome (19)

This syndrome means yin is deficient but yang is excessive. Common signs are excessive sex drive in men, insomnia, and jumpiness. To treat this syndrome, it is necessary to tone yin and sedate yang, in other words, make yin stronger and yang weaker. Diseases and symptoms treated under this syndrome include arteriosclerosis (hardening of blood vessels), dizziness, and hypertension.

Deficiency cold (deficient and cold) syndrome (20)

This syndrome means pathogenic cold attacks the body while the body is deficient. Common signs are abdominal pain, excessive perspiration, cold limbs, pale complexion, short breath, and menstrual pain. To treat this syndrome, it is necessary to tone the energy and expel cold. Diseases and symptoms treated under this syndrome include abdominal pain, gastroptosis (falling of the stomach), stomachache, and infertility in women.

Yang deficiency (yang energy deficiency) syndrome (21)
Common signs are excessive perspiration, cold limbs, urine of pale color, diarrhea, constipation, fatigue, edema, and excessive sleepiness. To treat this syndrome, it is necessary to tone yang energy. Diseases and symptoms treated under this syndrome include chronic fatigue syndrome, hiccups, and vomiting.

Yin deficiency (yin energy deficiency) syndrome (22)
Common signs are dizziness, constipation, insomnia, night sweats, fatigue, pain in the throat, and toothache. To treat this syndrome, it is necessary to tone yin energy. Diseases and symptoms treated under this syndrome include chronic fatigue syndrome, cough, hiccups, infertility in women, stomachache, and vomiting.

Yin deficiency with abundant fire syndrome (23)
Fire attacks the body while yin energy in the body is deficient. Common signs are dry throat, toothache, night sweats, coughing blood, and fever. To treat this syndrome, it is necessary to tone yin energy and sedate fire. Diseases and symptoms treated under this syndrome include arrhythmia (irregular heartbeat), bronchiectasis (dilation of bronchi), and prostatitis (inflammation of the prostate gland).

Energy, Blood, Body Fluids, and Phlegm

Energy

Energy is called "Qi" (pronounced *chi*) in Chinese medicine. It is a unique term and often mystifying. Energy is the motor of all human activities. If we ask why the heart is able to contract, we say it is because the heart has energy in it; if the contraction of the heart stops, we say it is because there is no energy in the heart. Although we do not see energy as such, we do know whether it is working or not, like electricity. When energy is disordered, it can cause various types of observable symptoms. Syndromes related to energy are generally divided into energy deficiency, energy stagnation (or energy congestion), and energy upsurging (energy rebellion).

Energy deficiency syndrome (24)
Energy deficiency refers to functional decline in internal organs and low resistance of the organism to attack by climatic factors. It may be seen in a chronic symptom, weakness due to aging, or during the recuperating stage of an acute symptom. The general signs of energy deficiency include white or pale complexion, fatigue, weak-

ness, low spirits, shortness of breath, speaking in a low and feeble voice, and excessive perspiration. To treat energy deficiency, it is necessary to tone up energy.

Diseases and symptoms treated under this syndrome include chronic fatigue syndrome, constipation, diminished urination, leukorrhea (vaginal discharge), menorrhagia (excessive menstrual bleeding), and metrorrhagia (uterine bleeding).

Energy stagnation syndrome (25)

Energy stagnation means energy fails to travel smoothly throughout the body. Various types of factors, including emotional stress, irregular eating, attack by climatic energies, external injuries, etc., can impair energy circulation to cause congestion. The common signs of energy stagnation are pain and swelling, such as chest pain and swelling of breasts in women. To treat energy stagnation, it is necessary to promote the flow of energy and break up stagnated energy. Diseases and symptoms treated under this syndrome include abdominal pain, amenorrhea (absent period), constipation, dysmenorrhea (period pain), irritable bowel, and metrorrhagia (uterine bleeding).

Energy upsurging syndrome (26)

Energy upsurging means energy is moving upward instead of downward as it should. This applies to the lungs and stomach in particular. Energy in the stomach should move downward; if it moves upward, it is called upsurging energy of the stomach, which causes nausea and vomiting. Energy in the lungs should also move downward; if it moves upward, it is called upsurging energy of the lungs and causes coughing and hiccups. In a broad sense, energy upsurging applies to any movement of energy that is contrary to normal patterns, which is why it is also called energy uprising or energy rebellion. For another example, the energy in the liver may act up and move fiercely to the top of head, which is called energy upsurging of the liver.

Deficiency of energy and yin syndrome (27)

Four substances in the body are blood, energy, yin, and yang. Although yin means yin energy, it is different from energy itself. Because blood and energy work together, yin energy and yang energy work together. This syndrome means both energy and yin are deficient. Common signs are constipation, dizziness, dry cough, fatigue, stomachache, thirst, and poor appetite. To treat this syndrome, it is necessary to tone both energy and yin. Diseases and symptoms treated under this syndrome include arrhythmia (irregular heartbeat), hyperthyroidism, hypotension (low blood pressure), and pulmonary tuberculosis.

Blood

Blood is a product of water and grains undergoing energy transformation. Put another way, energy transforms water and grains into blood. Syndromes related to the blood may be divided into blood deficiency, blood coagulation (blood stasis), hot blood, cold blood, dry blood, and so on.

Blood deficiency syndrome (28)

Blood deficiency refers to a shortage of blood due to loss or insufficient production. The common signs of blood deficiency are pale complexion, light finger and/or toenail color, dizziness, and constipation. To treat blood deficiency, it is necessary to tone the blood. Diseases and symptoms treated under this syndrome include amenorrhea (absent period), chronic fatigue, constipation, dysmenorrhea (period pain), eczema (a cutaneous inflammatory skin disease with erythema, papular vesicles, or scales), oligomenorrhea (scanty or infrequent menstrual flow), osteoporosis (reduction in the mass of bone), and shortage of milk in nursing mothers.

Blood coagulation syndrome (29)

Blood coagulation refers to an impairment in blood circulation. Common signs are acute, mostly pricking pain in a fixed region, pain that gets worse on pressure, local swelling with lumps, and pain in the lower abdomen before a period. To treat this syndrome, it is necessary to "activate" the blood. Diseases and symptoms treated under this syndrome include abdominal pain, amenorrhea (absent period), diminished urination, dysmenorrhea (period pain), metrorrhagia (uterine bleeding), oligomenorrhea (scanty or infrequent menstrual flow), osteoporosis, psoriasis (a skin disease with silvery scales but no itching), and stomachache.

Hot blood syndrome (30)

The blood, like anything else, can get too hot. Common signs of hot blood are red swelling, bleeding, skin eruptions, premature period, excessive menstrual flow of bright-red color, mental depression, chronic thirst, reddish urine, and fever. To treat hot blood, it is necessary to cool the blood. Diseases and symptoms treated under this syndrome include hemorrhoids, infertility in women, menorrhagia (excessive menstrual bleeding), metrorrhagia (uterine bleeding), premature gray hair, and psoriasis.

Cold blood (internal cold) syndrome (31)

This syndrome means the internal region is cold. Common signs are cold limbs, diarrhea, and aversion to cold. To treat this syndrome, it is necessary to warm up the internal region. Diseases and symptoms treated under this syndrome include oligomenorrhea (scanty or infrequent menstrual flow).

Dry blood (internal dryness) syndrome (32)

This syndrome means an exhaustion of internal body fluids. Common signs are constipation with dry stools, dry skin, dry throat, fatigue, night sweats, and thirst. To treat this syndrome, it is necessary to moisten the internal region and tone yin. Psoriasis is treated under this syndrome.

Deficiency of energy and blood syndrome (33)

Both energy and blood are deficient in this syndrome. Common signs are blurred vision, dizziness, insomnia, low voice, pale complexion, and palpitation. To treat this syndrome, it is necessary to tone both energy and blood. Diseases and symptoms under this syndrome include high cholesterol, blood in urine, dizziness, infertility in women, nephritis (inflammation of the kidney), and oligomenorrhea (scanty or infrequent menstrual flow).

Energy congestion and blood coagulation syndrome (34)

Energy congestion means energy fails to flow smoothly, while blood coagulation means blood stagnates and fails to circulate smoothly. Common signs of this syndrome are blood clots in menstrual flow, congested chest, and abdominal distention. To treat this syndrome, it is necessary to disperse the energy and blood to make them circulate optimally again. Diseases and symptoms treated under this syndrome include prostatitis (inflammation of the prostate gland), Alzheimer's disease (a chronic mental disorder normally attacking people aged 40 to 60 and over), coronary heart disease, hepatitis, premenstrual syndrome (PMS or premenstrual tension), simple obesity, urinary stones, and arrhythmia (irregular heartbeat).

Body Fluids

Body fluids refer to the water in the body under normal circumstances. The functions of body fluids are to lubricate internal organs, muscles, skin, hair, membranes and cavities, and the joints, as well as to moisten and nourish the brain and marrow, the bones, and other body parts. Body fluids may be further divided into clear fluids and turbid fluids (also called muddy fluids). Clear fluids are spread in the muscles and membranes to moisten the muscles, the skin and hair, and the cavities of four of the five senses, namely, the eyes, the ears, the mouth, and the nose. Sweat and urine are products of clear fluids. Turbid fluids are spread in the internal organs to nourish them as well as the brain, marrow, and bones. Turbid fluids also lubricate the joints and nourish the muscles.

Syndromes of body fluids may be divided into "harmed fluids" and exhausted fluids (or "harmed yin").

Harmed fluids syndrome (35)

"Harmed fluids" is due to a temporary excessive consumption of body fluids that results in a reduction in the watering and moistening functions. Primary signs are chronic thirst, dry skin, dry stools, and short streams of urination with scanty urine.

Exhausted fluids syndrome (36)

Exhausted fluids, or "harmed yin," indicates a severe shortage of body fluids. It is more severe than harmed fluids. The common signs include a general deterioration in the whole body, accompanied by widespread dryness.

Phlegm/Sputum

Phlegm/sputum syndrome (37)

Production of phlegm can be traced back not only to the inability of the lungs to expand and clean the air inhaled, but also to the inability of the spleen to adequately transport and distribute body fluids, resulting in the accumulation of water to become phlegm that causes such symptoms as coughing. This is why there is a saying about phlegm in Chinese medicine that "the spleen produces phlegm and the lungs store it away." Leukorrhea (vaginal discharge) is a symptom treated under this syndrome.

Damp phlegm syndrome (38)

Damp phlegm means presence of sputum due to an accumulation of excessive dampness in the body. Common signs are coughing out copious, whitish, watery phlegm, dizziness, chest pain, excessive sleeping, hiccups, and vomiting. To treat this syndrome, it is necessary to remove dampness from the body and transform phlegm (make phlegm disappear). Diseases and symptoms treated under this syndrome include amenorrhea (absent period), arrhythmia (irregular heartbeat), cough, goiter, infertility in women, menorrhagia (excessive menstrual bleeding), oligomenorrhea (scanty or infrequent menstrual flow), ringing in the ears and deafness, and vomiting.

Hot phlegm syndrome (39)

Hot phlegm (or hot sputum) means presence of phlegm due to an accumulation of excessive heat in the body. Common signs are hard, yellowish phlegm in lumps, blood in sputum, insomnia, coughing out yellowish phlegm, wheezing, and fever. To treat this syndrome, it is necessary to clear heat and transform sputum. Alzheimer's disease is treated under this syndrome.

Internal phlegm syndrome (40)

Internal phlegm means that dampness in the spleen has become sputum. Common signs are obesity with poor appetite, secretion of excessive saliva in the mouth, and fatigue. To treat this syndrome, it is necessary to tone spleen energy and dry dampness. Simple obesity is a symptom treated under this syndrome.

Sputum congestion syndrome (41)

Sputum congestion means sputum gets congested in a particular internal region. Common signs are chest congestion, chest pain, and the subjective sensation of something getting stuck in the throat. To treat this syndrome, it is necessary to promote energy circulation and dissolve congestion. Diseases and symptoms treated under this syndrome include arteriosclerosis (hardening of blood vessels), metrorrhagia (uterine bleeding), and morning sickness.

Sputum congestion and blood coagulation syndrome (42)

Common signs include the signs of sputum congestion and those of blood coagulation. Since this syndrome is a combination of two syndromes, both should be treated simultaneously. Alzheimer's disease is treated under this syndrome.

Sputum energy heat (sputum heat obstructing the lungs) syndrome (43)

This syndrome refers to hot sputum obstructing the lungs. Common signs are coughing and panting; copious yellowish, sticky sputum; fever; and congested chest. To treat this syndrome, it is necessary to clear heat and transform sputum. Pneumonia is the disease to be treated under this syndrome.

Sputum fire syndrome (44)

When hot sputum bursts into fire, it is called sputum fire. Common signs are palpitation, headache, ringing in the ears, hiccups, dizziness, belching, and hunger with no appetite. To treat this syndrome, it is necessary to clear heat and transform sputum. Hyperthyroidism and insomnia are the disease and symptom to be treated under this syndrome.

Internal Organs

There are a total of twelve internal organs in Chinese medicine, divided into yin and yang organs. The six yin organs are called viscera, the six yang organs are called bowels. Yin organs and yang organs are formed into six pairs as follows: 1) the heart (yin) paired with the small intestine (yang), 2) the liver (yin) paired with the gallbladder (yang), 3) the lungs (yin) paired with the large intestine (yang), 4) the kidneys (yin) paired with the bladder (yang), 5) the pericardium (yin) paired with the *sanjiao* (yang). *Sanjiao* means the triple cavity—the upper cavity (thoracic), the middle cavity (abdominal), and the lower cavity (pelvic)—and is treated as an internal organ also. The following are the twelve organs and their associated syndromes.

Heart

The heart is the master of the human body and in control of human activities; it is in charge of various parts of the body and coordinates the functions of other internal organs. The heart is also the master of spirits, which includes mental condition, consciousness, thought, etc. The next twelve syndromes are associated with the heart.

Heart blood deficiency syndrome (45)

Blood deficiency of the heart means insufficient blood in the heart. Common signs are palpitation, depression, insomnia, dream-filled sleep, forgetfulness, being easily shocked, and pale complexion and tongue. To treat this syndrome, it is necessary to tone blood in the heart and calm the spirits.

Heart yin deficiency syndrome (46)

Heart yin deficiency means insufficient yin energy in the heart. Common signs are palpitation, depression, insomnia, dream-filled sleep, forgetfulness, being easily distressed, low fever, night sweats, red appearance of zygoma (cheek region), depression, and hot, dry mouth with reddish tongue. To treat this syndrome, it is necessary to tone yin energy in the heart and calm the spirits.

Heart energy deficiency syndrome (47)

Heart energy deficiency means there is insufficient energy in the heart. Common signs are palpitation, shortness of breath, excessive perspiration, fatigue, weakness, and pale complexion. To treat this syndrome, it is necessary to tone the energy in the heart. Arrhythmia (irregular heartbeat) is treated under this syndrome.

Heart yang deficiency syndrome (48)

Heart yang deficiency means there is insufficient yang energy in the heart. Common signs are chest pain, profuse perspiration, fatigue, cold sensations, and cold limbs. To treat this syndrome, it is necessary to tone yang energy in the heart. Hypotension is treated under this syndrome.

Heart yang prolapse syndrome (49)

Prolapse means to fall. Heart yang prolapse means yang energy in the heart falls. Common signs are excessive perspiration, chest pain, and pain in the heart. To treat this syndrome, it is necessary to tone yang energy in the heart. Arteriosclerosis (hardening of blood vessels) is treated under this syndrome.

Heart blood coagulation syndrome (50)

Heart blood coagulation means the blood in the heart gets coagulated. Common signs are pricking pain or dull pain in front of the heart or behind the chest bone, acute pain extending to the back and shoulders, palpitation, nervousness, purple-blue nails and lips, and cool sensations in the four limbs. To treat this syndrome, it is necessary to "activate the blood," or promote circulation. Coronary heart disease is treated under this syndrome.

Heart fire (heart fire flaming upward) syndrome (51)

Heart fire flaming upward means the heart is under the attack of fire (heat) moving upward to the throat and mouth. Common signs are insomnia, thirst, yellowish-red urine, dribbling of urine, pricking pain on urination, and blood in urine. To treat this syndrome, it is necessary to "clear the heart" (extinguish heat in the heart), push down fire, and promote urination. Blood in urine and diminished urination are the two symptoms treated under this syndrome.

Heart-gallbladder energy deficiency syndrome (52)

Both the heart and gallbladder are underfunctioning. Common signs are a bitter taste in the mouth, nausea, feelings of panic, and aversion to light. To treat this syndrome, it is necessary to tone the energy in the heart and gallbladder. Insomnia is the symptom treated under this syndrome.

Heart-kidney yin deficiency (heart and kidneys unable to communicate with each other) syndrome (53)

The heart is a fire organ, the kidney is a water organ. Fire and water must stay in balance so that the body will not be too cold or too hot; this is called communication between the heart and the kidney. When water is deficient, it may fail to control fire, which is called "heart and kidneys unable to communicate with each other." Common signs are dizziness, aversion to light, forgetfulness, fever, nervousness, night sweats, and seminal emission. To treat this syndrome, it is necessary to tone yin energy in the kidneys so that they can control heart fire. Insomnia is the symptom treated under this syndrome.

Heart-kidney yang deficiency syndrome (54)

Yang energy in the heart and kidneys is deficient. Common signs are cold limbs, edema, chest pain, palpitation, and nervousness. To treat this syndrome, it is necessary to tone yang energy in the heart and kidneys. Hypotension and hypothyroidism are two diseases treated under this syndrome.

Heart-spleen deficiency syndrome (55)

This is a combination of heart blood deficiency and spleen energy deficiency. Common signs are palpitation, insomnia, forgetfulness, dream-filled sleep, poor appetite, and fatigue. To treat this syndrome, it is necessary to tone heart blood and spleen energy. Diseases and symptoms treated under this syndrome include anemia, arrhythmia (irregular heartbeat), and insomnia.

Sputum-fire-disturbing-the-heart syndrome(56)

"Sputum fire disturbing the heart" means fire burning the phlegm that has accumulated in the heart. Common signs are mental confusion, incoherent speech, inappropriate laughter and crying, abnormal behavior, angry-looking eyes, violent behavior, and reddish color of the tongue. To treat this syndrome, it is necessary to calm the heart, expel sputum, and sedate fire.

Small Intestine

The primary function of the small intestine is that of receiving water and food from the stomach. It is in charge of transforming foods and differentiating clear energy from turbid energy.

Small-intestine-energy-pain syndrome (57)

"Small intestine energy pain" refers to pain in the scrotum and groin due to energy stagnation in the small intestine. Common signs are pain in the small intestine, abdominal swelling, intestinal rumbling, and hernia pain in the scrotum. To treat this syndrome, it is necessary to regulate the energy of the small intestine.

Pericardium

The pericardium forms the external defense of the heart; before a pathogen can attack the heart, it must first pass through the pericardium.

Pericardium heat (heat entering the pericardium) (58)

The common signs of pericardium heat are high fever, coma, and delirium. To treat this syndrome, it is necessary to clear heat in the pericardium. Pneumonia is the disease to be treated under this syndrome.

Triple cavity (*sanjiao*; triple burning space)

Triple cavity refers to the thoracic cavity, the abdominal cavity, and the pelvic cavity. The major function of the triple cavity is to transport water and warm the whole body. When the triple cavity breaks down, it may affect different internal organs.

Lower-cavity damp heat (lower burning space damp heat) syndrome (59)

Diseases and symptoms to be treated under this syndrome include urinary infections (pyelonephritis, urethritis, cystitis, prostatitis), and urinary stones.

Liver

The liver takes charge of storing and regulating the blood in the whole body, and is also in control of flexing and extending joints and muscles. The liver loves to disperse and grow, but hates to be inhibited and oppressed. When the liver is inhibited by the emotion of anger, it will be harmed as a result. Common syndromes of the liver are as follows:

Liver energy congestion syndrome (60)

Liver energy congestion means the energy in the liver becomes congested. Common signs are pain and swelling of the ribs on both sides, and wandering pain in the chest, back of the shoulders, or lower abdomen. Sometimes, there may be discomfort in the chest, jumpiness, sensations of something in the throat, abdominal obstructions and lumps, swelling of the liver and spleen, and irregular menstruation. To treat this syndrome, it is necessary to disperse and regulate the energy in the liver. Diseases and symptoms to be treated under this syndrome include hepatitis, frigidity (absence of sexual desire and orgasm in women), goiter, hyperthyroidism, infertility in women, shortage of milk in nursing mothers, simple obesity, and stomachache.

Liver fire syndrome (61)

Liver fire means the liver is under attack by fire. Common signs are headache, dizziness, ringing in the ears, deafness, jumpiness, red complexion, burning pain in the rib region, dry sensations and bitter taste in the mouth, vomiting of blood or nosebleed in severe cases, yellowish urine, and dry stools. To treat this syndrome, it is necessary to clear heat and sedate fire in the liver. Hypertension is the disease treated under this syndrome.

Liver yin deficiency syndrome (62)

Liver yin deficiency means there is insufficient yin energy in the liver. Common signs are dry eyes, decreased visual acuity, tremors and numbness of limbs, dizziness, ringing in the ears, dry and shriveled nails, jumpiness, and scanty menstrual flow or suppression of menses. To treat this syndrome, it is necessary to tone yin energy in the liver.

Liver yang upsurging (liver yang moving fiercely upward) syndrome (63)

"Liver yang upsurging" refers to yang energy in the liver that moves fiercely upward to the head. Common signs are vertigo, headache, burning sensations in the face, dry sensations in the mouth and throat, and heavy sensations in the head with light sensations in the legs. To treat this syndrome, it is necessary to clear heat in the liver, since excessive heat is the cause of the liver's yang energy rising upward.

Liver wind (liver wind blowing internally) syndrome (64)

Liver wind refers to the liver under attack by wind. Common signs are high fever with twitching, spasms of the four limbs, sudden fainting, dry mouth and eyes, numbness of limbs, shaking of the head, trembling, and tremors of the hands and feet. To treat this syndrome, it is necessary to calm the liver and dispel the wind.

Extreme-heat-generating-wind-in-the-liver syndrome (65)

Extreme heat in the internal region causes liver wind. Common signs are high fever, spasms of the four limbs, and stiff neck. To treat this syndrome, it is necessary to clear heat and cool the blood. Pneumonia is treated under this syndrome.

Hot liver syndrome (66)

Liver is under attack by heat. Common signs are a bitter taste in the mouth, dry throat, twitching, vomiting of blood, and nosebleed. To treat this syndrome, it is necessary to clear heat and calm the liver. Diseases and symptoms treated under this syndrome include morning sickness, nosebleed, and ringing in the ears and deafness.

Liver-energy-attacking-the-spleen (disharmony of liver and spleen) syndrome (67)

Because the energy of the liver is getting too strong and attacking the spleen, disharmony results. Common signs are swelling in the rib region, poor appetite, congested sensations in the stomach, stomachache, belching, acid swallowing, nausea, vomiting, abdominal swelling, intestinal rumbling, and discharge of watery stools. To treat this syndrome, it is necessary to disperse the energy in the liver and strengthen the spleen. Diseases and symptoms treated under this syndrome include hepatitis, irritable bowels, and diarrhea.

Liver-energy-attacking-the-stomach (disharmony of liver and stomach) syndrome (68)

Because the liver is getting too strong and attacking the stomach, disharmony results. Common signs are abdominal rumbling, vomiting, belching, irregular bowel movement, and discomfort in the chest. To treat this syndrome, it is necessary to disperse the energy in the liver and harmonize the stomach. Gastroptosis (falling of the stomach) and gastroduodenal ulcers are two diseases treated under this syndrome.

Liver-fire-attacking-the-lungs syndrome (69)

When the liver is under attack by fire, the fire may spread to the lungs. Common signs are coughing, coughing out blood, blood in sputum, and vomiting of blood. To treat this syndrome, it is necessary to clear the liver, sedate the fire, and relieve cough. Bronchitis and bronchiectasis (dilation of bronchi) are two diseases treated under this syndrome.

Liver fire upsurging syndrome (70)

When the liver is under attack by fire, the fire may move upward. Common signs are headache, ringing in the ears, deafness, a bitter taste in the mouth, vomiting of blood, and yellowish urine. To treat this syndrome, it is necessary to sedate fire in the liver. Cough, dizziness, and high cholesterol are symptoms treated under this syndrome.

Liver-kidney yin deficiency syndrome (71)

Yin energy in the liver and kidneys is deficient. Common signs are dizziness, ringing in the ears, numbness of limbs, muscular spasms, night blindness, lumbago, and reddish tongue. To treat this syndrome, it is necessary to tone energy in the liver and kidneys. Diseases and symptoms treated under this syndrome include Alzheimer's disease, anemia, coronary heart disease, hepatitis, hyperthyroidism, menopausal symptoms, nephritis, and cirrhosis.

Liver-kidney yin deficiency with liver yang upsurging syndrome (72)

When yin energy in the liver and kidneys is deficient, it may cause a yin-yang imbalance in the liver so that yang energy in the liver moves upward to affect the head. Common signs are headache, dizziness, and heavy sensations in the head. To treat this syndrome, it is necessary to tone yin and moderate yang energy in the liver. Hypertension is treated under this syndrome.

Gallbladder

The gallbladder is situated below the right lobe of the liver. Since the gallbladder stores bile from the liver, when the gallbladder is diseased, the patient will have a bitter taste in the mouth, vomiting of bitter water, jaundice, etc. The gallbladder is paired with the liver, which is why the syndrome of the gallbladder is associated with the liver.

Liver-gallbladder damp heat syndrome (73)

Liver and gallbladder damp heat refers to an excessive amount of dampness and heat accumulating in the liver and the gallbladder simultaneously. The common signs are yellowish appearance of sclera (white fibrous tissue covering the white of the eye), apparent pain in the ribs, scanty urine of yellowish-red color, fever, thirst, nausea, vomiting, poor appetite, and abdominal swelling. To treat this syndrome, it is necessary to clear heat and remove dampness from both the liver and gallbladder.

Spleen

The stomach receives nutrients and digests them first, then the spleen digests them for the second time before sending them to the lungs for transmitting throughout the body. Common syndromes of the spleen are as follows:

Falling-of-the-middle-energy (collapse of the middle energy) syndrome (74)

This syndrome refers to a severe case of energy deficiency. "Falling of the middle energy" means the young energy in the spleen is not sufficient or strong enough to hold up the internal organs. Common signs are shortness of breath, disinclination to talk, falling and swelling of the lower abdomen, and chronic diarrhea. To treat this syndrome, it is necessary to tone up the middle energy of the spleen.

Spleen-unable-to-govern-the-blood syndrome (75)

One function of the spleen is to make certain that the blood stays within the vessels so that bleeding will not occur. When the spleen is short of energy, it may become incapable of governing the blood so that various types of bleeding occur, such as functional bleeding from the uterus and bleeding from the anus. To treat this syndrome, it is necessary to tone up the energy and stop bleeding. Blood in the stools is a symptom treated under this syndrome.

Spleen dampness (spleen deficiency with an attack of dampness) syndrome (76)

When the spleen is short of energy, it is vulnerable to the invasion of dampness. The common signs are heavy sensations in the head (as if being wrapped in a wet towel), sticky or dry sensations in the mouth with no thirst, decreased appetite, dull sensations in the stomach, nausea, diarrhea, swelling of limbs, excessive white vaginal discharge, and heavy sensations in the body. To treat this syndrome, it is necessary to expel dampness and strengthen the spleen. Diseases and symptoms treated under this syndrome include cirrhosis, diarrhea, hepatitis, oligomenorrhea (scanty or infrequent menstrual flow), and simple obesity.

Spleen-dampness-attacking-the-lungs syndrome (77)

When dampness attacks the spleen, it may transform into phlegm and affect the lungs. Common signs are coughing, whitish and watery phlegm, shortness of breath, and limb fatigue. To treat this syndrome, it is necessary to dry dampness in the spleen and relieve cough. Bronchitis and nephritis are two diseases treated under this syndrome.

Spleen damp heat syndrome (78)

Spleen damp heat means the spleen is under attack by dampness and heat simultaneously. Common signs are sallow appearance of the face and eyes, congested sensations in the stomach and abdomen, no appetite, aversion to greasy foods, nausea, vomiting, reddish and scanty urine, itching, fever, a bitter taste and dry sensations in the mouth, constipation, and difficult bowel movement. To treat this syndrome, it is necessary to clear dampness and heat from the spleen.

Cold spleen syndrome (79)

When the spleen is under attack by cold, common signs are chronic abdominal pain, cold hands and feet, indigestion, poor appetite, and vomiting. To treat this syndrome, it is necessary to warm the spleen and expel cold. Abdominal pain is treated under this syndrome.

Spleen deficiency syndrome (80)

Spleen deficiency refers to a general weakness of the spleen. Common signs are clear and long streams of urine, abdominal pain and distention, diarrhea, copious sputum, poor appetite, fatigue, cold limbs, and indigestion. To treat this syndrome, it is necessary to tone up the spleen. Amenorrhea (absent period), gastroptosis (falling of the stomach), impotence in men, metrorrhagia (uterine bleeding), and urinary infections (pyelonephritis, urethritis, cystitis, prostatitis) are treated under this syndrome.

Spleen energy deficiency syndrome (81)

When energy in the spleen is deficient, common signs are abdominal pain, diarrhea, stomachache, vomiting of blood, and falling of internal organs. To treat this syndrome, it is necessary to tone the energy in the spleen. Hemorrhoids are treated under this syndrome.

Spleen-kidney deficiency syndrome (82)

This refers to a general deficiency in the spleen and kidneys. Common signs are diarrhea, hearing difficulties, insomnia, and blurred vision. To treat this syndrome, it is necessary to tone the spleen and kidneys. Hypotension is treated under this syndrome.

Spleen-kidney yang deficiency syndrome (83)

When yang energy in the spleen and kidneys is deficient, common signs are shivering with cold, cold limbs, diarrhea early in the morning, poor appetite, fatigue, and aversion to cold. To treat this syndrome, it is necessary to warm the spleen and kidneys. Diseases and symptoms treated under this syndrome include Alzheimer's disease, anemia, arrhythmia (irregular heartbeat), high cholesterol, hypothyroidism, nephritis, simple obesity, urinary stones, cirrhosis, and diarrhea.

Spleen-lung energy deficiency syndrome (84)

When energy in the spleen and lungs is deficient, common signs are abdominal swelling, cough, shortness of breath, poor appetite, and thinness. To treat this syndrome, it is necessary to tone up the energy in the spleen and lungs. Enuresis (incontinence of urine) and respiratory allergies are treated under this syndrome.

Spleen sputum syndrome (85)

Dampness in the spleen may become sputum. Common signs are excessive saliva, sudden outburts of crying and laughing, dizziness, headache, palpitation, and nausea. To treat this syndrome, it is necessary to dry the spleen and eliminate sputum. Diseases and symptoms treated under this syndrome include Alzheimer's disease, dizziness, and high cholesterol.

Spleen yang deficiency syndrome (86)

When yang energy in the spleen is deficient, common signs are excessive saliva, abdominal pain, diarrhea, stomachache, and excessive whitish vaginal discharge. To treat this syndrome, it is necessary to warm the spleen. Dysentery is treated under this syndrome.

Stomach

The stomach performs the functions of receiving and digesting foods. It is also in charge of pushing down turbid substances. When stomach energy moves downward, water and grains will also move downward, contributing to digestion, absorption, and excretion. If instead of moving downward, stomach energy moves upward, then it will cause such symptoms as belching, hiccups, nausea, and vomiting, etc. As the stomach is paired with the spleen, some common syndromes of the stomach also involve the spleen.

Spleen-stomach energy deficiency syndrome (87)

Spleen-stomach energy deficiency means there is insufficient energy in the spleen and the stomach. Common signs are poor appetite, belching, swallowing of acid, nausea, vomiting, stomachache with fondness for massage, pain getting better after eating a meal, fullness of stomach, and abdominal swelling with discharge of watery stools. To treat this syndrome, it is necessary to strengthen the spleen and harmonize the stomach. Irritable bowels and morning sickness are treated under this syndrome.

Spleen-stomach damp heat syndrome (88)

When dampness and heat attack the spleen and stomach, common signs are yellowish appearance of sclera, pain in the ribs, scanty urine, poor appetite, thirst, and diarrhea. To treat this syndrome, it is necessary to clear heat and eliminate dampness. Simple obesity is a symptom treated under this syndrome.

Spleen-stomach yang deficiency syndrome (89)

When there is insufficient yang energy in the spleen and the stomach, common signs are abdominal pain, desire for warmth and heat, clear saliva, hiccups, vomiting, poor appetite, abdominal swelling after a meal, fatigue, weakness, cold or puffy limbs, scanty urine, and whitish vaginal discharge. To treat this syndrome, it is necessary to warm and tone up yang energy of the spleen and the stomach. Diseases and symptoms treated under this syndrome include gastroduodenal ulcers, gastroenteritis, hypotension, and morning sickness.

Stomach fire syndrome (90)

Stomach fire means the stomach is under attack by fire. The common signs are thirst with desire for cold drinks, a bitter taste in the mouth, bleeding from gums with pain, toothache, sore throat, headache, nosebleed, and stomachache with burning sensations. To treat this syndrome, it is necessary to clear and sedate stomach fire. Diabetes mellitus is a disease treated under this syndrome.

Stomach yin deficiency syndrome (91)

Stomach yin deficiency means there is insufficient yin energy in the stomach. The common signs are dry lips and mouth, lack of appetite, abdominal swelling after a meal, discharge of dry stools, dry vomiting, hiccups, dry tongue, and burning pain in the stomach. To treat this syndrome, it is necessary to nourish yin energy and clear excessive heat in the stomach (heat may burn up yin energy). Gastroduodenal ulcers and gastroptosis (falling of the stomach) are treated under this syndrome.

Hot stomach (stomach heat) syndrome (92)

When the stomach is under attack by heat, common signs are bad breath, bleeding from gums, frequent feelings of hunger, hiccups, nosebleed, swelling of gums, stomachache, and thirst. To treat this syndrome, it is necessary to clear heat in the stomach. Diseases and symptoms to be treated under this syndrome include high cholesterol, hyperthyroidism, morning sickness, and nosebleed.

Stomach blood coagulation syndrome (93)

When coagulation of blood occurs in the stomach, common signs are pricking pain in the stomach with aversion to massage of the stomach, vomiting of blood, and pain that stays in region of the stomach. To treat this syndrome, it is necessary to disperse blood in the stomach. Gastroduodenal ulcers are treated under this syndrome.

Stomach energy upsurging syndrome (94)

When the energy of the stomach moves upward instead of downward as it should, common signs are dry vomiting, vomiting of foods, nausea, belching, and hiccups. To treat this syndrome, it is necessary to direct stomach energy downward. Vomiting is a symptom treated under this syndrome.

Stomach indigestion syndrome (95)

When there is poor digestive function of the stomach, common signs are swelling of the stomach and abdomen, belching of bad air from the stomach, discharge of stools with an offensive smell, diarrhea or constipation, and poor appetite. To treat this syndrome, it is necessary to promote digestion. Gastroduodenal ulcers and gastroenteritis are treated under this syndrome.

Lungs

The lungs are situated in the thoracic cavity and paired with the large intestine. When the lungs fail to control the respiratory energy properly, coughing, asthma, and difficult breathing will result. The lungs are also in charge of expansion so that air can go through the nose and mouth easily and push energy downward. When the lungs fail to expand, this will give rise to congested chest, coughing, and asthma. When the lungs fail to push energy downward, this will result in coughing, asthma, scanty urine, and edema. The common syndromes of the lungs are as follows:

Dry lungs syndrome (96)

"Dry lungs" refers to insufficient moisture in the lungs. The common signs are dry cough without sputum or with scanty phlegm not easily coughed out, dry sensations in the nose, dry throat, and coughing causing chest pain. To treat this syndrome, it is necessary to clear heat in the lungs and lubricate the lungs.

Cold lungs syndrome (97)

Cold lungs means there is insufficient yang energy in the lungs to make the lungs warm. The common signs are coughing with excessive thin, white phlegm, aversion to cold, absence of thirst, congested chest, and shortness of breath. To treat this syndrome, it is necessary to warm up the lungs and eliminate phlegm.

Hot lungs syndrome (98)

Hot lungs refers to excessive heat in the lungs. The common signs are coughing or panting, yellowish, sticky phlegm with an offensive smell, fever, chest pain, dry mouth, dry stools, and yellowish urine. To treat this syndrome, it is necessary to clear heat in the lungs, eliminate phlegm, and relieve coughing and asthma. Diminished urination and nosebleed are two symptoms treated under this syndrome.

Turbid-phlegm-obstructing-the-lungs syndrome (99)

Turbid phlegm refers to phlegm that looks like dirty water. When the lungs are full of turbid phlegm, the common signs are coughing, shortness of breath, congested chest, inability to lie on the back, noise of phlegm in the throat, and excessive phlegm. To treat this syndrome, it is necessary to clear heat and eliminate phlegm from the lungs.

Cold-phlegm-obstructing-the-lungs syndrome (100)

Internal cold may slow down water flow in the body to produce cold sputum, which obstructs the normal function of the lungs. Common signs are coughing, chest pain, shortness of breath, wheezing, and excessive clear and watery sputum. To treat this syndrome, it is necessary to warm the lungs and eliminate sputum. Bronchial asthma is a symptom treated under this syndrome.

Lung yin deficiency syndrome (101)

Lung yin deficiency means there is insufficient yin energy in the lungs. The common signs are a dry cough without phlegm or with scanty, sticky phlegm containing blood, night sweats, hot sensations in the palms of the hands and soles of the feet, and dry throat with hoarseness. To treat this syndrome, it is necessary to water yin energy in the lungs (like watering plants in your garden) and lubricate the lungs. Pulmonary tuberculosis is treated under this syndrome.

Lung energy deficiency syndrome (102)

Lung energy deficiency means there is insufficient energy in the lungs. The common signs are feeble coughing, excessive clear, thin phlegm, panting and shortness of breath in severe cases, pale complexion, fatigue, and excessive perspiration. To treat this syndrome, it is necessary to tone up energy in the lungs. Bronchial asthma is treated under this syndrome.

Lung energy deficiency and cold syndrome (103)

This syndrome is a combination of cold lungs and lung energy deficiency. Common signs are feeble coughing, excessive clear, thin phlegm, pale complexion, fatigue, excessive perspiration, aversion to cold, absence of thirst, congested chest, and shortness of breath. To treat this syndrome, it is necessary to tone the energy and warm the lungs. Respiratory allergies are treated under this syndrome.

Lung dampness syndrome (104)

When dampness attacks the lungs, common signs are congested chest, excessive sticky phlegm, nausea, palpitation, insomnia, and vomiting. To treat this syndrome, it is necessary to remove dampness from the lungs. Bronchial asthma is treated under this syndrome.

Lung fire syndrome (105)

When fire attacks the lungs, common signs are dry nose, pain in the throat, vomiting of blood, and chronic thirst. To treat this syndrome, it is necessary to sedate fire in the lungs. Diabetes mellitus (production of insufficient insulin by the pancreas) is a disease treated under this syndrome.

Lung-kidney yang deficiency syndrome (106)

When yang energy in the lungs and kidneys is deficient, common signs are clear, thin sputum, feeble coughing, shortness of breath, cold limbs, and excessive perspiration. To treat this syndrome, it is necessary to tone yang energy in the lungs and kidneys. Emphysema is treated under this syndrome.

Lung-kidney yin deficiency syndrome (107)

When yin energy in the lungs and kidneys is deficient, common signs are coughing, blood in sputum, diminished urination, dry sensations in the mouth at night, night sweats, insomnia, and chronic thirst. To treat this syndrome, it is necessary to tone yin energy in the lungs and kidneys. Emphysema is treated under this syndrome.

Lung energy upsurging (lungs unable to direct energy downward) syndrome (108)

Normally lung energy moves downward; when it moves upward, it is called "lung energy upsurging." Common signs are coughing, pain in the throat, difficulty lying on the back, aversion to cold, and wheezing. To treat this syndrome, it is necessary to direct lung energy downward. Bronchial asthma is treated under this syndrome.

Hot-sputum-obstructing-the-lungs syndrome (109)

Excessive heat in the body may produce hot sputum that obstructs the lungs. Common signs are fever, blood in sputum, yellowish sputum, wheezing, shortness of breath, and coughing. To treat this syndrome, it is necessary to clear heat in the lungs and transform sputum. Bronchiectasis (dilation of bronchi) and bronchial asthma are treated under this syndrome.

Wind-heat-attacking-the-lungs syndrome (110)

When the lungs are under attack by wind and heat, common signs are coughing, chest pain, pain in the throat, blood in sputum, thirst with a desire for cold drinks, and reddish tongue. To treat this syndrome, it is necessary to disperse wind and clear heat in the lungs. Bronchiectasis is treated under this syndrome.

Large Intestine

The function of the large intestine is to excrete waste matter. The lungs and the large intestine are paired, so that some syndromes of the lungs may be corrected through the treatment of the large intestine. For example, cough and asthma due to hot lungs may be treated by clearing excessive heat in the large intestine.

Large intestine damp heat syndrome (111)

Large intestine damp heat means there is an excessive amount of dampness and heat in the large intestine. The common signs are abdominal pain, diarrhea with discharge of pus and blood, burning sensations in the anus, reddish short streams of urine, and fever. To treat this syndrome, it is necessary to clear up heat and eliminate dampness from the lungs. Blood in stools is a symptom treated under this syndrome.

Large intestine heat syndrome (112)

When excessive heat accumulates in the large intestine, it may hinder normal movement within. Common signs are pain in the lower abdomen, discharge of solid, hard stools or sticky stools with an offensive smell, short streams of urine, swelling of gums, and dry sensations in the mouth. To treat this syndrome, it is necessary to clear heat in the large intestine. Constipation is a symptom treated under this syndrome.

Cold large intestine syndrome (113).

When excessive cold accumulates in the large intestine, it may hinder normal functioning. Common signs are abdominal pain with rumbling; clear, long streams of urine; cold limbs; and discharge of sticky, muddy stools. To treat this syndrome, it is necessary to warm the large intestine. Constipation is a symptom treated under this syndrome.

Kidneys

The kidneys are important organs in charge of growth, reproduction, and maintenance of the metabolic balance of water. The kidneys are believed to store pure essence, which is closely related to reproduction, growth, and aging. For that reason, when pure essence of the kidneys is in short supply, a man may suffer from shortage of semen and infertility while a woman may suffer from suppression of menses and infertility, slow growth, and premature aging. The kidneys and the bladder are a pair; conditions of kidney energy have a direct bearing on the capacity of the bladder in urination. Some common syndromes of the kidneys are as follows:

Kidney deficiency syndrome (114)

This syndrome refers to a general deficiency in the kidneys. Common signs are chronic backache, diarrhea, frequent miscarriage, large quantities of urine, ringing in the ears, and seminal emission. To treat this syndrome, it is necessary to tone up the kidneys. Diseases and symptoms treated under this syndrome include blood in urine, dysmenorrhea (period pain), metrorrhagia (uterine bleeding), oligomenorrhea (scanty or infrequent menstrual flow), ringing in the ears and hearing impairment, and urinary infections (pyelonephritis, urethritis, cystitis, prostatitis).

Kidney energy deficiency syndrome (115)

When kidney energy is deficient, common signs are dizziness, fatigue, headache, impotence, lumbago, ringing in the ears, and seminal emission. To treat this syndrome, it is necessary to tone up kidney energy. Diseases and symptoms to be treated under this syndrome include enuresis (incontinence of urine) and seminal emission and premature ejaculation.

Kidney yin deficiency syndrome (116)

Kidney yin deficiency means there is insufficient yin energy in the kidneys. The common signs are soreness across the loins, weak legs, dizziness, ringing in the ears, hearing difficulty, seminal emission, suppression of menses, infertility, night sweats, and dry sensations in the mouth with no desire to drink. To treat this syndrome, it is necessary to tone up yin energy in the kidneys. Diseases and symptoms treated under this syndrome include: arteriosclerosis (hardening of blood vessels), diabetes mellitus (production of insufficient insulin by the pancreas), frigidity (absence of sexual desire and orgasm in women), respiratory allergies, and seminal emission and premature ejaculation in men.

Kidney yang deficiency syndrome (117)

Kidney yang deficiency means there is insufficient yang energy in the kidneys. The common signs are lumbago, cold sensations in the knees, decreased sexual desire, impotence, premature ejaculation, scanty urine, edema, decreased appetite, watery stools, cold limbs, and unusually pale or dark complexion. To treat this syndrome, it is necessary to warm and tone up yang energy in the kidneys. Diseases and symptoms treated under this syndrome include diminished urination, frigidity, impotence, menopause syndrome, and respiratory allergies.

Deficiency of kidney yin and kidney yang syndrome (118)

When both yin energy and yang energy in the kidneys are deficient, common signs are coughing, decreased sexual desire in men, infertility in women, impotence, irregular menstruation, shortness of breath, premature ejaculation, and chronic thirst. To treat this syndrome, it is necessary to tone up yin and yang in the kidneys. Hypothyroidism (a condition caused by an insufficient secretion in the thyroid gland) is treated under this syndrome.

Kidney-energy-not-solid (looseness of kidney energy) syndrome (119)

"Kidney energy not solid" means the kidneys are losing control of semen and urine due to lack of energy. The common signs are premature ejaculation, "sliding" (very weak) ejaculation, frequent urination, incontinent urination with dribbling, and frequent urination at night. To treat this syndrome, it is necessary to tone up and constrict kidney energy. Enuresis is treated under this syndrome.

Loss-of-kidneys'-capacity-for-absorbing-inspiration syndrome (120)

The lungs inhale air and send it downward to the lower abdomen so that the kidneys can absorb it; this is the normal pattern of deep breathing. When the kidneys lose their capacity for absorbing air due to deficiency, common signs are breathing difficulty, aversion to cold, cold limbs, shortness of breath, and wheezing. To treat this syndrome, it is necessary to tone the kidneys. Bronchial asthma is treated under this syndrome.

Bladder

The bladder stores urine and is in control of urination. When the bladder does not function properly, it will cause urinary disorders, including difficult urination. A common syndrome of the bladder is called bladder damp heat.

Bladder damp heat syndrome (121)

Bladder damp heat refers to excessive dampness and heat accumulated in the bladder. The common signs are frequent and difficult urination, pain on urination, and sudden interruption during urination. To treat this syndrome, it is necessary to clear heat and eliminate dampness from the bladder. A disease treated under this syndrome is cystitis (infection of the bladder).

Excessive-heat-in-the-bladder syndrome (122)

When the bladder is under the attack of excessive heat, common signs are cloudy urine, urination difficulty, pain in the lower abdomen, bladder stones, and yellowish urine. To treat this syndrome, it is necessary to clear heat in the bladder. Diminished urination is a symptom treated under this syndrome.

CHAPTER 2

Diseases and Symptoms

The following are diseases and symptoms listed for treatment in this book. They are arranged in alphabetical order along with the syndromes to be treated. This list serves two major purposes:

One, since most symptoms or diseases can arise from a number of different syndromes, it is wise to check against the signs for each syndrome involved to see which particular one is more likely to be responsible for the disease or symptom that interests you.

Two, if you find you have two or more diseases or symptoms that fall under a given syndrome, most probably that syndrome is responsible for your diseases or symptoms and should be treated accordingly. Supposing that you suffer from arteriosclerosis (hardening of blood vessels) and diabetes mellitus (production of insufficient insulin by the pancreas) at the same time, you will find that kidney yin deficiency is a syndrome common to both. This being the case, chances are that kidney yin deficiency is responsible for your arteriosclerosis and diabetes, and your treatment should be directed to this particular syndrome. If, on top of that, you also have respiratory allergies which also fall under kidney yin deficiency, you have one more reason to believe that kidney yin deficiency should be treated to correct your health problems.

abdominal pains
cold spleen (79), deficiency cold (20), excess heat (15), stomach indigestion (95), energy stagnation (25), blood coagulation (29).

Alzheimer's disease
spleen sputum (85), sputum congestion and blood coagulation (42), hot phlegm (39), spleen-kidney yang deficiency (83), liver-kidney yin deficiency (71), energy congestion and blood coagulation (34).

amenorrhea (absent period)
wind cold (2), damp phlegm (38), internal heat (17), energy stagnation (25), blood deficiency (28), blood coagulation (29), spleen deficiency (80).

anemia
heart-spleen deficiency (55), liver-kidney yin deficiency (71), spleen-kidney yang deficiency (83).

arrhythmia (irregular heartbeat)
heart energy deficiency (47), deficiency of energy and yin (27), energy congestion and blood coagulation (34), yin deficiency with abundant fire (23), heart-spleen deficiency (55), damp phlegm (38), spleen-kidney yang deficiency (83).

arteriosclerosis (hardening of blood vessels)
deficient yin with excessive yang (19), kidney yin deficiency (116), sputum congestion (41), heart yang prolapse (49).

arthritis and rheumatoid arthritis
wind (1), cold (5), dampness (8), heat (6).

blood in stool
spleen-unable-to-govern-the-blood (75), large intestine damp heat (111).

blood in urine
heart fire (51), damp heat (10), deficiency of energy and blood (33), kidney deficiency (114).

bronchial asthma
cold-phlegm-obstructing-the-lungs (100), hot-sputum-obstructing-the-lungs (109), lung dampness (104), lung energy upsurging (108), lung energy deficiency (103), loss-of-kidneys'-capacity-for-absorbing-inspiration (120).

bronchiectasis (dilatation of bronchi)
wind-heat-attacking-the-lungs (110), liver-fire-attacking-the-lungs (69), hot-sputum-obstructing-the-lungs (109), yin deficiency with abundant fire (23).

bronchitis
spleen-dampness-attacking-the-lungs (77), liver-fire-attacking-the-lungs (69).

cancers of various kinds
no specific syndromes mentioned.

chronic fatigue syndrome
energy deficiency (24), blood deficiency (28), yang deficiency (21), yin deficiency (22).

cirrhosis
dampness (8), damp heat (10), spleen dampness (76), spleen-kidney yang deficiency (83), liver-kidney yin deficiency (71).

common acne
heat (6).

common cold and flu
wind cold (2), wind heat (3), summer heat (7).

constipation
large intestine heat (112), energy stagnation (25), cold large intestine (113), energy deficiency (24), blood deficiency (28).

coronary heart disease
heart blood coagulation (50), energy congestion and blood coagulation (34), liver-kidney yin deficiency (71), deficiency of yin and yang (18).

cough
wind cold (2), wind heat (3), dry heat (14), damp phlegm (38), liver fire upsurging (70), yin deficiency (22).

cystitis (infection of the bladder)
bladder damp heat (121).

diabetes mellitus (production of insufficient insulin by the pancreas)
lung fire (105), stomach fire (90), kidney yin deficiency (116).

diarrhea
cold dampness (13), superficial damp heat (10), stomach indigestion (95), liver-energy-attacking-the-spleen (67), spleen dampness (76), spleen-kidney yang deficiency (83).

diminished urination
hot lungs (98), heart fire (51), superficial damp heat (10), energy deficiency (24), excessive-heat-in-the-bladder (122), blood coagulation (29), kidney yang deficiency (117).

dizziness
liver fire upsurging (70), yin deficiency with yang excess (19), deficiency of yin and yang (18), spleen sputum (85), deficiency of energy and blood (33).

dysentery
superficial damp heat (10), toxic-heat-penetrating-into-the-deep-region (16), spleen yang deficiency (86).

dysmenorrhea (period pain)
wind cold (2), cold dampness (11), energy stagnation (25), blood deficiency (28), blood coagulation (29), kidney deficiency (114).

eczema
wind (1), blood deficiency (28), hot fire (13).

emphysema
lung-kidney yang deficiency (106), lung-kidney yin deficiency (107).

enuresis (incontinence of urine)
spleen-lung energy deficiency (84), kidney energy deficiency (115), looseness of kidney energy (119).

frigidity (absence of sexual desire and orgasm in women)
liver energy congestion (60), kidney yang deficiency (117), kidney yin deficiency (116).

gallstones
heat (6), cold (5).

gastroduodenal ulcer
stomach indigestion (95), liver-energy-attacking-the-stomach (68), stomach yin deficiency (91), spleen-stomach yang deficiency (89), stomach blood coagulation (93).

gastroenteritis
cold dampness (11), summer heat and dampness (9), stomach indigestion (95), spleen-stomach yang deficiency (89).

gastroptosis (falling of the stomach)
spleen deficiency (80), deficiency cold (20), disharmony of liver and stomach (68), stomach yin deficiency (91).

goiter
liver energy congestion (60), damp phlegm (38).

hemorrhoid
damp heat (10), hot blood (30), spleen energy deficiency (81).

hepatitis
superficial damp heat (10), spleen dampness (76), liver energy congestion (60), energy congestion and blood coagulation (34), disharmony of liver and spleen (67), liver-kidney yin deficiency (71).

hiccups
cold (5), heat (6), stomach indigestion (95), yin deficiency (22), yang deficiency (21).

high cholesterol
superficial damp heat (10), spleen dampness (76), hot stomach (92), liver fire upsurging (70), spleen-kidney yang deficiency (83), deficiency of energy and blood (33).

hypertension
liver fire (61), liver-kidney yin deficiency with liver yang upsurging (72), deficiency of yin and yang (18).

hyperthyroidism
hot stomach (92), liver energy congestion (60), sputum fire (44), liver-kidney yin deficiency (71), deficiency fire (11), deficiency of energy and yin (27).

hypotension
heart yang deficiency (48), spleen stomach yang deficiency (89), spleen-kidney deficiency (82), deficiency of yin and energy (18), heart-kidney yang deficiency (54).

hypothyroidism
spleen-kidney yang deficiency (83), heart-kidney yang deficiency (54), deficiency of kidney yin and kidney yang (118).

impotence in men
deficiency fire (12), spleen deficiency (80), kidney yang deficiency (117).

infertility in women
deficiency of energy and blood (33), yin deficiency (22), deficiency cold (20), hot blood (30), liver energy congestion (60), damp phlegm (38).

insomnia
heart-spleen deficiency (55), heart-kidney yin deficiency (53), heart-gallbladder de-

ficiency (52), sputum fire (44), stomach indigestion (95).

irritable bowel
liver-energy-attacking-the-spleen (67), spleen-stomach energy deficiency (87), cold dampness (11), energy stagnation (25).

leukorrhea (vaginal discharge)
energy deficiency (24), sputum (37).

menopause syndrome
kidney yang deficiency (117), liver-kidney yin deficiency (71).

menorrhagia (excessive menstrual bleeding)
damp sputum (38), energy deficiency (24), hot blood (30).

metrorrhagia (uterine bleeding)
sputum congestion (41), energy deficiency (24), energy stagnation (25), hot blood (30), blood coagulation (29), spleen deficiency (80), kidney deficiency (114).

morning sickness
sputum congestion (41), spleen-stomach yang deficiency (89), hot stomach (92), hot liver (66) spleen-stomach energy deficiency (87).

nephritis (infection of the kidneys)
spleen-dampness-attacking-the-lungs (77), spleen-kidney yang deficiency (83), deficiency of energy and blood (33), liver-kidney yin deficiency (71).

nosebleed
hot lungs (98), hot stomach (92), hot liver (66).

oligomenorrhea (scanty or infrequent menstrual flow)
blood deficiency (28), damp sputum (38), spleen dampness (76), cold blood (31), blood deficiency (28), deficiency of energy and blood (33), blood coagulation (29), kidney deficiency (114).

osteoporosis
blood deficiency (28), blood coagulation (29).

pneumonia
wind warm superficial (4), sputum energy heat (43), heat entering the pericardium (58), extreme-heat-generating-wind-in-the-liver (65).

premature gray hair
innate deficiency (0), hot blood (30).

premenstrual syndrome (PMS or premenstrual tension)
energy congestion and blood coagulation (34), cold dampness (13).

prostatitis (inflammation of the prostate gland)
damp heat (10), yin deficiency with abundant fire (23), energy congestion and blood coagulation (34), deficiency of yin and yang (18).

psoriasis
dry blood (32), hot blood (30), blood coagulation (29).

pulmonary tuberculosis
lung yin deficiency (101), deficiency fire (11), deficiency of energy and yin (27).

respiratory allergies
lung energy deficiency and cold (103), spleen-lung energy deficiency (84), kidney yang deficiency (117), kidney yin deficiency (116).

ringing in ears and hearing difficulties
wind heat (3), hot liver (66), damp phlegm (38), kidney deficiency (114).

seminal emission and premature ejaculation in men
deficiency fire (12), superficial damp heat (10), kidney yin deficiency (116), kidney energy deficiency (115).

shortage of milk in nursing mothers
blood deficiency (28), liver energy congestion (60).

simple obesity
spleen dampness (76), spleen-stomach damp heat (88), liver energy congestion (60), energy congestion and blood coagulation (34), internal phlegm (40), spleen-kidney yang deficiency (83).

smoking and intoxication
no specific syndrome.

stomachache
liver energy congestion (60), blood coagulation (29), stomach indigestion (95), deficiency cold (20), yin deficiency (22).

urinary infections (pyelonephritis, urethritis, cystitis, prostatitis)
lower-burning-space damp heat (59), spleen deficiency (80), kidney deficiency (114).

urinary stones
lower-burning-space damp heat (59), energy congestion and blood coagulation (34), spleen-kidney yang deficiency (83).

vomiting
cold dampness (11), stomach indigestion (95), damp phlegm (38), stomach energy upsurging (94), yang deficiency (21), yin deficiency (22).

CHAPTER 3 Cooking of Foods and Herbs

How to Decoct Herbs

The most common way of using herbs in cooking is first to decoct herbs to obtain herbal soup, and then mix the herbal soup with the foods already cooked. For this reason, it is important to know how to decoct herbs.

Pot Used for Decoction

The pot to be used for decoction should be made of something other than iron or bronze in order to prevent chemical changes; an earthenware pot is recommended. Place the herbs in the pot, add just enough cold water to cover the herbs plus an additional cup so that the water level will be slightly higher than the herbs to be decocted. Stir a little bit and let the herbs soak for about 20 minutes, then bring the water to a boil and reduce to low heat. During decoction, the pot should remain covered in order to retain the volatile properties of the herbs.

Decoction Time

The total decoction time depends upon the herbs being decocted. For example, leaves may be decocted over high heat for less than 10 minutes after the water starts boiling, then they are removed from heat and strained to obtain herbal soup; roots and barks may be decocted for as long as an hour over low heat.

Decoction Varies with Different Herbs

If two or more herbs are to be decocted together as in a recipe, in general the heavy or hard herbs like barks or roots should first be decocted over low heat for 10 to 20 minutes so that their properties may become fully soluble in boiling water. After heavy and hard herbs have been boiled for 10 to 20 minutes, add the aromatic herbs and then the very light herbs like leaves and flowers, which should be decocted for only about 5 minutes or so in order to prevent evaporation of some properties.

Dosages of Herbs

The quantity of herbs to be taken each time depends upon the effects of herbs, the severity of the disease under treatment, the type of recipe, and the physical conditions of the patient.

Diseases and Dosages

A light or chronic disease may be treated with a smaller dosage while a severe or acute disease may be treated with a larger dosage. This is due to the fact that body energy and disease are two opposing sides in the treatment; they are each other's enemies, so to speak. In a light disease body energy is still fairly strong, so that the body needs only a little bit of help from the herbs to successfully resist the attack of disease. But in a severe and acute disease life may be in danger, and the body needs more assistance from herbs to resist the attack of the disease, which is why a larger dosage of herbs is required.*

---

* As an example, if we cook 7 g fresh ginger to treat a common cold at the beginning when the disease is still light, we may have to cook 12 g fresh ginger to treat the same common cold after it gets worse. However, dosages suggested in the recipes for health and healing are approximate only; they may fluctuate from individual to individual. In my clinic, when I (or other doctors in the office) prescribe a herbal formula for patients to take, I will explain to them how much to take each time and how often. Having said that, however, I always make a point of reminding them, "You are taking natural herbs, not chemical drugs. You should not have to follow rigid rules or worry about one gram too much or too little."

Physical Conditions and Dosages

The physical condition of the patient, including body size, age, sex, and body strength, should be taken into account in determination of dosages. Children and older patients should take smaller dosages than strong and middle-aged patients; stronger patients should take larger dosages than weaker patients; men should take larger dosages than women; pregnant women and women right after childbirth should take smaller dosages than other women. In addition, larger dosages may be taken in cold winter and smaller dosages taken in hot summer.

Composition of a Recipe

A recipe is composed of different herbs and foods, each ingredient playing a specific role in the recipe. In a standard recipe, there are four kinds of ingredients: master ingredient, associate ingredient, assistant ingredient, and seasoning ingredient. However, a substantial number of recipes do not have all four ingredient types; some recipes may contain only two ingredients while others may contain as many as eight ingredients. In general, there should not be too many ingredients in each recipe in order that they do not cancel out each other's effects. The precise roles played by the ingredients are as follows:

Master ingredients

A master ingredient is intended to treat the primary symptoms. Many recipes have only one master ingredient; other recipes have two to five master ingredients. For example, if you have a headache, you may want to select one or more ingredients to deal with the headache.

Associate ingredients

An associate ingredient plays the supporting role: it supports the master ingredient in achieving its primary therapeutic objective. For example, having selected the master ingredient to deal with your headache, you may want to select an associate ingredient to reinforce the master ingredient.

Assistant ingredients

An assistant ingredient assists the master and associate ingredients in treating the symptoms which may or may not be covered by the master and associate ingredients. For example, having selected the master and associate ingredients to treat your headache, you may want to select an assistant ingredient to treat your nasal discharge. If you have no symptoms to treat other than the key one, your assistant ingredient may also assist the master ingredient in achieving its objective.

Seasoning ingredient

A seasoning ingredient plays two different roles in the recipe: some seasoning is there just to improve the taste of the recipe, whereas other seasoning may be intended to facilitate the action of the recipe. For example, in cooking fish, fresh ginger is often used to remove the fishy smell and improve its taste; in cooking mutton, we may add wine to speed up its actions.

As a general rule, the master ingredients should be in larger quantity than other ingredients, but this is no more than a general rule—many exceptions exist.

Five Kinds of Seasoning Ingredients

There are five common kinds of seasoning ingredients, all of which are discussed in the list of health foods and herbs. Their uses may be summarized as follows. Note that when seasoning ingredients are needed in a recipe to speed up the functions of other ingredients, their amounts are specified. If seasoning ingredients are not included in a recipe, it means that they are not required either to improve the taste or to speed up the effects. Some recipes include seasoning ingredients without specified amounts. Such seasoning ingredients are included simply to improve the taste of the recipe, and as such should be adjusted to suit individual taste. As a rule, however, seasonings should be kept to a minimum so that they do not interfere with other ingredients, and should be added right after removing from heat.

Simple carbohydrates (white sugar, honey, rock sugar, maltose or malt sugar, and other sweeteners)

Simple carbohydrates can slow down acute symptoms in general and relieve pain. Such sweet seasonings are good for the spleen and stomach, and ideal for those with weak stomach, poor appetite, and abdominal pain. For example, a patient recuperating from a chronic illness may be wise to use such seasonings because their digestive system has been weakened by illness.

Liquids (such as wine, vinegar, and soy sauce)

Wine can raise spirits and promote blood circulation. Vinegar can promote blood circulation and stop bleeding, but it is extremely sour and should be avoided by those with ulcers. Soy sauce can counteract fish, meat, vegetable, and mushroom poisoning.

Oils (vegetable and animal oils)

Oils are important to the human body; they can make skin moist and smooth and also promote bowel movement. An excessive consumption of oils, however, may increase the burden on the heart, and it may also cause diarrhea. Sesame, soybean, peanut, rapeseed, corn, sunflower, and tea oils can lower the level of cholesterol in the blood, minimizing the chances of developing arteriosclerosis.

Salt

Salt is indispensable for life due to the important roles it plays in the functions of cells. Kelp and seaweed, which are salty, are often used to treat hard symptoms such as constipation, hard lesions as in tuberculosis, and hard swelling as in goiter. People with constipation are often advised to drink a cup of salty water first thing in the morning, because salt can push downward to promote bowel movement. Duck meat and pork, which are salty, can lubricate the internal region, and are good for yin deficiency and internal dryness. In addition, salty foods in general are cold and act on the kidney; they can thus extinguish fire, particularly in the kidneys, and cool the blood. However, they should be avoided by those with edema, nephritis, and hypertension.

Spices (including onions and garlic)

Spices in general can excite the spirits, resist cold sensations, induce perspiration, and effectively promote blood circulation and digestion. Spices are good for indigestion, low body temperature, poor blood circulation, and rheumatoid arthritis, but they should be avoided by those with eye diseases, hemorrhoids, infectious diseases, and mental depression. The following are a list of common spices: chili pepper (cayenne pepper), Chinese chive, cinnamon, clove, fresh and dried ginger, garlic, green onion (green and white parts), mustard seed, nutmeg, onion, black pepper, and white pepper. "Five spices" is most often used in Chinese cooking. This seasoning is composed of prickly ash, star anise, cinnamon, clove, and fennel, and is good for cold liver.

Herbal Wine

Herbal wine is widely consumed by the Chinese people. Wine has been called the friend of herbs because it is a good solvent. When herbs are immersed in wine, the wine can facilitate the release of their active ingredients. Here is how to make a "medicated" wine:

1 Boil herbs in water for two minutes, then remove from water to cool.

2 Immerse boiled herbs in wine and store in a bottle (500 g wine for 50 g herbs).

3 Add white sugar if you want to make a sweet wine, seal and let sit for over three months.

Herbal Congee

Herbal congee (porridge or gruel) is another popular way of consuming herbs with rice, wheat, millet, etc. The following are four common ways of cooking medicated congee:

1 Decoct herbs first to obtain an herbal soup, then boil rice, wheat, or millet in water with the soup. This is the most common way of cooking herbs with rice.

2 Boil herbs with rice, wheat, millet, etc. This method of cooking is applied to herbs that can be eaten.

3 Grind herbs into powder to cook with rice, etc. This method of cooking is applicable to herbs that are easily ground into powder.

4 Most common seasonings for an herbal congee include brown sugar, white sugar, rock sugar, or honey, fresh ginger, green onion, and salt. Other seasonings may be added provided you know what properties they have.

Identifying the Type of Disease

Before you create a recipe, you must have a clear idea of the ailment to be treated. But an ailment may belong to many different syndromes, which is why you need to identify that first. Follow the steps below:

First, identify your chief complaint or complaints. When you are ill, the symptom or symptoms that trouble you most are your chief complaints, such as headache, numbness, ringing in the ears, etc. You may have one chief complaint or three or more chief complaints.

Second, read through the symptoms under each syndrome in this book and mark off your chief complaints. The type of disease under which your chief complaints fall is the syndrome to be treated.

Take gallstones as an example. There are two different types, or syndromes, namely, hot and cold:

Hot syndrome

SYMPTOMS AND SIGNS:

- **Bitter taste in the mouth.**
- Hearing impairment.
- Frequent sighing.
- **Pain in the rib region**.

Cold syndrome

SYMPTOMS AND SIGNS:

- **Cold limbs**.
- Falling of scrotum with hardness, swelling, and pain.
- Sensitive to cold.
- Pain in the lower abdomen affecting the testes.

When you want to treat gallstones, you must determine the syndrome. To do this, you simply read through the symptoms and signs under each type and highlight your chief complaints. The more symptoms/signs applicable to you, the more likely that your gallstones belong to that syndrome. Now, assuming that pain in the rib region is your chief complaint, which falls under the hot syndrome, then this syndrome should be treated. But let us suppose that pain in the rib region and pain in the lower abdomen affecting the testes are your chief complaints; one falls under the hot syndrome, the other under the cold syndrome. Under such circumstances, you should determine your chief complaint: pain in the rib region or pain in the lower abdomen? If pain in the rib region troubles you more, then the hot syndrome should be treated; if pain in the lower abdomen affecting the testes troubles you more, then the cold syndrome should be treated. If two chief complaints trouble you almost equally, you can treat both types of gallstones.

Sometimes, determination of which type of disease, or syndrome, to treat is not so critical, but sometimes it is very important—even crucial—in treatment. Take the three types of hypertension listed below as an example. If you have noticed that your blood pressure rises easily due to anger and stress, then you definitely belong to the "liver fire" syndrome, because only this type of hypertension involves this symptom. Again, if severe headache is your chief complaint, you would definitely want to treat the liver fire syndrome. To treat other types will not produce good results. This means that determination of the syndrome of the disease is important and crucial in this case. On the other hand, some hypertension patients have no chief complaints; they feel nothing particularly wrong with themselves, but when the doctor took their blood pressure it was found to be too high. Under such circumstances, they can still read through the symptoms and signs under each type to see which type of disease has more applicable symptoms, and treat their condition accordingly.

Let us assume that the following minor symptoms, which may not be properly called chief complaints, are applicable to you as highlighted. The result shows that four symptoms are highlighted under the first syndrome, three symptoms under the second syndrome, and eight symptoms under the third syndrome. We may conclude that the third syndrome should be treated.

Three types of hypertension:

Liver Fire Syndrome (61)

SYMPTOMS AND SIGNS:

- **Bitter taste in the mouth.**
- Blood pressure rises easily due to anger or stress.
- Discharge of yellowish, scanty urine.
- **Dry mouth.**
- **Hot temper.**
- **Red eyes.**
- Red face.
- Vertigo.
- Severe headache.

Liver-Kidney Yin Deficiency with Liver Yang Upsurging Syndrome (72)

SYMPTOMS AND SIGNS:

- Blood pressure rises easily due to fatigue and stress.
- Discharge of reddish, scanty urine.
- **Hot temper.**
- **Insomnia.**
- Lumbago.
- **Dream-filled sleep.**
- Numbness of the four limbs.
- Pain in the legs.
- Ringing in the ears.
- Seminal emission in men.
- Vertigo.

Deficiency of Yin and Yang Syndrome (18)

SYMPTOMS AND SIGNS:

- **Blurred vision.**
- **Cold limbs.**
- **Dry mouth.**
- **Frequent urination at night.**
- Heavy breathing on walking.
- **Insomnia.**
- Light headache.
- Lumbago.
- **Dream-filled sleep.**
- **Perspiration.**
- Ringing in the ears.
- **Slightly red face.**
- Twitching of muscles.
- Vertigo.
- Weak legs.

If, having highlighted all applicable symptoms, you still cannot decide on the type of disease (syndrome) to be treated, chances are that your symptoms/signs belong to the "ambiguous type," in which case its determination is not crucial and you can treat any syndrome based upon guesswork. In point of fact, even an experienced doctor of traditional Chinese medicine very often has to rely on educated guesses in clinical practice, particularly when patients do not have any chief complaints.

Creating a Recipe

After you have decided on the syndrome to be treated, you are ready to create a recipe. In the earlier example, assuming that you have decided that your gallstones belong to the hot syndrome, you are ready to select ingredients. You will see instructions similar to the following:

INGREDIENTS FOR CREATING RECIPES

FOODS FOR EXCESS: chicory, celery.

FOODS FOR DEFICIENCY: walnut, sesame oil, rock sugar, polished rice, cuttlefish.

HERBS: Ji-nei-jin, Jin-qian-cao, Yu-mi-xu, Yi-yi-ren, Yin-chen. (See Chapter 5.)

Syndromes of disease and herbs to use:

1. **HOT:** Ji-nei-jin, Jin-qian-cao, Yu-mi-xu, Yin-chen; cook with foods for excess.
2. **COLD:** Yi-yi-ren; cook with foods for excess or foods for deficiency.

There are four herbs listed for the hot syndrome; all of them may be selected as ingredients in your recipe, depending on your preference and availability of herbs. Let us select 5 g Ji-nei-jin as the master ingredient. The dosage may be increased or reduced. Some herbs have a strong odor and taste unpleasant, so you may reduce the amount.

Foods are classified into foods for excess and foods for deficiency, the former being good for an excessive type of disease while the latter are good for a deficiency type of disease. A deficiency syndrome normally contains the word "deficiency" such as "spleen deficiency" or "liver deficiency" or "yin deficiency." When the word "deficiency" does not appear, it is an excessive disease, such as a hot syndrome, hot phlegm syndrome, indigestion, or wind heat syndrome.

As a general rule, foods for excess are used as associate ingredients in a recipe to treat that syndrome, and foods for deficiency are used as associate ingredients to treat a deficiency syndrome. Foods for excess may be used as assistant ingredients in a recipe to treat a deficiency syndrome, and foods for deficiency may be used as assistant ingredients to treat an excess syndrome. This is due to the fact that it is desirable to have both foods for excess and foods for deficiency to strike a balance in a recipe.

In the recipe we are trying to create, we may select some foods for excess as associate ingredients, but we don't have to. So, let us select polished rice as our assistant ingredient to nourish the body, and select white sugar as a seasoning ingredient. (Use rock sugar instead of white sugar if weight control is desired, since rock sugar does not increase weight.) We now have a list of ingredients for a hot syndrome of gallstones as in Recipe 28 (see Chapter 7):

MASTER: 5 g Ji-nei-jin.

ASSOCIATE: none.

ASSISTANT: 100 g polished rice.

SEASONING: white sugar.

The ingredients we have selected for the hot syndrome of gallstones may be cooked in the following way:

Fry Ji-nei-jin over low heat until brown, then grind into powder (with a miller or food processor).

Boil polished rice together with the sugar in water, add the Ji-nei-jin powder about 2 minutes before the rice is cooked, and bring to a brief boil again.

CONSUMPTION: serve as a side dish or as a dessert. (Virtually all the recipes can be served at mealtimes as a main dish if the quantity is large or your appetite is small. How and when to serve depends on your preference and should not make any difference in the medicinal effects).

INDICATIONS: hot syndrome of gallstones.

ANALYSIS: Ji-nei-jin (membrane of chicken gizzard) has a neutral energy, which is why it is good for the hot syndrome of gallstones. Polished rice (white rice) also has neutral energy and sweet flavor, which promotes urination and assists the master ingredient in dissolving the gallstones. White sugar is used to improve the taste.

Deciding on the Cooking Method

After you have selected the ingredients, you must decide how to cook them.

There are four different ways to cook herbs to be mixed with foods: first, you can decoct herbs first, then strain to obtain an herbal soup to be mixed with foods; second, you can wrap herbs in gauze to be boiled together with foods; third, you can bake or roast or dry fry the herbs to grind into powder to be mixed with foods; fourth, you can boil herbs with foods if the herbs are edible; if not, they should be removed from foods before eating.

You can cook foods the way you want to, such as steaming, boiling, frying, or roasting.

Steaming

Put water in a saucepan. Place the food in a steamer, in a bowl or plate or on a rack over the water and cover. Bring water to a boil and periodically check the level of the water so you don't burn the saucepan. This is to use the heat of steam to cook food. The food cooked by steaming is more yin in nature, which is good for those with too much heat or fire in the body.

Boiling

Boiling means to cook food in water, and there are two ways. One is to put the water and food in a pot, and bring to a boil until the food is cooked; or two, put the water in a pot and bring to a boil, then add the food to cook.

Beans will feature prominently in the recipes, so a word about cooking them: to save time, rinse the beans and soak them in a large amount of boiled water for 2 to 3 hours. Change the water prior to cooking them with other ingredients.

Fat Frying, Stir Frying, Dry Frying

The Chinese are in the habit of using a wok to fry food. A wok is a large steel pan with a round or flat bottom, with high sloping sides and two handles, used for cooking over high heat. Many people use an electric wok nowadays.

Fat frying is frying food in oil which has been preheated in a pan or wok. Stir frying is frying chopped foods in small amounts of oil over high heat quickly to avoid overcooking.

Dry frying is frying foods without oil or water until foods are charred in order to grind the foods into powder. Many foods are too wet to grind into powder easily, but after they have been fried until yellowish or charred, they are easily crushed and ground into powder. Dry frying is a useful technique in cooking for health because some foods, such as seaweed and garlic, are not palatable to some people no matter how they are cooked, while others can only be eaten after they are ground into powder (such as orange or banana peel and litchi nut seeds).

Roasting or Baking

Foods may be roasted by application of heat in a closed oven or exposed directly to the heat source over fresh cinders. Roasting is more likely to change cold and cool foods into warm foods. Some foods may be roasted in order to grind into powder for consumption.

Cooking Rice

The proper way to cook rice is to first rinse it thoroughly in cold water three or four times; soak in cold water for approximately thirty minutes, then apply heat to cook. The quantity of water used should be in proportion to the quantity of rice, depending on whether you intend to cook rice gruel or regular steamed rice. In general, when you are cooking steamed rice, a ratio of 2 cups of water to 1 cup of rice should do (the rice will be ready when the water has evaporated), but if you are cooking porridge, the ratio of water should be increased, so that when the rice is cooked, a desirable quantity of water is still left. Most people use rice cookers nowadays, which is indeed very convenient. Porridge is consumed as a tonic food, especially suitable for someone recuperating from an illness and also for those with diarrhea, fever, or indigestion.

PART II

HEALTH FOODS AND HERBS FOR COOKING

CHAPTER 4 Foods

In this chapter you will find an analysis of common foods that can be combined with herbs for the most efficacious treatment of symptoms and ailments. A few notes are in order on the analysis of the foods listed and odd terms of expression.

- When a listed food is missing a particular property, such as "meridians" or "energy" or "nutrients," it is due to lack of information. We do not know everything about foods and herbs. "Meridians" are pathways by which different reqions of the body are connected with internal organs. They are similar to the nerves in Western medicine, but the two are not identical.
- "Benefit water," perhaps a literal translation from the Chinese, means good for water in the body in promoting water flow. Why is this good? Because it is the nature of water to run; anything that can promote its flow is considered clean and good, and in the human body, water should be constantly flowing. Since we are dealing with traditional Chinese medicine, "diuretic" is not used. The terms may not be the same after all.
- Some properties listed under "nutrients" may seem odd. For example, "soft and bland." This is because it is a quality of food, important to patients recuperating from illness or surgery. On the other hand, I have made a note of such properties as "phosphorous-rich," because an excessive intake may cause calcium deficiency in the blood. "Purine-rich" is another example, since a person with gout should not consume purine-rich foods.
- "Secure the fetus" is another uniquely Chinese term. When the fetus is in motion, it is called "insecure fetus." Thus to secure the fetus is to stop its motion in the womb.
- "To water yin" is a poetic Chinese expression, meaning to increase yin energy in the body, like watering a plant.

- "Steaming bones" refers to hot sensations deep inside the body, as if steam were arising from the bone.
- The "middle region" of the body refers to the stomach and spleen, thus, "to tone the middle region" means to increase the energy there.
- Blood, like other physical properties, may get too hot. To "cool the blood" means to reduce its temperature.
- In some ailments, particularly skin infections, there is pus deep under the skin, called "poison" in Chinese. To "draw out poison" thus means to remove the pus from the deep region of the skin.
- To "solidify or constrict semen" means to make kidney energy solid and constrict the movement of semen as a way of preventing and checking premature ejaculation and incontinence of urine.

Please remember that if you see such terms as "deficiency fatigue" or "irregular periods due to cold," both the "deficiency" and "cold" are referring to syndromes, explained in Chapter 1. Thus, for example, "deficiency fatigue" means chronic fatigue due to body deficiency, which includes energy deficiency, blood deficiency, etc.

■ anchovy, long-tailed

CHINESE: ji-yu.

SCIENTIFIC: Coilia ectenes Jordan et Seale.

FLAVOR: sweet.

ENERGY: warm.

ACTIONS: tones up energy deficiency.

■ apple

CHINESE: ping-guo.

SCIENTIFIC: Malus pumila Mill.

FLAVOR: sweet and sour.

ENERGY: cool.

NUTRIENTS: high-fiber; phosphorus-free; low-sodium.

ACTIONS: produces and nourishes fluids; lubricates the lungs; relieves mental depression or stress; clears summer heat; improves appetite; relieves intoxication.

INDICATIONS: intoxication, thirst, mental depression.

■ apricot

CHINESE: xing-zi.

SCIENTIFIC: Prunus armeniaca L./P. armeniaca L. var. ansu Maxim.

FLAVOR: sweet and sour.

ENERGY: neutral.

NUTRIENTS: high-fiber; iron; vitamin A.

ACTIONS: lubricates the lungs; relieves asthma; produces or nourishes fluids; quenches thirst.

INDICATIONS: excessive thirst, cough, asthma.

■ asparagus

CHINESE: xiao-bai-bu, lu-yu, long-xu-cai.

SCIENTIFIC: Asparagus officinalis L.

FLAVOR: slightly pungent and bitter.

ENERGY: warm.

NUTRIENTS: fiber; iron; phosphorus; vitamin B_1; vitamin E; vitamin K; folic acid.

ACTIONS: lubricates the lungs; relieves cough; expels sputum; destroys worms.

INDICATIONS: dry cough, lung heat, lymphatic tuberculosis.

■ azuki

CHINESE: chi-xiao-dou.

SCIENTIFIC: Phaseolus calcaratus Roxb./ Phaseolus angularis Wight.

FLAVOR: sweet and sour.

ENERGY: neutral.

MERIDIAN: heart and small intestine.

ACTIONS: benefits water; expels dampness; harmonizes the blood; drains off pus; heals swelling; counteracts toxic effects.

NOTE: Azuki bean is used both as a herb in Chinese medicine and as a food in Chinese food cures.

■ banana

CHINESE: xiang-jiao.

SCIENTIFIC: Musa paradisiaca L. var. sapientum O.Ktze.

FLAVOR: sweet.

ENERGY: cold.

NUTRIENTS: chromium; copper; high-fiber; potassium; vitamin B.

ACTIONS: clears heat; lubricates intestines; counteracts toxic effects.

INDICATIONS: intoxication, constipation, chronic thirst, bleeding piles (hemorrhoids), diarrhea due to spleen fire.

■ barley

CHINESE: da-mai.

SCIENTIFIC: Hordeum vulgare L.

FLAVOR: sweet and salty.

ENERGY: cool.

MERIDIAN: spleen and stomach.

NUTRIENTS: carbohydrate-rich; phosphorus-rich.

ACTIONS: harmonizes the stomach; benefits intestines; benefits water.

INDICATIONS: indigestion, diarrhea, pain on urination, edema, burns.

■ beef and veal

CHINESE: niu-rou.

SCIENTIFIC: Bos taurus domesticus Gmelin/ Bubalus bubalis L.

FLAVOR: sweet.

ENERGY: neutral.

MERIDIAN: spleen and stomach.

NUTRIENTS: low-carbohydrate; anti-stress and nerve-calming; cholesterol-rich; iron; nicotinic acid; phosphorus-rich; potassium; low-sodium; vitamin B; biotin; folic acid; zinc.

ACTIONS: tones the spleen; tones the stomach; benefits blood; benefits energy; strengthens tendons and bones.

INDICATIONS: diabetes, edema, general weakness, poor digestion.

■ beef liver

CHINESE: niu-gan.

SCIENTIFIC: Bos taurus domesticus Gmelin/ Bubalus bubalis L.

FLAVOR: sweet.

ENERGY: neutral.

MERIDIAN: liver.

NUTRIENTS: choline; pantothenic acid; vitamin B; vitamin K.

ACTIONS: nourishes blood; tones the liver; sharpens vision.

INDICATIONS: night blindness, glaucoma, blurred vision, anemia.

■ beef stomach (beef tripe)

CHINESE: niu-du.

SCIENTIFIC: Bos taurus domesticus Gmelin/ Bubalus bubalis L.

FLAVOR: sweet.

ENERGY: neutral.

ACTIONS: to benefit semen; to benefit the stomach; to tone up deficiency.

INDICATIONS: diabetes, dizziness, anemia.

■ beetroot (sugar beet)

CHINESE: tian-cai-gen, hong-cai-tou.

SCIENTIFIC: Beta vulgaris L.

FLAVOR: sweet.

ENERGY: neutral.

ACTIONS: pushes down energy and facilitates menstruation.

INDICATIONS: congested chest, hiccups.

■ bird's nest 燕窩

CHINESE: yan-wo.

SCIENTIFIC: Collocalia esculenta L.

FLAVOR: sweet.

ENERGY: neutral.

MERIDIAN: kidneys, stomach, and lungs.

ACTIONS: nourishes yin; lubricates dryness; tones the middle region; benefits energy.

INDICATIONS: asthma, cough, vomiting of blood, discharge of blood from the mouth, hiccups, weakness.

NOTE: Esculent swifts make nests by regurgitating gelatinous substances. The nests are called bird's nest and are sold in virtually all Chinese food stores. Rinse nests in cold water, changing the water once, and soak in water for 5 to 6 hours. Remove to dry, then cut up and place in a saucepan with one cup of water for every 20 g. Boil over medium heat for 15 minutes, then add rock sugar to season.

■ bitter gourd

CHINESE: ku-gua.

SCIENTIFIC: Momordica charantia L.

FLAVOR: bitter.

ENERGY: cold.

MERIDIAN: spleen, heart, and stomach.

ACTIONS: clears heat or summer heat; counteracts toxic effects; sharpens vision.

INDICATIONS: sunstroke, dysentery, pink eyes with pain, carbuncle swelling, erysipelas, boils.

■ broomcorn 黍米 (broomcorn millet)

CHINESE: shu-mi.

SCIENTIFIC: Panicum miliaceum L.

FLAVOR: sweet.

ENERGY: neutral.

MERIDIAN: spleen, stomach, lungs, large intestine.

ACTIONS: tones the middle region; pushes down energy.

INDICATIONS: cough, diarrhea, thirst, mouth cankers in children.

NOTE: Cook and eat like rice.

■ buckwheat

CHINESE: qiao-mai.

SCIENTIFIC: Fagopyrum esculentum Moench.

FLAVOR: sweet.

ENERGY: cool.

NUTRIENTS: pantothenic acid.

ACTIONS: improves appetite; enlarges intestines; pushes energy downward; eliminates congestion or coagulation.

INDICATIONS: indigestion, abdominal distention, chronic diarrhea, scrofula (tuberculosis of the lymph nodes), burns.

■ burdock

CHINESE: niu-bang-zi.

SCIENTIFIC: Arctium lappa L.

FLAVOR: pungent and bitter.

ENERGY: cool.

MERIDIAN: stomach and lungs.

ACTIONS: disperses wind; clears heat; expands the lungs; heals swelling; counteracts toxic effects.

INDICATIONS: common cold, sore throat, measles, carbuncles, swelling.

■ cantaloupe or muskmelon

CHINESE: tian-gua, xiang-gua, gan-gua.

SCIENTIFIC: Cucumis melo L.

FLAVOR: sweet.

ENERGY: cold.

MERIDIAN: heart and stomach.

NUTRIENTS: vitamin A; vitamin C.

ACTIONS: clears summer heat; promotes urination; quenches thirst.

INDICATIONS: chronic thirst, diminished urination, general pain in the four limbs, rheumatism, numbness.

■ carp, common

CHINESE: li-yu.

SCIENTIFIC: Cyprinus carpio L.

FLAVOR: sweet.

ENERGY: neutral.

MERIDIAN: kidneys and spleen.

ACTIONS: benefits water; heals swelling; pushes energy downward; promotes lactation.

INDICATIONS: edema, beriberi, jaundice, cough, shortage of milk secretion in nursing mother.

■ carp, gold

CHINESE: ji-yu.

SCIENTIFIC: Carassius auratus (L.).

FLAVOR: sweet.

ENERGY: neutral.

MERIDIAN: spleen, stomach, and large intestine.

ACTIONS: strengthens the spleen; benefits dampness.

INDICATIONS: poor appetite, dysentery, discharge of blood from the anus, edema, urinary problems, carbuncles.

■ carrot

CHINESE: hu-luo-bo.

SCIENTIFIC: Daucus carota L. var. sativa DC.

FLAVOR: sweet.

ENERGY: neutral.

MERIDIAN: spleen and lungs.

NUTRIENTS: calcium; low-calorie; chromium; low-fat; high-fiber; potassium; low-protein; vitamin A; vitamin K.

ACTIONS: strengthens the spleen.

INDICATIONS: indigestion, chronic diarrhea, cough.

■ cashew nut

CHINESE: du-xian-zi.

SCIENTIFIC: Anacardium occidentale L.

FLAVOR: sweet.

ENERGY: neutral.

ACTIONS: pushes down energy; quenches chronic thirst.

INDICATIONS: cough, hiccups, excessive thirst, depression.

■ celery

CHINESE: han-qin, qin-cai.

SCIENTIFIC: Apium graveolens L. var. dulce DC.

FLAVOR: sweet and bitter.

ENERGY: neutral.

MERIDIAN: liver and stomach.

NUTRIENTS: calcium; low-calorie; high-fiber; iron; phosphorus-rich; potassium.

ACTIONS: clears heat; calms the liver; benefits dampness; expels wind.

INDICATIONS: hypertension, headache, dizziness, red complexion, red eyes, blood in urine, carbuncle swelling.

■ celery root

CHINESE: qin-cai-gen.

SCIENTIFIC: Apium graveolens L. var. dulce DC.

ACTIONS: eliminates damp heat.

INDICATIONS: jaundice, gallstone.

■ cherry

CHINESE: ying-tao.

SCIENTIFIC: Prunus pseudocerasus Lindl.

FLAVOR: sweet.

ENERGY: warm.

NUTRIENTS: vitamin A.

ACTIONS: benefits energy; relieves rheumatism.

INDICATIONS: paralysis, rheumatism, numbness, frostbite; paralysis and numbness (soak in wine to take internally).

■ chestnut

CHINESE: li-zi.

SCIENTIFIC: Castanea mollissima Bl.

FLAVOR: sweet.

ENERGY: warm.

MERIDIAN: kidneys, spleen, and stomach.

NUTRIENTS: carbohydrate-rich.

ACTIONS: strengthens the spleen; tones kidneys; strengthens tendons; activates the blood; arrests bleeding.

INDICATIONS: upset stomach, diarrhea, weak loins and legs, vomiting of blood, nosebleed, stool with blood, pain and swelling due to injuries, scrofula (tuberculosis).

■ chicken

CHINESE: ji-rou.

SCIENTIFIC: Gallus gallus domesticus Brisson.

FLAVOR: sweet.

ENERGY: warm.

MERIDIAN: spleen and stomach.

NUTRIENTS: low fiber; nicotinic acid; phosphorus-rich; potassium; low-sodium; vitamin B; biotin.

ACTIONS: benefits energy; warms the middle region; nourishes semen.

INDICATIONS: deficiency fatigue, skinniness, poor appetite, diarrhea, dysentery, edema, diabetes, frequent urination, vaginal bleeding and discharge, shortage of milk secretion in nursing mother, weakness after childbirth.

■ chicken egg

CHINESE: ji-zi, ji-dan.

SCIENTIFIC: Gallus gallus domesticus Brisson.

FLAVOR: sweet.

ENERGY: neutral.

MERIDIAN: lungs.

NUTRIENTS: high-fat; phosphorus-rich; high-protein; low-sodium.

ACTIONS: lubricates dryness; "waters yin" (increases yin energy); nourishes the blood; secures the fetus.

INDICATIONS: hot disease, depression, dry cough, hoarseness, pink eyes, sore throat, insecure fetus, thirst after childbirth, diarrhea, burns.

■ chickpea (garbanzo bean)

CHINESE: hui-hui-dou.

SCIENTIFIC: Cicer arietinum L.

FLAVOR: sweet.

ENERGY: warm.

ACTIONS: relieves diabetes.

INDICATIONS: diabetes, high cholesterol.

■ chicory

CHINESE: ju-qu.

SCIENTIFIC: Cichorium intybus L.

MERIDIAN: liver and gallbladder.

ACTIONS: benefits the liver and gallbladder; removes damp heat from liver and gallbladder.

INDICATIONS: jaundice-type hepatitis.

■ chili pepper

CHINESE: la-jiao.

SCIENTIFIC: Capsicum frutescens L.

FLAVOR: pungent.

ENERGY: hot.

MERIDIAN: spleen and heart.

NUTRIENTS: selenium; vitamin C.

ACTIONS: warms the middle region; disperses cold; improves appetite; promotes digestion.

INDICATIONS: cold abdominal pain, vomiting, diarrhea, frostbite, carbuncles. Chili pepper should be avoided by those with cough and eye diseases.

■ chive, Chinese

CHINESE: jiu-cai.

SCIENTIFIC: Allium tuberosum Rottler.

FLAVOR: pungent.

ENERGY: warm.

MERIDIAN: liver, kidneys, and stomach.

NUTRIENTS: low-calorie; high-fiber.

ACTIONS: warms the middle region; promotes energy circulation; disperses blood coagulation; counteracts toxic effects.

INDICATIONS: chest pain, hiccups, swallowing difficulty, upset stomach, vomiting of blood, nosebleed, urine in blood, dysentery, hemorrhoids, prolapse of rectum and uterus, injuries from falls.

■ clam, freshwater

CHINESE: bang-rou.

SCIENTIFIC: Anodonta oodiana Lea/Cristaria plicata Lea/Hyriopsis cumingii Lea.

FLAVOR: sweet and salty.

ENERGY: cold.

MERIDIAN: liver and kidneys.

ACTIONS: clears heat; counteracts toxic effects; waters yin; sharpens vision.

INDICATIONS: depression, diabetes, vaginal bleeding and discharge, hemorrhoids, pink eyes, eczema.

■ coconut juice

CHINESE: ye-zi-jiang.

SCIENTIFIC: Cocos nucifera L.

FLAVOR: slightly sweet.

ENERGY: warm.

ACTIONS: clears summer heat; quenches thirst.

INDICATIONS: diabetes, vomiting of blood, edema.

■ coconut meat

CHINESE: ye-zi-rang, ye-rou.

SCIENTIFIC: Cocos nucifera L.

FLAVOR: sweet.

ENERGY: neutral.

ACTIONS: improves energy; expels wind.

INDICATIONS: malnutrition in children, excessive thinness (to be consumed with honey).

■ coconut oil

CHINESE: ye-zi-you.

SCIENTIFIC: Cocos nucifera L.

INDICATIONS: diseases of the teeth, summer heat, nervous dermatitis.

■ coriander (Chinese parsley)

CHINESE: hu-sui, xiang-cai, yuan-sui.

SCIENTIFIC: Coriandrum sativul Linne.

FLAVOR: pungent.

ENERGY: warm.

MERIDIAN: spleen and lungs.

ACTIONS: induces perspiration; promotes digestion; pushes energy downward.

INDICATIONS: measles not erupting, indigestion.

■ corn leaf 玉蜀黍葉

CHINESE: yu-mi-ye, yu-shu-shu-ye.

SCIENTIFIC: Zea mays L.

ACTIONS: expels urinary stones.

INDICATIONS: urinary stones with pain.

■ corn root 玉蜀黍根

CHINESE: yu-mi-gen, yu-shu-shu-gen.

SCIENTIFIC: Zea mays L.

ACTIONS: relieves lin syndrome (urinary problem); promotes urination; eliminates congestion or coagulation.

INDICATIONS: urinary stones with pain, diminished urination, vomiting of blood.

■ corn, sweet or Indian

CHINESE: yu-mi, yu-shu-shu.

SCIENTIFIC: Zea mays L.

FLAVOR: sweet.

ENERGY: neutral.

MERIDIAN: stomach and large intestine.

NUTRIENTS: carbohydrate-rich; iron; nicotinic acid; phosphorus-rich; high-protein; low-sodium; vitamin A; vitamin B.

ACTIONS: regulates the middle energy; improves appetite.

INDICATIONS: weak stomach, diminished urination.

■ cow marrowbone

CHINESE: niu-gu.

SCIENTIFIC: Bos taurus domesticus Gmelin/ Bubalus bubalis L.

FLAVOR: sweet.

ENERGY: warm.

ACTIONS: none.

INDICATIONS: vomiting of blood, profuse nosebleed, vaginal bleeding and discharge, discharge of blood from the anus in hemorrhoids and diarrhea, watery diarrhea.

■ crab

CHINESE: xie, pang-xie.

SCIENTIFIC: Eriocheir sinensis H. Milne-Edwards.

FLAVOR: salty.

ENERGY: cold.

MERIDIAN: liver and stomach.

NUTRIENTS: selenium; vitamin A; vitamin B; zinc.

ACTIONS: clears heat; disperses or expels blood coagulations.

INDICATIONS: fracture and jaundice (by internal consumption), scabies and tinea (by external application of powder).

■ cucumber

CHINESE: huang-gua.

SCIENTIFIC: Cucumis sativus L.

FLAVOR: sweet.

ENERGY: cool.

MERIDIAN: spleen, stomach, and large intestine.

NUTRIENTS: low-calorie; low-carbohydrate; iron; phosphorus-rich.

ACTIONS: clears heat; counteracts toxic effects; benefits water (promotes water flow).

INDICATIONS: diabetes, sore throat with swelling, pink eyes, burns.

■ cuttlefish

CHINESE: wu-zei-yu-rou, mo-yu.

SCIENTIFIC: Sepiella maindroni de Rochebrune/Sepia esculenta Hoyle.

FLAVOR: salty.

ENERGY: neutral.

MERIDIAN: liver and kidneys.

NUTRIENTS: low phosphorus.

ACTIONS: nourishes the blood; waters yin (increase yin energy).

INDICATIONS: amenorrhea (suppression of menstruation), unusual vaginal bleeding and discharge, blurred vision.

NOTE: Cuttlefish (sepia) is not the same as squid (loligo), but they look similar, which is why cuttlefish is often substituted for squid in Chinese restaurants.

■ date

CHINESE: wu-lou-zi.

SCIENTIFIC: Phoenix dactylifera L.

FLAVOR: sweet.

ENERGY: warm.

ACTIONS: warms the middle region; benefits

energy; eliminates sputum; tones up deficiency.

INDICATIONS: indigestion, cough with sputum, weakness, skinniness.

■ day lily 金針菜

CHINESE: jin-zhen-cai.

SCIENTIFIC: Hemerocallis fulva L./H. flava L./H. minor mill.

FLAVOR: sweet.

ENERGY: cool.

NUTRIENTS: vitamin B.

ACTIONS: benefits damp heat; expands the chest and diaphragm.

INDICATIONS: difficult, reddish urination, jaundice, hot sensation and congestion in the chest, insomnia, hemorrhoidal bleeding.

■ day lily root 金針根

CHINESE: xuan-cao-gen, jin-zhen-gen.

SCIENTIFIC: Hemerocallis fulva L./H. flava L./H. minor mill.

FLAVOR: sweet.

ENERGY: cool.

MERIDIAN: spleen and lungs.

ACTIONS: benefits water; cools the blood.

INDICATIONS: edema, diminished urination, urinary problems, unusual vaginal discharge or bleeding, jaundice, nosebleed, anal bleeding, mastitis.

■ duck

CHINESE: ya-rou, bai-ya-rou.

SCIENTIFIC: Anas domestica L.

FLAVOR: sweet, salty.

ENERGY: neutral.

MERIDIAN: kidneys and lungs.

NUTRIENTS: iron; phosphorus-rich.

ACTIONS: waters yin (promotes water flow); heals swelling.

INDICATIONS: "steaming bones," cough, edema.

■ duck egg

CHINESE: ya-dan, ya-luan.

SCIENTIFIC: Anas domestica L.

FLAVOR: sweet.

ENERGY: cool.

NUTRIENTS: anti-stress and nerve-calming; cholesterol-rich.

ACTIONS: clears the lungs; waters yin.

INDICATIONS: cough, sore throat, toothache, diarrhea.

■ duck egg, preserved

CHINESE: bian-dan, pi-dan.

SCIENTIFIC: n/a.

FLAVOR: pungent, sweet, and salty.

ENERGY: cold.

ACTIONS: stabilizes and obstructs; clears the lungs; alleviates intoxication; clears large intestine heat.

INDICATIONS: intoxication, diarrhea.

■ eel

CHINESE: shan-yu, huang-shan.

SCIENTIFIC: Monopterus albus (Zuiew).

FLAVOR: sweet.

ENERGY: warm.

MERIDIAN: liver, kidneys, and spleen.

NUTRIENTS: vitamin B.

ACTIONS: tones up deficiency; relieves rheumatism; strengthens tendons and bones.

INDICATIONS: fatigue, wind-cold-damp rheumatism (a combination of wind, cold, and dampness syndromes), continual bleeding after childbirth, bloody dysentery, hemorrhoids.

■ eggplant (aubergine)

CHINESE: qie-zi, ai-gua.

SCIENTIFIC: Solanum melongena L.

FLAVOR: sweet.

ENERGY: cool.

MERIDIAN: spleen, stomach, and large intestine.

NUTRIENTS: low-calorie; low-carbohydrate.

ACTIONS: clears heat; activates the blood; relieves pain; heals swelling.

INDICATIONS: discharge of blood from the anus, carbuncles, skin eruptions.

■ fennel seed

CHINESE: hui-xiang, xiao-hui-xiang.

SCIENTIFIC: Foeniculum vulgare Mill.

FLAVOR: pungent.

ENERGY: warm.

MERIDIAN: bladder, kidneys, and stomach.

ACTIONS: warms kidneys; disperses cold; harmonizes the stomach; regulates energy.

INDICATIONS: hernia, pain in the lower abdomen, intestinal rumbling, lumbago, stomachache, vomiting, beriberi.

■ fig

CHINESE: wu-hua-guo.

SCIENTIFIC: Ficus carica L.

FLAVOR: sweet.

ENERGY: neutral.

MERIDIAN: spleen, large intestine.

NUTRIENTS: calcium; low-calorie; phosphorus-rich.

ACTIONS: strengthens the stomach; clears intestines; heals swelling; counteracts toxic effects.

INDICATIONS: enteritis, dysentery, constipation, hemorrhoids, sore throat, carbuncles, boils, scabies, tinea.

■ frog, river or pond

CHINESE: qing-wa.

SCIENTIFIC: Rana nigromaculata Hallowell/ Rana plancyi Lataste.

FLAVOR: sweet.

ENERGY: cool.

MERIDIAN: stomach, large intestine, and small intestine.

ACTIONS: clears heat; counteracts toxic effects; tones up energy deficiency; benefits water; heals swelling.

INDICATIONS: hot sensations, edema, malnutrition in children, tympanitis (middle-ear infection), hiccup, pyogenic (pus-producing) inflammation of cheeks, mumps, erysipelas of the face, hot boils in children.

■ fungus, black

CHINESE: hei-mu-er, mu-er.

SCIENTIFIC: Auricularia auricula (L. ex Hook.).

FLAVOR: sweet.

ENERGY: neutral.

MERIDIAN: stomach and large intestine.

NUTRIENTS: carbohydrate-rich; vitamin B.

SCTIONS: cools the blood; arrests bleeding.

INDICATIONS: discharge of blood from the anus, bloody dysentery, unusual vaginal bleeding, hemorrhoids.

■ fungus, white

CHINESE: bai-mu-er, yin-er, xue-er.

SCIENTIFIC: Tremella fuciformis Berk.

FLAVOR: sweet.

ENERGY: neutral.

NUTRIENTS: carbohydrate-rich.

ACTIONS: waters yin; lubricates the lungs; produces and nourishes fluids.

INDICATIONS: dry cough, blood in phlegm, intestinal bleeding, peptic ulcers.

■ garlic

CHINESE: da-suan.

SCIENTIFIC: Allium sativum L.

FLAVOR: pungent.

ENERGY: warm.

MERIDIAN: spleen, stomach, and lungs.

NUTRIENTS: high-fiber; selenium.

ACTIONS: promotes energy circulation; warms the spleen; warms the stomach; counteracts toxic effects.

INDICATIONS: amebic dysentery, tapeworms, trichomonas vaginitis, fish and crab poisoning, edema, beriberi, whooping cough, diarrhea, cold abdominal pain.

■ ginger, fresh

CHINESE: sheng-jiang.

SCIENTIFIC: Zingiber officinale Rose.

FLAVOR: pungent.

ENERGY: warm.

MERIDIAN: spleen, stomach, and lungs.

ACTIONS: clears heat in the superficial region; disperses cold; relieves vomiting; eliminates sputum.

INDICATIONS: common cold due to wind and cold, vomiting, sputum, cough and asthma, diarrhea, relieves various types of poisoning including ban-xia (half-summer hinellia; see under Herbs, chapter 5) poisoning, tian-nan-xing poisoning, crab poisoning, bird and meat poisoning.

■ grape

CHINESE: pu-tao.

SCIENTIFIC: Vitis vinifera L.

FLAVOR: sweet and sour.

ENERGY: neutral.

MERIDIAN: kidneys, spleen, and lungs.

NUTRIENTS: carbohydrate-rich; vitamin P.

ACTIONS: tones energy deficiency; tones blood deficiency; strengthens tendons and bones.

INDICATIONS: diminished urination, cough due to lung deficiency, palpitation, night sweats, rheumatism, urinary problems, edema.

■ grapefruit

CHINESE: you, you-zi.

SCIENTIFIC: Citrus grandis (L.) Osbeck/Citrus grandis (L.) Osbeck var. tomentosa Hort.

FLAVOR: sweet and sour.

ENERGY: cold.

NUTRIENTS: vitamin C.

ACTIONS: counteracts alcoholism; promotes digestion.

INDICATIONS: alcoholism, high blood sugar, cough with sputum, bad breath, indigestion.

■ grapevine leaf and stem

CHINESE: pu-tao-teng-ye, pu-tao-ye.

SCIENTIFIC: Vitis vinifera L.

FLAVOR: sweet and neutral.

ENERGY: neutral.

ACTIONS: heals swelling; promotes urination.

INDICATIONS: edema, diminished urination, pink eyes, carbuncles with swelling.

■ green onion leaf

CHINESE: cong-ye, xiang-cong.

SCIENTIFIC: Allium fistulosum L.

FLAVOR: pungent.

ENERGY: warm.

ACTIONS: expels wind; induces perspiration; counteracts toxic effects; heals swelling.

INDICATIONS: common cold due to wind cold, headache, nasal congestion, fever without perspiration, stroke, puffy face and eyes, swelling carbuncles and pain, fall injuries.

■ guava

CHINESE: fan-shi-liu.

SCIENTIFIC: Psidium guajava L.

FLAVOR: sweet.

ENERGY: warm.

ACTIONS: constricts intestines; relieves diarrhea.

INDICATIONS: diarrhea, chronic dysentery, eczema, bleeding due to external wounds.

■ ham

CHINESE: huo-tui.

SCIENTIFIC: Sus scrofa domestica Brisson.

FLAVOR: salty.

ENERGY: warm.

NUTRIENTS: calorie-rich; low-carbohydrate; anti-stress and nerve-calming; cholesterol-rich; nicotinic acid; potassium; vitamin B.

ACTIONS: strengthens the spleen; improves appetite; produces and nourishes fluids; benefits the blood.

INDICATIONS: deficiency fatigue, nervousness, poor appetite, dysentery due to deficiency (spleen yang deficiency), chronic diarrhea.

■ honey

CHINESE: feng-mi.

SCIENTIFIC: Apis cerana Fabricius.

FLAVOR: sweet.

ENERGY: neutral.

MERIDIAN: spleen, lungs, and large intestine.

NUTRIENTS: carbohydrate-rich; low-sodium.

ACTIONS: tones the middle region; lubricates dryness; relieves pain; counteracts toxic effects.

INDICATIONS: dry constipation, cough due to dry lungs, sinusitis, mouth canker, burns, aconite poisoning.

■ horse bean (broad or fava bean)

CHINESE: can-dou.

SCIENTIFIC: Vicia faba L.

FLAVOR: sweet.

ENERGY: neutral.

MERIDIAN: spleen and stomach.

NUTRIENTS: low-carbohydrate; low-fat; high-fiber; vitamin B.

ACTIONS: strengthens the spleen; benefits dampness.

INDICATIONS: indigestion, edema, diminished urination, bleeding.

■ jellyfish 海蜇

CHINESE: hai-zhe.

SCIENTIFIC: Rhopilema esculenta Kishinouye.

FLAVOR: salty.

ENERGY: neutral.

MERIDIAN: liver and kidneys.

NUTRIENTS: iodine.

ACTIONS: clears heat; transforms sputum; eliminates congestion or coagulation; lubricates intestines.

INDICATIONS: cough with sputum, asthma, chest congestion, constipation, swelling of foot, swelling of lymph nodes.

■ jellyfish skin 海蜇皮

CHINESE: hai-zhe-pi.

SCIENTIFIC: Rhopilema esculenta Kishinouye.

FLAVOR: salty.

ENERGY: warm.

MERIDIAN: liver.

ACTIONS: transforms sputum; eliminates congestion or coagulation; expels wind; removes dampness.

INDICATIONS: lump, headache, whitish vaginal discharge, arthritis of the knees, erysipelas.

NOTE: There are two parts of a jellyfish: the umbrellalike body which is called jellyfish skin, and the mouth or neck which is called jellyfish head. Jellyfish should be washed before cooking.

■ Job's tears (coix seed)

CHINESE: yi-yi-ren.

SCIENTIFIC: Coix lachryma-jobi L.

FLAVOR: sweet.

ENERGY: cool.

MERIDIAN: kidneys, spleen, and lungs.

NUTRIENTS: vitamin B_1.

ACTIONS: strengthens the spleen; tones the lungs; clears heat; benefits dampness.

INDICATIONS: diminished urination, edema, diarrhea, twitching, beriberi, rheumatism, high blood sugar, consumptive lung disease, pulmonary abscess, acute appendicitis.

NOTE: Job's tears are white beadlike seeds of a grass of tropical Asia with the hard husk removed. Having been found to be anticancerous and antitumoral, the seeds are used both as an herb in Chinese medicine and as a food in Chinese food cures.

■ kelp

CHINESE: kun-bu.

SCIENTIFIC: Laminaria japonica Aresch.

FLAVOR: salty.

ENERGY: cold.

MERIDIAN: stomach.

NUTRIENTS: carbohydrate-rich; iodine.

ACTIONS: softens hardness; promotes water flow.

INDICATIONS: goiter, tuberculosis of lymph node, hernia, abdominal obstructions, hypertension.

■ kidney bean

CHINESE: bai-fan-dou, cai-dou.

SCIENTIFIC: Phaseolus vulgaris L.

FLAVOR: sweet.

ENERGY: neutral.

NUTRIENTS: calcium.

ACTIONS: nourishes yin; promotes urination; heals swelling.

INDICATIONS: edema, beriberi.

NOTE: To treat edema, boil 130 g kidney beans, 16 g garlic, and 35 g white sugar in water for internal consumption.

■ kiwi fruit

CHINESE: mi-hou-tao, teng-li.

SCIENTIFIC: Actinidia chinensis Planch.

FLAVOR: sweet and sour.

ENERGY: cold.

MERIDIAN: kidneys and stomach.

ACTIONS: quenches thirst; relieves lin syndrome (urinary problem).

INDICATIONS: mental depression, diabetes, jaundice, urinary stones, hemorrhoids.

■ lard

CHINESE: zhu-zhi-gao, zhu-you.

SCIENTIFIC: Sus scrofa domestica Brisson.

FLAVOR: sweet.

ENERGY: cool.

NUTRIENTS: calorie-rich; anti-stress and nerve-calming; cholesterol-rich; high-fat; low-purine.

ACTIONS: tones up deficiency; lubricates dryness; counteracts toxic effects.

INDICATIONS: difficult bowel movements, dryness in the internal organs (manifesting in dry cough, skin, eyes, nose, and stool; scanty urine; and frequent thirst).

■ laver

CHINESE: zi-cai.

SCIENTIFIC: Porphyra tenera Kjellm.

FLAVOR: sweet and salty.

ENERGY: cold.

MERIDIAN: lungs.

NUTRIENTS: iodine.

ACTIONS: transforms sputum; softens hardness; clears heat; promotes urination.

INDICATIONS: goiter, beriberi, edema, lin syndrome.

■ leaf beet (spinach beet or Swiss chard)

CHINESE: jun-da-cai.

SCIENTIFIC: Beta vulgaris L. var. cicla L.

FLAVOR: sweet.

ENERGY: cool.

MERIDIAN: stomach and large intestine.

ACTIONS: clears heat and eliminates toxic effects; disperses or expels blood coagulations; arrests bleeding.

INDICATIONS: measles that fail to erupt on time, hot diarrhea, suppression of menses, swelling in furuncles.

■ lemon

CHINESE: ning-meng.

SCIENTIFIC: Citrus limonia Osbeck/Citrus limon Burm.

FLAVOR: extremely sour.

NUTRIENTS: calcium; low-calorie; low-carbohydrate; low-sodium; vitamin C.

ACTIONS: quenches thirst; produces and nourishes fluids; clears summer heat.

INDICATIONS: thirst, sunstroke, consumption by pregnant women to "secure the fetus."

■ lettuce stalk and leaf

CHINESE: wo-ju.

SCIENTIFIC: Lactuca sativa L.

FLAVOR: sweet and bitter.

ENERGY: cool.

MERIDIAN: stomach and large intestine.

ACTIONS: promotes urination and milk secretion.

INDICATIONS: diminished urination, blood in urine, shortage of milk secretion in nursing mother.

■ ling, cooked 熟菱

CHINESE: ling, ling-jiao.

SCIENTIFIC: Trapa bispinosa Roxb.

FLAVOR: sweet.

ENERGY: cool.

MERIDIAN: stomach, large intestine, and small intestine.

ACTIONS: benefits energy; strengthens the spleen.

INDICATIONS: weakness, fatigue, weak spleen (symptoms manifesting from spleen deficiency syndrome).

■ ling, fresh 鲜菱

FLAVOR: sweet.

ENERGY: cold.

ACTIONS: clears summer heat; quenches thirst.

INDICATIONS: mental depression, thirst.

■ litchi nut

CHINESE: li-zhi.

SCIENTIFIC: Litchi chinensis Sonn.

FLAVOR: sweet and sour.

ENERGY: warm.

MERIDIAN: liver and spleen.

ACTIONS: produces and nourishes fluids; benefits the blood; regulates energy; relieves pain.

INDICATIONS: depression, thirst, hiccups, vomiting, stomachache, scrofula, boils, swelling, toothache.

■ loach

CHINESE: ni-qiu, qiu-yu.

SCIENTIFIC: Misgurnus anguillicaudatus (Cantor).

FLAVOR: sweet.

ENERGY: neutral.

MERIDIAN: spleen.

ACTIONS: tones the middle region; benefits energy; expels dampness.

INDICATIONS: diabetes, impotence, viral hepatitis, hemorrhoids, tinea, scabies.

■ lobster

CHINESE: hai-xia, da-hong-xia, long-xia.

SCIENTIFIC: Penaeus orientalis Kishinouye (dui-xia)/Panulirus (long-xia).

FLAVOR: sweet and salty.

ENERGY: warm.

NUTRIENTS: copper; pantothenic acid; selenium.

ACTIONS: tones kidneys; strengthens yang; transforms sputum; improves appetite.

INDICATIONS: impotence, itch, symptoms manifesting from sputum fire, pain in tendons and bones.

■ longan nut 龍眼

CHINESE: long-yan, long-yan-rou, gui-yuan.

SCIENTIFIC: Euphoria longan (Lour.) Steud.

FLAVOR: sweet.

ENERGY: warm.

MERIDIAN: spleen and heart.

ACTIONS: benefits the heart and spleen; tones blood deficiency; tones energy deficiency; calming.

INDICATIONS: blood deficiency, palpitation, insomnia, forgetfulness, chronic bleeding, excessive menstrual flow.

■ lotus root, cooked

CHINESE: ou, lian, lian-ou.

SCIENTIFIC: Nelumbo nucifera Gaertn.

FLAVOR: sweet.

ENERGY: warm.

MERIDIAN: spleen, heart, and stomach.

ACTIONS: strengthens the spleen; benefits the blood; improves appetite; relieves diarrhea; nourishes muscles.

INDICATIONS: poor appetite, diarrhea.

NOTE: If you eat lotus root on a regular basis, you can reduce your anger and promote calmness and joy.

■ lotus root, fresh

FLAVOR: sweet.

ENERGY: cold.

MERIDIAN: spleen, heart, and stomach.

ACTIONS: clears heat; cools the blood; disperses coagulations.

INDICATIONS: thirst in a hot disease, vomiting of blood, nosebleed, urinary problems, intoxication.

■ mango

CHINESE: mang-guo.

SCIENTIFIC: Mangifera indica L.

FLAVOR: sweet and sour.

ENERGY: cool.

NUTRIENTS: vitamin C.

ACTIONS: benefits the stomach; relieves vomiting; quenches thirst; promotes urination.

INDICATIONS: thirst, vomiting, diminished urination.

■ milk, cow's

CHINESE: niu-ru.

SCIENTIFIC: Bos taurus domesticus Gmelin/ Bubalus bubalis L.

FLAVOR: sweet.

ENERGY: neutral.

MERIDIAN: heart, stomach, and lungs.

NUTRIENTS: calcium; calorie-rich; low fiber; liquid food; pantothenic acid; phosphorus-rich; potassium; high-protein; low-purine; soft and bland; vitamin A; vitamin B; vitamin B; vitamin D; biotin.

ACTIONS: tones deficiency; benefits the lungs; benefits kidneys; lubricates intestines; produces and nourishes fluids.

INDICATIONS: deficiency fatigue, upset stomach, hiccups, swallowing difficulty, diabetes, constipation.

■ millet

CHINESE: su-mi, xiao-mi.

SCIENTIFIC: Setaria italica (L.) Beauv.

FLAVOR: sweet and salty.

ENERGY: cool.

MERIDIAN: kidneys, spleen, and stomach.

NUTRIENTS: carbohydrate-rich; high-protein; low-sodium; vitamin B.

ACTIONS: harmonizes the middle region; benefits kidneys; counteracts toxic effects; clears heat.

INDICATIONS: upset stomach with vomiting, diabetes, diarrhea.

NOTE: Old millet is good for dysentery and mental depression.

■ mung bean

CHINESE: lü-dou, qing-xiao-dou.

SCIENTIFIC: Phaseolus radiatus L.

FLAVOR: sweet.

ENERGY: cold.

MERIDIAN: heart and stomach.

NUTRIENTS: carbohydrate-rich; low-fat.

ACTIONS: clears heat; counteracts toxic effects; clears summer heat; benefits water.

INDICATIONS: summer heat, thirst, edema, diarrhea, erysipelas, furuncles, poisoning by regular consumption of herbs with a hot energy (not included in this book).

■ mung bean sprouts

CHINESE: lü-dou-ya.

SCIENTIFIC: Phaseolus radiatus L.

FLAVOR: sweet.

ENERGY: cold.

ACTIONS: counteracts alcoholism; clears heat; benefits the triple burning space or *sanjiao*.

INDICATIONS: alcoholism.

■ mushroom, common button

CHINESE: mo-gu.

SCIENTIFIC: Agaricus campestris L. ex Fr.

FLAVOR: sweet.

ENERGY: cool.

MERIDIAN: stomach, lungs, large intestine, and small intestine.

ACTIONS: soothes the spirits; improves appetite; relieves diarrhea; relieves vomiting; transforms sputum; regulates energy.

INDICATIONS: diarrhea, vomiting, poor spirits and appetite.

■ mussel

CHINESE: dan-cai.

SCIENTIFIC: Mytilus crassitesta Lischke.

FLAVOR: salty.

ENERGY: warm.

MERIDIAN: liver and kidneys.

ACTIONS: waters and nourishes the liver and kidneys; benefits semen; relieves goiter.

INDICATIONS: deficiency fatigue, skinniness, dizziness, night sweats, impotence, lumbago, vomiting of blood, vaginal bleeding and discharge, goiter, hernia and abdominal obstructions.

■ octopus

CHINESE: zhang-yu.

SCIENTIFIC: Octopus vulgaris Lamarck.

FLAVOR: sweet and salty.

ENERGY: cold.

ACTIONS: stabilizes and obstructs; benefits energy; benefits the blood; nourishes muscles.

INDICATIONS: energy deficiency, blood deficiency, chronic skin eruptions that fail to heal.

■ olive

CHINESE: gan-lan, qing-gan-lan.

SCIENTIFIC: Canarium album (Lour.) Raeusch.

FLAVOR: sweet and sour.

ENERGY: neutral.

MERIDIAN: stomach and lungs.

NUTRIENTS: calcium.

ACTIONS: stabilizes and obstructs; clears the lungs; counteracts toxic effects; produces and nourishes fluids.

INDICATIONS: coughing out blood, vomiting of blood, sore throat with swelling, epilepsy, alcoholism, bacillary dysentery.

■ onion

CHINESE: yang-cong.

SCIENTIFIC: Allium cepa L.

NUTRIENTS: low-calorie; low-carbohydrate; high-fiber; low-protein; vitamin C.

ACTIONS: heals inflammation.

INDICATIONS: wounds, ulcers, and trichomonal vaginitis.

NOTE: Crush fresh onion for external applications to treat these conditions.

■ oyster

CHINESE: mu-li-rou, sheng-hao.

SCIENTIFIC: Ostrea rivularis Gould/Ostrea gigas Thunb./Ostrea talienwhanensis Crosse.

FLAVOR: sweet and salty.

ENERGY: neutral.

NUTRIENTS: calcium; copper; iron; selenium; vitamin A; vitamin B; vitamin D; zinc.

ACTIONS: nourishes the blood; waters yin.

INDICATIONS: depression, hot sensations, insomnia, nervousness, erysipelas, lack of determination, thirst, aftereffects of intoxication.

■ papaya

CHINESE: fan-mu-gua.

SCIENTIFIC: Carica papaya L.

FLAVOR: sweet.

ENERGY: neutral.

NUTRIENTS: low-calorie; low-carbohydrate; vitamin C.

ACTIONS: disperses blood coagulations.

INDICATIONS: stomachache, dysentery, diminished urination, wind rheumatism.

NOTE: Unripe fruits are particularly good for indigestion and promoting milk secretion; ripe fruits are particularly good for promoting urination and bowel movements and also for dysentery.

■ pea

CHINESE: wan-dou.

SCIENTIFIC: Pisum sativum L.

FLAVOR: sweet.

ENERGY: neutral.

MERIDIAN: spleen and stomach.

NUTRIENTS: calcium; low cholesterol; chromium; low-fat; iron; nicotinic acid; pantothenic acid; phosphorus-rich; vitamin B; vitamin K;

ACTIONS: harmonizes the middle region; pushes energy downward; promotes urination.

INDICATIONS: beriberi, furuncle swelling.

■ peach

CHINESE: tao-zi.

SCIENTIFIC: Prunus persica (L.) Batsch/ Prunus davidiana (Carr.) Franch.

FLAVOR: sweet and sour.

ENERGY: warm.

NUTRIENTS: low-calorie; iron; potassium; low-sodium; vitamin A.

ACTIONS: produces and nourishes fluids; lubricates intestines; activates the blood; eliminates congestion or coagulation.

INDICATIONS: constipation, suppression of menstruation.

■ peanut

CHINESE: luo-hua-sheng, hua-sheng.

SCIENTIFIC: Arachis hypogaea L.

FLAVOR: sweet.

ENERGY: neutral.

MERIDIAN: spleen and lungs.

NUTRIENTS: calorie-rich; choline; high-fat; high-fiber; iron; nicotinic acid; pantothenic acid; phosphorus-rich; potassium; high-protein; vitamin B; vitamin E; biotin; zinc.

ACTIONS: lubricates the lungs; harmonizes the stomach.

INDICATIONS: dry cough, upset stomach, beriberi, shortage of milk secretion in nursing mother.

■ pear

CHINESE: li, bai-li, xue-li.

SCIENTIFIC: Pyrus bretschneideri Rehd.

FLAVOR: sweet.

ENERGY: cool.

MERIDIAN: stomach and lungs.

NUTRIENTS: low-calorie; high-fiber; low-phosphorus.

ACTIONS: produces and nourishes fluids; lubricates dryness; clears heat; sedates sputum.

INDICATIONS: thirst in a hot disease, diabetes, hot cough, mental instability with hot phlegm (39) or sputum fire (44), dysphagia, constipation.

■ pepper, black

CHINESE: hu-jiao, hei-hu-jiao.

SCIENTIFIC: Piper nigrum L.

FLAVOR: pungent.

ENERGY: hot.

MERIDIAN: stomach and large intestine.

NUTRIENTS: copper.

ACTIONS: warms the middle region; pushes energy downward; eliminates sputum; counteracts toxic effects.

INDICATIONS: damp sputum, asthma and cough, cold abdominal pain, vomiting and diarrhea.

■ pepper, white

CHINESE: hu-jiao, bai-hu-jiao.

SCIENTIFIC: Piper nigrum L.

FLAVOR: pungent.

ENERGY: hot.

MERIDIAN: stomach, large intestine, and small intestine.

NUTRIENTS: calcium; phosphorus; iron; potassium.

ACTIONS: warms the middle region; pushes energy downward; eliminates sputum; counteracts toxic effects.

INDICATIONS: nephritis, indigestion and diarrhea in children, chronic tracheitis and asthma, neurasthenia.

■ persimmon

CHINESE: shi-zi, shi.

SCIENTIFIC: Diospyros kaki L. f.

FLAVOR: sweet.

ENERGY: cold.

MERIDIAN: heart, lungs, and large intestine.

NUTRIENTS: potassium.

ACTIONS: clears heat; lubricates the lungs; quenches thirst.

INDICATIONS: thirst, cough, vomiting of blood, mouth canker.

■ persimmon cake 柿餅

CHINESE: shi-bing.

SCIENTIFIC: Diospyros kaki L. f.

FLAVOR: sweet.

ENERGY: cold.

ACTIONS: stabilizes and obstructs; arrests bleeding.

INDICATIONS: vomiting of blood, discharge of blood from the mouth, blood in urine, discharge of blood from the anus, hemorrhoids, dysentery.

■ pistachio

CHINESE: wu-ming-zi.

SCIENTIFIC: Pistacia vera L.

FLAVOR: pungent.

ENERGY: warm.

ACTIONS: stabilizes and obstructs; warms the spleen and kidneys.

INDICATIONS: impotence, diarrhea due to cold.

■ plum

CHINESE: li-zi.

SCIENTIFIC: Prunus salicina Lindl.

FLAVOR: sweet and sour.

ENERGY: neutral.

MERIDIAN: liver and kidneys.

ACTIONS: promotes energy circulation; warms the middle region; disperses rheumatism (due to wind and dampness syndromes); activates the blood; heals swelling.

INDICATIONS: deficiency fatigue, "steaming bones," diabetes.

■ pork

CHINESE: zhu-rou.

SCIENTIFIC: Sus scrofa domestica Brisson.

FLAVOR: sweet and salty.

ENERGY: neutral.

MERIDIAN: kidneys, spleen, and stomach.

NUTRIENTS: low-carbohydrate; iron; potassium; low-sodium; vitamin B; biotin; vitamin K; zinc.

ACTIONS: waters yin; lubricates dryness.

INDICATIONS: diabetes, skinniness, dry cough, constipation.

■ pork gallbladder

CHINESE: zhu-dan.

SCIENTIFIC: Sus scrofa domestica Brisson.

FLAVOR: bitter.

ENERGY: cold.

MERIDIAN: liver, lungs, and large intestine.

ACTIONS: clears heat; lubricates dryness; counteracts toxic effects.

INDICATIONS: thirst, constipation, jaundice, whooping cough, asthma, diarrhea, dysentery, pink eyes, sore throat, otitis media suppurativa, boils, carbuncle swelling.

NOTE: Pork gallbladder can be processed and used as eye drops to treat eye infections and trachoma (a chronic contagious form of conjunctivitis).

■ pork liver

CHINESE: zhu-gan.

SCIENTIFIC: Sus scrofa domestica Brisson.

FLAVOR: sweet and bitter.

ENERGY: warm.

MERIDIAN: liver.

NUTRIENTS: anti-stress and nerve-calming; cholesterol-rich; choline; vitamin K.

ACTIONS: tones the liver; nourishes the blood; sharpens vision.

INDICATIONS: night sweats, withered and yellowish complexion, night blindness, pink eye, puffiness around the eyes, beriberi.

■ pork marrowbone

CHINESE: zhu-gu.

SCIENTIFIC: Sus scrofa domestica Brisson.

ACTIONS: relieves diarrhea.

INDICATIONS: internal consumption due to diarrhea.

NOTE: Ground marrowbone is effective when applied externally to scabies and tinea.

■ pork pancreas

CHINESE: zhu-yi.

SCIENTIFIC: Sus scrofa domestica Brisson.

FLAVOR: sweet.

ENERGY: neutral.

ACTIONS: benefits the lungs; tones the spleen; lubricates dryness.

INDICATIONS: cough due to lung deficiency (101), discharge of blood from the mouth, asthma with swelling of the lungs, diarrhea due to spleen deficiency, shortage of milk secretion in nursing mothers, cracked skin around hands and feet, chronic tracheitis.

■ pork skin

CHINESE: zhu-fu.

SCIENTIFIC: Sus scrofa domestica Brisson.

FLAVOR: sweet.

ENERGY: cool.

MERIDIAN: kidneys.

ACTIONS: relieves diarrhea.

INDICATIONS: diarrhea, sore throat.

■ pork stomach (pork tripe)

CHINESE: zhu-du.

SCIENTIFIC: Sus scrofa domestica Brisson.

FLAVOR: sweet.

ENERGY: warm.

ACTIONS: tones up deficiency; strengthens the spleen; strengthens the stomach.

INDICATIONS: fatigue due to various kinds

of deficiency, skinniness, diarrhea, dysentery, diabetes, frequent urination, malnutrition in children.

■ pork trotter

CHINESE: zhu-ti.

SCIENTIFIC: Sus scrofa domestica Brisson.

FLAVOR: sweet and salty.

ENERGY: neutral.

MERIDIAN: stomach.

ACTIONS: tones blood deficiency; promotes milk secretion.

INDICATIONS: shortage of milk secretion in nursing mothers, furuncle, boils.

■ potato, Irish

CHINESE: yang-yu, ma-ling-shu.

SCIENTIFIC: Solanum tuberosum L.

FLAVOR: sweet.

ENERGY: neutral.

NUTRIENTS: carbohydrate-rich; choline; low fiber; iron; low-protein; soft and bland; vitamin B; vitamin C; vitamin K; folic acid.

ACTIONS: strengthens the spleen; tones energy deficiency; heals inflammation.

INDICATIONS: parotitis, burns.

■ potato, sweet

CHINESE: fan-shu.

SCIENTIFIC: Ipomoea batatas Lam.

FLAVOR: sweet.

ENERGY: neutral.

MERIDIAN: kidneys and spleen.

NUTRIENTS: carbohydrate-rich; low-fat; low-phosphorus; potassium; low-protein; vitamin A.

ACTIONS: tones the middle region; harmonizes the middle region; benefits energy; produces and nourishes fluids; enlarges intestines; induces bowel movements.

INDICATIONS: constipation, thirst, jaundice due to damp heat.

■ prickly ash 花椒

CHINESE: hua-jiao, chuan-jiao.

SCIENTIFIC: Amaranthus mangostanus L.

FLAVOR: pungent.

ENERGY: warm.

MERIDIAN: kidneys, spleen, and lungs.

ACTIONS: warms the middle region; disperses cold; removes dampness; relieves pain; destroys worms; counteracts poisoning by fish, crab, etc.

INDICATIONS: glaucoma, corneal opacity, blurred vision, hematochyluria, constipation, difficult urination.

■ prunes

CHINESE: mei.

SCIENTIFIC: Prunus mume (Sieb.) Sieb. et Zucc.

FLAVOR: sweet and sour.

ENERGY: neutral.

NUTRIENTS: high-fiber; iron; phosphorus-rich; potassium.

ACTIONS: produces body fluids; checks diarrhea.

INDICATIONS: thirst, diarrhea, indigestion.

■ rabbit

CHINESE: tu-rou.

SCIENTIFIC: Lepus tolai Pallas/Lepus mandschuricus Badde/Lepus oiostolus Hodgson/Lepus sinensis Gray/Oryctolagus cuniculus domesticus (Gmelin).

FLAVOR: sweet.

ENERGY: cool.

MERIDIAN: liver, and large intestine.

NUTRIENTS: low-carbohydrate; anti-stress and nerve-calming; cholesterol-rich; nicotinic acid.

ACTIONS: tones the middle region; benefits energy; cools the blood; counteracts toxic effects.

INDICATIONS: diabetes, skinniness, vomiting

due to hot stomach, discharge of blood from the anus.

■ radish

CHINESE: lai-fu, bai-luo-bo, luo-bo.

SCIENTIFIC: Raphanus sativus L.

FLAVOR: pungent and sweet.

ENERGY: cool.

MERIDIAN: stomach and lungs.

NUTRIENTS: low-calorie; low-carbohydrate; low-fat; iron; low-phosphorus; potassium; low-protein.

ACTIONS: eliminates congestion or coagulation; clears sputum fire; pushes energy downward; expands the middle region; counteracts toxic effects.

INDICATIONS: abdominal distension due to indigestion, loss of voice due to sputum in the lungs, vomiting of blood, nosebleed, diabetes, dysentery, headache.

■ radish leaf

CHINESE: lai-fu-ye, hu-luo-bo-ying, luo-bo-ying.

SCIENTIFIC: Raphanus sativus L.

FLAVOR: sweet and bitter.

ENERGY: neutral.

ACTIONS: promotes digestion; regulates energy.

INDICATIONS: congestion in the chest and diaphragm regions with a tendency to hiccup, indigestion, diarrhea, sore throat, swelling of nipples in women, shortage of milk secretion.

■ red bayberry

CHINESE: yang-mei.

SCIENTIFIC: Myrica rubra Sieb. et Zucc.

FLAVOR: sweet and sour.

ENERGY: warm.

MERIDIAN: stomach and lungs.

ACTIONS: produces and nourishes fluids; quenches thirst; harmonizes the stomach; promotes digestion.

INDICATIONS: thirst, vomiting and diarrhea, dysentery, abdominal pain.

■ rice, glutinous ("sweet rice")

CHINESE: nuo-mi.

SCIENTIFIC: Oryza sativa L.

FLAVOR: sweet.

ENERGY: warm.

MERIDIAN: stomach and lungs.

ACTIONS: tones the middle region; benefits energy.

INDICATIONS: diabetes, urine in large quantity, excessive perspiration during the day, diarrhea.

■ rice, polished

CHINESE: jing-mi, da-mi.

SCIENTIFIC: Oryza sativa L.

FLAVOR: sweet.

ENERGY: neutral.

MERIDIAN: spleen and stomach.

ACTIONS: tones the middle region; benefits energy; strengthens the spleen; harmonizes the stomach; quenches thirst.

INDICATIONS: diarrhea, thirst, diminished urination.

■ rice bran

CHINESE: mi-pi-kang, mi-kang.

SCIENTIFIC: Oryza sativa L.

FLAVOR: pungent and sweet.

ENERGY: neutral.

MERIDIAN: stomach and large intestine.

NUTRIENTS: choline; pantothenic acid; phosphorus; potassium; vitamin B_6.

ACTIONS: improves appetite; pushes energy downward.

INDICATIONS: dysphagia, beriberi.

■ rock sugar 冰糖

CHINESE: bing-tang.

FLAVOR: sweet.

ENERGY: neutral.

MERIDIAN: spleen and lungs.

ACTIONS: tones the middle region; benefits energy; harmonizes the stomach; lubricates the lungs; relieves cough; transforms sputum.

INDICATIONS: fasting dysentery (characterized by inability to eat or drink), cough, vomiting of blood.

NOTE: Rock sugar, also called candy sugar, is considered the best quality of sugar in traditional Chinese medicine. To make it, boil white sugar and form a lump. It is sold in most Chinese herb shops.

■ rooster

CHINESE: gong-ji

ACTIONS: tones yang energy, particularly good for young and middle-aged men.

INDICATIONS: impotence, weakness, bronchitis, bronchial asthma.

NOTE: The rooster (cock), the male domestic fowl, is considered a very yang creature, producing yang energy in the human body when consumed.

■ rose

CHINESE: mei-gui-hua.

SCIENTIFIC: Rosa rugosa Thunb.

FLAVOR: sweet and bitter.

ENERGY: warm.

MERIDIAN: liver and spleen.

ACTIONS: regulates energy; disperses liver energy congestion; harmonizes the blood; disperses or expels blood coagulations.

INDICATIONS: acute and chronic wind rheumatism, vomiting of blood, discharge of blood from the mouth, irregular menstruation, unusual reddish or whitish vaginal discharge, dysentery, mastitis, swelling.

■ rose, Chinese

CHINESE: yue-ji-hua.

SCIENTIFIC: Rosa chinensis Jacq.

ACTIONS: activates the blood; regulates menstruation; heals swelling; counteracts toxic effects.

INDICATIONS: irregular menstruation, period pain, external injuries, swelling and pain due to blood coagulation, carbuncles.

■ royal jelly

CHINESE: feng-ru, wang-jiang, ru-jiang.

SCIENTIFIC: Apis cerana Fabricius.

FLAVOR: sweet and sour.

ENERGY: neutral.

ACTIONS: waters yin; tones deficiency; nourishes the liver; strengthens the spleen.

INDICATIONS: general weakness after a prolonged illness, malnutrition in children, weakness in the elderly, viral hepatitis, hypertension, arthritis, duodenal ulcer.

■ salt

CHINESE: shi-yan.

SCIENTIFIC: salt.

FLAVOR: salty.

ENERGY: cold.

MERIDIAN: kidneys, stomach, large intestine, and small intestine.

ACTIONS: induces vomiting; clears fire; cools the blood; counteracts toxic effects.

INDICATIONS: indigestion, swelling and pain in the chest and abdomen, sputum in the chest, difficult urination and bowel movements, bleeding from gums, sore throat, toothache, corneal opacity, boils, insect bites.

NOTE: The amount of salt one should consume each day varies from individual to individual. For example, if one exercises and perspires a lot, one should consume more salt in order to compensate for the loss, but elderly people in general are less active and also more susceptible to the attack of hypertension and heart disease.

For that reason, it is necessary for them to take a more cautious attitude toward salt consumption.

■ scallion bulb

CHINESE: xie-bai.

SCIENTIFIC: Allium macrostemon Bge.

FLAVOR: pungent and bitter.

ENERGY: warm.

MERIDIAN: liver, heart, and large intestine.

ACTIONS: regulates energy; expands the chest; connects or facilitates yang; disperses energy congestion.

INDICATIONS: chest pain and heart pain affecting the back, stomach discomfort, diarrhea, nausea without vomiting, boils and carbuncles.

■ sea cucumber 海參

CHINESE: hai-shen.

SCIENTIFIC: Stichopus japonicus Selenka.

FLAVOR: salty.

ENERGY: warm.

MERIDIAN: kidneys and heart.

NUTRIENTS: cholesterol; high-protein.

ACTIONS: tones kidneys; benefits semen; nourishes the blood; lubricates dryness.

INDICATIONS: deficiency fatigue, impotence, seminal emission with erotic dreams, frequent urination, dry intestines with difficult bowel movements.

■ seagrass

CHINESE: hai-zao.

SCIENTIFIC: Sargassum fusiforme (Harv.) Setch.

FLAVOR: bitter and salty.

ENERGY: cold.

MERIDIAN: kidneys, spleen, and lungs.

NUTRIENTS: iodine.

ACTIONS: softens hardness; eliminates sputum; benefits water; sedates heat.

INDICATIONS: scrofula, goiter, tumor, accumulations, edema, beriberi, swelling and pain in the testes.

■ seaweed

CHINESE: hai-dai

SCIENTIFIC: Zostera marina L.

FLAVOR: salty.

ENERGY: cold.

NUTRIENTS: calcium; carbohydrate-rich; high-fiber; iodine; potassium.

ACTIONS: softens hardness; transforms sputum; benefits water; sedates heat.

INDICATIONS: goiter, tuberculosis, hernia, abdominal obstructions, edema, beriberi.

■ sesame oil

CHINESE: ma-you, zhi-ma-you, xiang-you.

SCIENTIFIC: Sesamum indicum DC.

FLAVOR: sweet.

ENERGY: cool.

MERIDIAN: stomach.

NUTRIENTS: vitamin E.

ACTIONS: lubricates dryness; induces bowel movements; counteracts toxic effects; nourishes muscles.

INDICATIONS: chronic simple rhinitis (bring sesame oil to a boil, let it cool, and store in a jar to use as nose drops), constipation with dry intestines, roundworm, abdominal pain due to indigestion, carbuncle swelling, tinea, cracked skin, ulcers.

■ sesame seed, black

CHINESE: hei-zhi-ma, zhi-ma.

SCIENTIFIC: Sesamum indicum DC.

FLAVOR: sweet.

ENERGY: neutral.

MERIDIAN: liver and kidneys.

NUTRIENTS: calorie-rich; high-protein.

ACTIONS: tones kidneys and liver.

INDICATIONS: dizziness, rheumatism, paralysis, constipation, weakness after illness, premature gray hair, shortage of milk secretion in nursing mothers.

■ sheep or goat liver

CHINESE: yang-gan.

SCIENTIFIC: Capra hircus L./Ovis aries L.

FLAVOR: sweet and bitter.

ENERGY: cool.

MERIDIAN: liver.

NUTRIENTS: phosphorus-rich.

ACTIONS: benefits blood; tones the liver; sharpens vision.

INDICATIONS: anemia, blurred vision, night blindness, glaucoma, corneal opacity.

■ sheep or goat meat (mutton)

CHINESE: yang-rou.

SCIENTIFIC: Capra hircus L./Ovis aries L.

FLAVOR: sweet.

ENERGY: warm.

MERIDIAN: kidneys and spleen.

ACTIONS: benefits energy; tones deficiency; warms the middle and lower regions.

INDICATIONS: skinniness, sore loins, abdominal swelling, cold hernia, upset stomach.

■ shepherd's purse 薺菜

CHINESE: ji-cai.

SCIENTIFIC: Capsella bursa-pastoris (L.) Medic.

FLAVOR: sweet.

ENERGY: neutral.

MERIDIAN: liver.

NUTRIENTS: calcium; high-fiber; vitamin A; vitamin B_2.

ACTIONS: harmonizes the spleen; benefits water; arrests bleeding; sharpens vision.

INDICATIONS: dysentery, edema, chyluria (presence of chyle or fat globules in the urine), vomiting of blood, discharge of blood from the anus, unusual vaginal or heavy menstrual bleeding, pink eyes with pain.

■ shiitake mushroom

CHINESE: xiang-xun, xiang-gu.

SCIENTIFIC: Lentinus edodes (Berk.) Sing.

FLAVOR: sweet.

ENERGY: neutral.

MERIDIAN: stomach.

NUTRIENTS: vitamin D.

ACTIONS: benefits the stomach; facilitates eruption of measles.

INDICATIONS: hunger, prevention of rickets, anemia.

■ shrimp

CHINESE: xia, qing-xia.

SCIENTIFIC: Macrobrachium nipponense (de Haan).

FLAVOR: sweet.

ENERGY: warm.

MERIDIAN: liver and kidneys.

NUTRIENTS: calcium; anti-stress and nerve-calming; cholesterol-rich; low fiber;

ACTIONS: tones kidneys; strengthens yang; promotes milk secretion; draws out poison.

INDICATIONS: impotence, shortage of milk secretion, erysipelas, carbuncle, ecthyma.

■ snail

CHINESE: tian-luo.

SCIENTIFIC: Cipangopaludina chinensis (Gray).

FLAVOR: sweet and salty.

ENERGY: cold.

MERIDIAN: stomach, bladder, large intestine, and small intestine.

ACTIONS: clears heat; benefits water.

INDICATIONS: diminished urination due to heat, jaundice, beriberi, edema, diabetes, hemorrhoids, discharge of blood from the anus, pink eyes with pain, boils.

■ sorghum

CHINESE: gao-liang.

SCIENTIFIC: Sorghum vulgare Pers.

FLAVOR: sweet.

ENERGY: warm.

MERIDIAN: spleen, stomach, lungs, and large intestine.

NUTRIENTS: carbohydrate-rich; high-protein.

ACTIONS: warms the middle region; constricts intestines.

INDICATIONS: indigestion, diarrhea, diminished urination due to damp heat.

■ soybean, black

CHINESE: hei-da-dou.

SCIENTIFIC: Glycine max (L.) Merr.

FLAVOR: sweet.

ENERGY: neutral.

MERIDIAN: kidneys and spleen.

ACTIONS: activates the blood; benefits water; expels wind; counteracts toxic effects.

INDICATIONS: edema, beriberi, jaundice, rheumatism, tendon spasms, spasms after delivery, lockjaw, carbuncles, herb poisoning.

■ soybean, fermented black 發酵黑大豆

CHINESE: dan-dou-chi, dou-chi.

SCIENTIFIC: Glycine max (L.) Merr.

FLAVOR: bitter.

ENERGY: cold.

MERIDIAN: stomach and lungs.

ACTIONS: disperses the vicious energy in the superficial region; relieves mental depression or stress; disperses liver energy congestion; counteracts toxic effects.

INDICATIONS: congested chest, depression, headache, alternating cold and hot sensations.

■ soybean, yellow

CHINESE: huang-dou, huang-da-dou.

SCIENTIFIC: Max (L.) Merr.

FLAVOR: sweet.

ENERGY: neutral.

MERIDIAN: spleen and large intestine.

ACTIONS: strengthens the spleen; expands the middle region; lubricates dryness; eliminates water.

INDICATIONS: malnutrition, diarrhea, abdominal swelling, carbuncle swelling, bleeding due to external injuries.

■ soybean curd (tofu)

CHINESE: dou-fu.

FLAVOR: sweet.

ENERGY: cool.

MERIDIAN: spleen, stomach, large intestine.

NUTRIENTS: calcium; low-calorie; low-carbohydrate; low-fat; low fiber; high-protein; low-sodium; soft and bland.

ACTIONS: benefits energy; harmonizes the middle region; produces or nourishes fluids; lubricates dryness; clears heat; counteracts toxic effects.

INDICATIONS: cough, poor appetite, frequent or diminished urination, pink eyes, thirst, abdominal bloating.

■ soybean oil

CHINESE: dou-you, jiang-you.

SCIENTIFIC: Glycine max (L.) Merr.

FLAVOR: pungent and sweet.

ENERGY: hot.

NUTRIENTS: high-fat; vitamin E; vitamin K.

ACTIONS: lubricates intestines; expels worms.

INDICATIONS: intestinal gas, constipation.

■ soybean paste, fermented (miso)

CHINESE: jiang.

SCIENTIFIC: n/a.

FLAVOR: salty.

ENERGY: cold.

MERIDIAN: kidneys, spleen, and stomach.

ACTIONS: clears heat; counteracts toxic effects.

INDICATIONS: insect bite, burn.

■ soy milk

CHINESE: dou-fu-jiang, dou-jiang.

SCIENTIFIC: Glycine max (L) Merr.

FLAVOR: sweet.

ENERGY: neutral.

NUTRIENTS: low fiber; low-protein; non-cholesterol; iron; calcium.

ACTIONS: tones up deficiency; lubricates dryness; clears the lungs; transforms sputum.

INDICATIONS: cough due to chronic fatigue, asthma due to sputum fire, constipation, urination disorders.

■ sparrow

CHINESE: que.

SCIENTIFIC: Passer montamus saturatus Stejneger.

FLAVOR: sweet.

ENERGY: warm.

MERIDIAN: kidneys, heart, and large intestine.

ACTIONS: strengthens yang; benefits semen; warms the loins and knees; checks or reduces urination.

INDICATIONS: impotence, skinniness, excessive urination, excessive vaginal bleeding and discharge.

■ spinach

CHINESE: bo-cai.

SCIENTIFIC: Spinacia oleracea L.

FLAVOR: sweet.

ENERGY: cool.

MERIDIAN: large intestine and small intestine.

NUTRIENTS: calcium; low-calorie; high-fiber; low-phosphorus; potassium; vitamin A; vitamin B; vitamin C; vitamin E; vitamin K; folic acid.

ACTIONS: cools the blood; arrests bleeding; lubricates dryness; constricts yin.

INDICATIONS: nosebleed, discharge of blood from anus, scurvy, thirst in diabetes, difficult bowel movements.

■ squash

CHINESE: nan-gua.

SCIENTIFIC: Curcurbita moschata Duch.

FLAVOR: sweet.

ENERGY: warm.

MERIDIAN: spleen and stomach.

NUTRIENTS: vitamin A.

ACTIONS: tones the middle region; benefits energy; heals inflammation; relieves pain; counteracts toxic effects.

INDICATIONS: pain, infection, diminished urination.

■ squash seed

CHINESE: nan-gua-zi.

SCIENTIFIC: see squash.

FLAVOR: sweet.

ENERGY: neutral.

NUTRIENTS: phosphorus-rich.

ACTIONS: expels worms.

INDICATIONS: tapeworms.

■ string bean (cowpea; black-eyed pea)

CHINESE: jiang-dou.

SCIENTIFIC: Vigna sinensis (L.) Savi.

FLAVOR: sweet.

ENERGY: neutral.

MERIDIAN: kidneys and spleen.

NUTRIENTS: low-calorie; low-carbohydrate; low-fat; phosphorus; low-protein; vitamin P.

ACTIONS: strengthens the spleen; tones kidneys.

INDICATIONS: weak stomach and spleen, diarrhea, vomiting, hiccups, diabetes, seminal emission, whitish or turbid vaginal discharge, frequent urination.

■ sugar, brown

CHINESE: chi-sha-tang, hong-tang.

SCIENTIFIC: Saccharum sinensis Roxb.

FLAVOR: sweet.

ENERGY: warm.

MERIDIAN: liver, spleen, stomach.

ACTIONS: tones the middle region; relaxes the liver; activates the blood by warming the meridians.

INDICATIONS: retention of lochia (discharge from the uterus and vagina following delivery), weakness, dry mouth, discharge of blood in dysentery.

■ sugar, white

CHINESE: bai-sha-tang, bai-tang.

SCIENTIFIC: Saccharum Sinensis Roxb.

FLAVOR: sweet.

ENERGY: neutral.

MERIDIAN: spleen.

NUTRIENTS: carbohydrate-rich; low-sodium.

ACTIONS: lubricates the lungs; produces and nourishes fluids.

INDICATIONS: dry cough, thirst, dry mouth, stomachache.

■ sugar cane

CHINESE: gan-zhe.

SCIENTIFIC: Saccharum sinensis Roxb.

FLAVOR: sweet.

ENERGY: cold.

MERIDIAN: stomach and lungs.

ACTIONS: clears heat; produces and nourishes fluids; pushes energy downward; lubricates dryness.

INDICATIONS: thirst, vomiting, dry cough, constipation, alcoholism.

■ sunflower

CHINESE: xiang-ri-kui-hua.

SCIENTIFIC: Helianthus annuus L.

MERIDIAN: undetermined.

ACTIONS: sharpens vision, reduces high blood pressure.

INDICATIONS: dim vision, hypertension. (Use dried flowers to inhale like a cigarette to heal toothache.)

■ sunflower disc or receptacle 向日葵花托

CHINESE: xiang-ri-kui-hua-tuo-pan.

SCIENTIFIC: see sunflower.

FLAVOR: sweet.

ENERGY: warm.

MERIDIAN: undetermined.

ACTIONS: promotes urination; reduces high blood pressure.

INDICATIONS: headache, hypertension, toothache, stomachache, abdominal pain, period pain, carbuncle swelling.

■ sunflower leaf 向日葵花葉

CHINESE: xiang-ri-kui-ye.

SCIENTIFIC: see sunflower.

FLAVOR: bitter.

ENERGY: undetermined.

ACTIONS: strengthens the stomach.

INDICATIONS: hypertension.

■ sunflower seed

CHINESE: xiang-ri-kui-zi.

FLAVOR: sweet.

ENERGY: warm.

NUTRIENTS: fatty acids; iron; nicotinic acid; pantothenic acid; phosphorus; potassium; protein; vitamin B_1; vitamin B_2; vitamin B_6; vitamin E.

ACTIONS: relieves diarrhea; reduces cholesterol.

INDICATIONS: dysentery, high cholesterol.

■ sunflower stem and pith 向日葵莖髓

CHINESE: xiang-ri-kui-jing-sui.

SCIENTIFIC: see sunflower.

ACTIONS: relieves lin syndrome.

INDICATIONS: chyluria, blood in urine, urinary stones, diminished urination, whooping cough, kidney stones.

■ sword bean (jack bean)

CHINESE: dao-dou.

SCIENTIFIC: Canavalia gladiata (Jacq.) DC.

FLAVOR: sweet.

ENERGY: warm.

MERIDIAN: stomach and large intestine.

NUTRIENTS: low-calorie; low-fat.

ACTIONS: warms the middle region; pushes energy downward; benefits kidneys; tones original energy.

INDICATIONS: hiccups due to cold and deficiency, vomiting, abdominal swelling, lumbago due to kidney deficiency, asthma with sputum.

■ tangerine leaf

CHINESE: ju-ye.

SCIENTIFIC: Citrus tangerina Hort. et Tanaka/ Citrus erythrosa Tanaka.

FLAVOR: pungent and bitter.

ENERGY: neutral.

MERIDIAN: liver.

ACTIONS: disperses liver energy congestion; promotes energy circulation; transforms sputum; heals swelling.

INDICATIONS: pain in the ribs, acute mastitis (inflammation of the breast involving bacterial infection), pulmonary abscess (pus in the lung tissues), cough, chest congestion, hernia.

■ tea

CHINESE: cha-ye.

SCIENTIFIC: Camellia sinensis O. Ktze.

FLAVOR: bitter.

ENERGY: cold or cool.

MERIDIAN: heart, stomach and lungs.

NUTRIENTS: low-carbohydrate; low fiber; fluorine; low-sodium; vitamin C; vitamin P.

ACTIONS: clears the head; relieves mental depression or stress; transforms sputum; promotes digestion; promotes urination; counteracts toxic effects.

INDICATIONS: headache, blurred vision, sleepiness, thirst, depression, sputum, diarrhea.

■ tomato

CHINESE: fan-qie, xi-hong-shi.

SCIENTIFIC: Lycopersicon esculentum Mill.

FLAVOR: sweet and sour.

ENERGY: cold.

NUTRIENTS: low-calorie; low-carbohydrate; iron; potassium; low-protein; vitamin A; vitamin C; vitamin K.

ACTIONS: produces and nourishes fluids; strengthens the stomach; quenches thirst; promotes digestion.

INDICATIONS: thirst, poor appetite.

■ torreyanut 榧子

CHINESE: fei-zi.

SCIENTIFIC: Torreya grandis Fort.

FLAVOR: sweet.

ENERGY: neutral.

MERIDIAN: stomach, lungs, and large intestine.

NUTRIENTS: high-calorie.

ACTIONS: destroys worms; eliminates congestion or coagulation; lubricates dryness.

INDICATIONS: tapeworms, hookworms, pinworms.

■ towel gourd 絲瓜

CHINESE: si-gua.

SCIENTIFIC: Luff cylindrica (L.) Roem.

FLAVOR: sweet.

ENERGY: cool.

MERIDIAN: liver and stomach.

ACTIONS: clears heat; transforms sputum; cools the blood; counteracts toxic effects.

INDICATIONS: fever in a hot disease, asthma, sputum, cough, hemorrhoids, unusual vaginal bleeding and discharge, shortage of milk secretion.

■ turnip leaf

CHINESE: wu-jing; wu-jing da-tou-cai.

SCIENTIFIC: Brassica rapa L.

FLAVOR: pungent, sweet, and bitter.

ENERGY: neutral.

NUTRIENTS: low-calorie; low-protein.

ACTIONS: improves appetite; pushes energy downward; benefits dampness; counteracts toxic effects.

INDICATIONS: indigestion, jaundice, diabetes, swelling with hot sensation, boils, mastitis.

■ vinegar

CHINESE: cu.

FLAVOR: sour and bitter.

ENERGY: warm.

MERIDIAN: liver and stomach.

ACTIONS: arrests bleeding; counteracts toxic effects; destroys worms.

INDICATIONS: fainting after childbirth, jaundice, yellowish sweat, vomiting of blood, nosebleed, discharge of blood from the anus, itch around the genitals, carbuncle swelling, fish and meat poisoning.

■ walnut

CHINESE: hu-tao-ren-rou, he-tao-ren.

SCIENTIFIC: Juglans regio L.

FLAVOR: sweet.

ENERGY: warm.

MERIDIAN: kidneys and lungs.

NUTRIENTS: calcium; calorie-rich; high-fat; high-fiber; phosphorus-rich; high-protein; vitamin B; vitamin E.

ACTIONS: tones kidneys; solidifies or constricts semen; warms the lungs; relieves asthma.

INDICATIONS: asthma and cough due to kidney deficiency, lumbago with weak limbs, impotence, seminal emission, frequent urination, urinary stones, dry stools.

■ water chestnut

CHINESE: bo-qi ma-ti.

SCIENTIFIC: Heleocharis dulcis (Burm. f.) Trin. ex Henschel.

FLAVOR: sweet.

ENERGY: cold.

MERIDIAN: stomach and lungs.

NUTRIENTS: low-protein.

ACTIONS: clears heat; transforms sputum; eliminates congestion or coagulation.

INDICATIONS: warm disease, diabetes, jaundice, pink eyes, sore throat, warts.

■ water spinach 蕹菜

CHINESE: weng-cai kong-xin-cai.

SCIENTIFIC: Ipomoea aquatica Forsk.

FLAVOR: sweet.

ENERGY: cold.

MERIDIAN: stomach, large intestine, and small intestine.

NUTRIENTS: low-calorie.

ACTIONS: tones the heart; induces bowel movements; promotes water flow.

INDICATIONS: nosebleed, constipation, lin syndrome, anal bleeding, hemorrhoids, carbuncle swelling, snake bites.

■ watercress

CHINESE: xi-yang-cai-gan.

SCIENTIFIC: Nasturtium officinale R. Br

NUTRIENTS: calcium; vitamin C; vitamin K.

ACTIONS: relieves cough; lubricates the lungs.

INDICATIONS: dry cough due to hot lungs, lung disease.

■ watermelon

CHINESE: xi-gua.

SCIENTIFIC: Citrullus vulgaris Schrad.

FLAVOR: sweet.

ENERGY: cold.

MERIDIAN: bladder, heart, and stomach.

NUTRIENTS: low-calorie; low-carbohydrate; vitamin A.

ACTIONS: clears heat and summer heat; relieves mental depression or stress; quenches thirst; promotes urination.

INDICATIONS: thirst, shortage of body fluids due to heat, diminished urination, sore throat, mouth canker.

■ wax gourd, Chinese 冬瓜

CHINESE: dong-gua.

SCIENTIFIC: Benincasa hispida (Thunb.) Cogn.

FLAVOR: sweet.

ENERGY: cool.

MERIDIAN: bladder, lungs, large intestine, and small intestine.

ACTIONS: benefits water; eliminates sputum; clears heat; counteracts toxic effects.

INDICATIONS: edema, swelling and fullness, beriberi, lin syndrome, sputum, cough and asthma, diarrhea, carbuncle swelling, hemorrhoids, fish poisoning, alcoholism.

■ wax gourd peel, Chinese 冬瓜皮

CHINESE: dong-gua-pi.

SCIENTIFIC: Benincasa hispida (Thunb.) Cogn.

FLAVOR: sweet.

ENERGY: cool.

MERIDIAN: spleen and lungs.

ACTIONS: benefits water; heals swelling.

INDICATIONS: edema, urination difficulty.

NOTE: Use as an external wash for skin itching.

■ wheat

CHINESE: xiao-mai.

SCIENTIFIC: Triticum aestivum L.

FLAVOR: sweet.

ENERGY: cool.

MERIDIAN: kidneys, spleen, and heart.

NUTRIENTS: carbohydrate-rich; low-fat; high-fiber; nicotinic acid; high-protein; vitamin E; vitamin K.

ACTIONS: nourishes the heart; benefits kidneys; clears heat; quenches thirst.

INDICATIONS: hysteria in women, depression, diabetes, diarrhea, carbuncle swelling, bleeding from external injuries, burn.

■ wheat bran

CHINESE: xiao-mai-fu.

SCIENTIFIC: see wheat.

FLAVOR: sweet.

ENERGY: cool.

MERIDIAN: stomach.

NUTRIENTS: choline; copper; iron; magnesium; nicotinic acid; pantothenic acid; phosphorus-rich; potassium; selenium; vitamin B; biotin; folic acid; zinc.

ACTIONS: checks perspiration; relieves diabetes; relieves diarrhea; relieves rheumatism.

INDICATIONS: deficiency perspiration, night sweats, diarrhea, diabetes, stomatitis, skin eruptions due to heat, fracture, rheumatism, beriberi.

■ wild cabbage 甘藍

CHINESE: gan-lan.

SCIENTIFIC: Brassica oleracea L. var. capiata L.

FLAVOR: sweet.

ENERGY: neutral.

NUTRIENTS: high-fiber.

ACTIONS: benefits kidneys; benefits the five viscera; regulates the six bowels.

INDICATIONS: insomnia, jaundice, general fatigue.

■ wild rice gall 筊白 (water oats gall)

CHINESE: jiao-bai.

SCIENTIFIC: Ustilago esculenta Henn.

FLAVOR: sweet.

ENERGY: cold.

MERIDIAN: liver and spleen.

ACTIONS: clears heat; counteracts toxic effects; relieves mental depression or stress; promotes urination; induces bowel movements.

INDICATIONS: diabetes, jaundice, difficult urination and bowel movement, dysentery, pink eyes.

■ wine

CHINESE: jiu.

FLAVOR: pungent, sweet, and bitter.

ENERGY: warm.

MERIDIAN: liver, stomach, and lungs.

ACTIONS: promotes blood circulation; disperses cold; speeds up effects of herbs.

INDICATIONS: wind cold rheumatism, spasms of tendons, chest pain, cold abdominal pain.

CHAPTER 5

Herbs

This chapter introduces some of the major herbs used in traditional Chinese medicine and their properties. The herbs are arranged alphabetically by Chinese name. When you purchase herbs at a Chinese herb shop, always use the Chinese name, since Chinese merchants will not be familiar with the botanical or pharmaceutical name.

Again, a few notes are in order on the odd terms of expression that you will encounter.

- To "constrict yin" means to retain yin energy and prevent it from wasting away.
- To "soften up the liver" means to relax it so that it will not act up. The liver can easily become tense.
- To "transform dampness" means to eliminate excessive water in the body by promoting urination that is as slow as seeping water. It is different from promoting urination in the usual sense.
- Sputum, like other things, may be relatively dry (sticky and difficult to cough out) or damp (watery), yellow or white, etc. This may be caused by a variety of syndromes. There is dry sputum, damp sputum, cold sputum (cold syndrome), and hot sputum (heat syndrome).
- To "activate the blood" refers to a way of correcting blood stasis so that the blood can circulate normally.
- To "sedate fire" means to reduce the strength of fire (as opposed to "toning up fire," which is to increase the strength of fire).
- To "harmonize the blood" means to regulate blood circulation so that it will not be too fast or too slow.
- To "expand the middle region" means to relax the chest to relieve chest congestion.

- The word "toxic" as it is used in Chinese medicine refers to almost anything that is extreme; thus, there is toxic fire, toxic dampness, and toxic heat, all of which cause disease.
- "Abdominal obstruction" means enlargement of the abdomen due to enlargement of the spleen, liver, or abdominal tumors, with the belly as distended as a drum with or without pain.

As in the previous chapter, the reference to a syndrome will be evident by such terms as "cold rheumatism," referring to an attack of coldness, or "cold diarrhea," referring to diarrhea due to a cold syndrome. Similarly, a term such as "hot diarrhea" refers to one due to a heat syndrome.

1. **CHINESE:** Ai-ye 艾葉 (mugwort).

BOTANICAL: Artemisia argyi Levl. et Vant.

PHARMACEUTICAL: Folium Artemisiae Argyi.

PART USED: leaf.

DOSAGES: 3 to 10 g.

FLAVOR: bitter and pungent.

ENERGY: warm.

ACTIONS: To warm up meridians, arrest bleeding, disperse cold, remove dampness.

INDICATIONS: Irregular periods due to the attack of coldness, menstrual pain, unusual vaginal bleeding, miscarriage, cold abdominal pain, bleeding.

2. **CHINESE:** Bai-bian-dou 白扁豆 (hyacinth bean).

BOTANICAL: Dolichos lablab L.

PHARMACEUTICAL: Semen Dolichoris Album.

PART USED: seed.

DOSAGES: 10 to 12 g.

FLAVOR: sweet.

ENERGY: neutral.

ACTIONS: To tone up spleen, remove dampness, clear up summer heat, counteract toxic effects.

INDICATIONS: Vomiting, diarrhea, thirst, alcoholism, fish and shellfish poisoning, unusual vaginal discharge.

3. **CHINESE:** Bai-bu 百部 (wild asparagus/stemona root).

BOTANICAL: Stemona japonica (Bl) Miq./- sessilifolia (Miq.) Franch. et Sav./- tuberosa Lour.

PHARMACEUTICAL: Radix Stemonae.

PART USED: tuberous root.

DOSAGES: 3 to 10 g.

FLAVOR: sweet and bitter.

ENERGY: slightly warm.

ACTIONS: To lubricate lungs, suppress cough, bring down energy, destroy parasites.

INDICATIONS: Cough due to deficiency fatigue, pulmonary tuberculosis, chronic bronchitis, whooping cough.

4. **CHINESE:** Bai-dou-kou 白豆蔻 (cardamom seed).

BOTANICAL: Amomum cardamomum Linne.

PHARMACEUTICAL: Fructus Amomi Cardamomi.

PART USED: seed.

DOSAGES: 1.5 to 5 g.

FLAVOR: pungent.

ENERGY: warm.

ACTIONS: To transform dampness, promote energy circulation, relieve pain, relieve vomiting.

INDICATIONS: Vomiting, stomachache, fullness and distension in the abdominal region.

5. **CHINESE:** Bai-guo 白果 (Yinxing; ginkgo).

BOTANICAL: Ginkgo biloba L.

PHARMACEUTICAL: Semen Ginkgo.

PART USED: ripe seed.

DOSAGES: 3 to 10 g.

FLAVOR: sweet and bitter.

ENERGY: neutral.

ACTIONS: To expel sputum, suppress cough, calm asthma, remove dampness, produce constrictive effects.

INDICATIONS: Chronic cough, asthma, leukorrhea, nocturia (excessive urination at night).

NOTE: Use cooked ginkgo.

6. **CHINESE:** Bai-he 百合 (lily).

BOTANICAL: Lilium brownii F. E. Brown var. viridulum Baker/- lancifolium Thunb./- pumilum DC.

PHARMACEUTICAL: Bulbus Lilii.

PART USED: bulb.

DOSAGES: 5 to 10 g.

FLAVOR: sweet and slightly bitter.

ENERGY: cold.

ACTIONS: To lubricate the lungs, suppress cough, promote urination, calm the spirits, clear heat.

INDICATIONS: Vomiting of blood, edema, hysteria.

7. **CHINESE:** Bai-hua-she-she-cao 白花蛇舌草 (spreading hedyotis).

BOTANICAL: none.

PHARMACEUTICAL: Herba Hedyotis Diffusae.

PART USED: whole plant, including root.

DOSAGES: 30 to 60 g.

FLAVOR: bitter and sweet.

ACTIONS: To clear heat, eliminate dampness, and detoxify.

INDICATIONS: Asthma, cancers, tonsillitis, jaundice.

8. **CHINESE:** Bai-ji 白芨 (amethyst orchid).

BOTANICAL: Bletilla striata (Thunb.) Reichb. f.

PHARMACEUTICAL: Rhizoma Bletillae Tuber Bletillae.

PART USED: tuberous root.

DOSAGES: 10 to 20 g.

FLAVOR: bitter.

ENERGY: neutral.

ACTIONS: To arrest bleeding, constrict lungs, nourish muscles, heal wounds.

INDICATIONS: Vomiting of blood, coughing out blood, nosebleed, ulcers, pulmonary tuberculosis.

9. **CHINESE:** Bai-jiang-cao 敗醬草 (scabiosa-leaved valerian).

BOTANICAL: Patrinia scabiosaefolia Fisch./- villosa Juss.

PHARMACEUTICAL: Herba Patriniae.

PART USED: whole plant.

DOSAGES: 10 to 30 g.

FLAVOR: pungent and bitter.

ENERGY: cool.

ACTIONS: To clear heat, counteract toxic effects, heal swelling, drain off pus.

INDICATIONS: Appendicitis, carbuncle, abdominal pain after childbirth.

10. **CHINESE:** Bai-mao-gen 白茅根 (cogon satintail).

BOTANICAL: Imperata cylindrica Beauv. var. major (Nees) C.E.Hubb.

PHARMACEUTICAL: Rhizoma Imperatae.

PART USED: rhizome.

DOSAGES: 10 to 30 g.

FLAVOR: sweet.

ENERGY: cold.

ACTIONS: To clear heat, cool the blood, arrest bleeding, promote urination.

INDICATIONS: Urination difficulty, urinary problems with urine containing blood, vomiting of blood, nosebleed, cough.

11. **CHINESE:** Bai-shao 白芍 (white peony).

BOTANICAL: Paeonia lactiflora Pall.

PHARMACEUTICAL: Radix Paeoniae Alba/-Lactiflorae.

PART USED: root.

DOSAGES: 5 to 15 g.

FLAVOR: bitter and sour.

ENERGY: slightly cold.

ACTIONS: To nourish blood, consolidate yin (retain yin energy), pacify the liver, relieve pain.

INDICATIONS: Chest and rib pain, muscle spasms of the limbs, diarrhea, abdominal pain, excessive perspiration, headache.

12. **CHINESE:** Bai-tou-weng 白頭翁 (Chinese pulsatilla).

BOTANICAL: Pulsatilla chinensis (Bge.) Regel.

PHARMACEUTICAL: Radix Pulsatillae.

PART USED: root

DOSAGES: 10 to 15 g.

FLAVOR: bitter.

ENERGY: cold.

ACTIONS: To clear up heat, detoxify, cool blood, relieve dysentery.

INDICATIONS: Dysentery, nosebleed, hemorrhoids.

13. **CHINESE:** Bai-wei 白薇 (white rose).

BOTANICAL: Cynanchum atratum Bge./-versicolor Bge.

PHARMACEUTICAL: Radix Cynanchi Atrati.

PART USED: root.

DOSAGES: 6 to 12 g.

FLAVOR: bitter and salty.

ENERGY: cold.

ACTIONS: To benefit yin, clear heat, and cool blood.

INDICATIONS: Periodic fever due to yin deficiency.

14. **CHINESE:** Bai-xian-pi 白鮮皮 (white bark).

BOTANICAL: Dictamnus dasycarpus Turcz.

PHARMACEUTICAL: Cortex Dictamni Radicis.

PART USED: root bark.

DOSAGES: 5 to 10 g.

FLAVOR: bitter.

ENERGY: cold.

ACTIONS: To clear heat, dry dampness.

INDICATIONS: Eczema, rheumatism from dampness, jaundice, scabies, skin rash.

15. **CHINESE:** Bai-ying 白英 (white nightshade).

BOTANICAL: Solanum lyratum Thunb.

PHARMACEUTICAL: Herba Solani Lyrati.

PART USED: aerial part.

DOSAGES: 10 to 15 g.

FLAVOR: bitter.

ENERGY: cold.

ACTIONS: To clear heat, counteract toxic effects.

INDICATIONS: Scabies, rhus dermatitis (skin inflammation caused by poison ivy), cancer of uterus.

16. **CHINESE:** Bai-zhi 白芷 (angelica).

BOTANICAL: Angelica dahurica (Fisch. ex Hoffm.) Benth. et Hook. f./- var. taiwaniana (Boiss.) Shan et Yuan.

PHARMACEUTICAL: Radix Angelicae Dahuricae.

PART USED: root.

DOSAGES: 3 to 10 g.

FLAVOR: pungent.

ENERGY: warm.

ACTIONS: To induce perspiration, expel wind, heal swelling, relieve pain.

INDICATIONS: Headache, toothache, pain in bony ridge of eye socket, sinusitis, anal bleeding, itch.

17. **CHINESE:** Bai-zhu 白朮 (white atractylodes).

BOTANICAL: Atractylodes macrocephala Koidz.

PHARMACEUTICAL: Rhizoma Atractylodis Macrocephalae.

PART USED: rhizome.

DOSAGES: 5 to 10 g.

FLAVOR: sweet and bitter.

ENERGY: warm.

ACTIONS: To tone up energy, strengthen spleen, dry dampness, benefit water, check perspiration.

INDICATIONS: Spleen deficiency, poor appetite, edema, excessive perspiration.

18. **CHINESE:** Bai-zi-ren 柏子仁 (oriental arborvitae kernel).

BOTANICAL: Biota orientalis (L.) Endl.

PHARMACEUTICAL: Semen Biotae.

PART USED: ripe kernel.

DOSAGES: 3 to 10 g.

FLAVOR: sweet.

ENERGY: neutral.

ACTIONS: To calm the heart and spirits, check perspiration, lubricate dryness, induce bowel movements.

INDICATIONS: Insomnia, palpitation, constipation, night sweats.

19. **CHINESE:** Ba-ji-tian 巴戟天 (morinda root).

BOTANICAL: Morinda officinalis How.

PHARMACEUTICAL: Radix Morindae Officinalis.

PART USED: root.

DOSAGES: 6 to 15 g.

FLAVOR: pungent and sweet.

ENERGY: warm.

ACTIONS: To warm kidneys, strengthen yang, strengthen tendons and bones.

INDICATIONS: Kidney yang deficiency, impotence, lumbago, dizziness, ringing in ears.

20. **CHINESE:** Ban-lan-gen 板藍根 (woad).

BOTANICAL: Isatis tinctoria L.

PHARMACEUTICAL: Radix Isatidis.

PART USED: root.

DOSAGES: 10 to 60 g.

FLAVOR: bitter.

ENERGY: cold.

ACTIONS: To clear heat, counteract toxic effects, cool the blood, heal swelling, benefit throat.

INDICATIONS: Scabies, erysipelas, sore throat, hepatitis, mumps.

21. **CHINESE:** Ban-xia 半夏 (half-summer pinellia).

BOTANICAL: Pinellia ternata (Thunb.) Breit.

PHARMACEUTICAL: Rhizoma Pinelliae Tuber Pinelliae.

PART USED: rhizome.

DOSAGES: 3 to 10 g.

FLAVOR: pungent.

ENERGY: warm.

ACTIONS: To dry dampness, transform sputum, bring down upsurging energy, relieve vomiting.

INDICATIONS: Asthma, cough, vomiting.

NOTE: For carbuncles and swelling, apply externally; use with care for pregnant women.

22. **CHINESE:** Ban-zhi-lian 半枝蓮 (barbed skullcap).

BOTANICAL: Scutellaria barbata D. Don.

PHARMACEUTICAL: Herba Scutellariae Barbatae.

PART USED: whole plant.

DOSAGES: 15 to 30 g.

FLAVOR: bitter.

ENERGY: cool.

ACTIONS: To clear heat, counteract toxic effects, promote urination, heal swelling.

INDICATIONS: Cancers of various kinds, appendicitis, hepatitis, cirrhosis (degeneration of the liver cells and thickening of the surrounding tissues), ascites (accumulation of fluid in the abdomen), snake bites, carbuncles.

23. **CHINESE:** Bei-sha-shen 北沙參 (straight ladybell north).

BOTANICAL: Glehnia littoralis Fr. Schmidt ex Miq.

PHARMACEUTICAL: Radix Glehniae.

PART USED: root.

DOSAGES: 6 to 15 g.

FLAVOR: sweet and slightly bitter.

ENERGY: slightly cold.

ACTIONS: To benefit energy, lubricate the lungs, suppress cough, nourish stomach, produce fluids.

INDICATIONS: Dry cough, lung disease, dehydration after a hot disease, dry throat, thirst.

24. **CHINESE:** Bian-xu 萹蓄 (knot grass).

BOTANICAL: Polygonum aviculare L.

PHARMACEUTICAL: Herba Polygoni Avicularis.

PART USED: whole plant.

DOSAGES: 3 to 10 g.

FLAVOR: bitter.

ENERGY: neutral.

ACTIONS: To clear heat, benefit water, relieve urinary problems.

INDICATIONS: Urinary problems, jaundice, bacillary dysentery, abdominal pain due to roundworms, eczema.

25. **CHINESE:** Bi-bo 蓽茇 (long pepper).

BOTANICAL: Piper longum L.

PHARMACEUTICAL: Fructus Piperis Longi.

PART USED: fruit/pike.

DOSAGES: 2 to 3 g.

FLAVOR: pungent.

ENERGY: extremely warm.

ACTIONS: To warm the internal region and the stomach.

INDICATIONS: Vomiting due to cold, abdominal swelling and pain, headache, diarrhea, toothache, sinusitis.

26. **CHINESE:** Bing-lang 檳榔 (areca nut).

BOTANICAL: Areca Catechu L.

PHARMACEUTICAL: Semen Arecae.

PART USED: ripe seed.

DOSAGES: 9 to 60 g.

FLAVOR: bitter and pungent.

ENERGY: warm.

ACTIONS: To destroy worms, eliminate accumulations, promote energy circulation, induce bowel movements.

INDICATIONS: Parasites in the intestines, hydatid disease, fasciolopsis, edema, constipation.

27. **CHINESE:** Bo-he 薄荷 (peppermint).

BOTANICAL: Mentha haplocalyx Briq.

PHARMACEUTICAL: Herba Menthae.

PART USED: stalk and leaf.

DOSAGES: 2 to 3 g.

FLAVOR: pungent.

ENERGY: cool.

ACTIONS: Induce perspiration; clear heat; disperse wind.

INDICATIONS: Mouth canker, toothache, full sensation and pain in the chest and abdominal region.

28. **CHINESE:** Bu-gu-zhi 補骨脂 (Poguzhi; psoralea).

BOTANICAL: Psoralea corylifolia L.

PHARMACEUTICAL: Fructus Psoraleae.

PART USED: ripe fruit.

DOSAGES: 3 to 10 g.

FLAVOR: pungent.

ENERGY: extremely warm.

ACTIONS: To warm and tone kidney yang.

INDICATIONS: Kidney deficiency, seminal emission, diarrhea, enuresis (incontinence of urine).

29. **CHINESE:** Cang-er-zi 蒼耳子 (achene of Siberian cocklebur).

BOTANICAL: Xanthium sibiricum Patr.

PHARMACEUTICAL: Fructus Xanthii.

PART USED: ripe fruit.

DOSAGES: 3 to 10 g.

FLAVOR: sweet and bitter.

ENERGY: warm.

ACTIONS: To expel wind and drive out dampness, facilite passages of cavities.

INDICATIONS: Common cold, sinusitis, rhinitis, ringing in ears, hearing difficulty, leprosy.

30. **CHINESE:** Cang-zhu 蒼朮 (gray atractylodes).

BOTANICAL: Atractylodes lancea (Thunb.) D.C./- chinensis (DC.) Koidz.

PHARMACEUTICAL: Rhizoma Atractylodis.

PART USED: rhizome.

DOSAGES: 3 to 10 g.

FLAVOR: pungent and bitter.

ENERGY: warm.

ACTIONS: To dry up dampness, expel wind, relieve pain, sharpen vision.

INDICATIONS: Rheumatism, weak legs, night blindness, skin itch.

31. **CHINESE:** Cao-dou-kou 草豆蔻 (alpinis seed).

BOTANICAL: Alpinia katsumadai Hayata.

PHARMACEUTICAL: Semen Alpiniae Katsumadai.

PART USED: ripe seed.

DOSAGES: 2.5 to 6 g.

FLAVOR: pungent.

ENERGY: warm.

ACTIONS: To strengthen spleen, dry dampness, warm the stomach, relieve vomiting.

INDICATIONS: Cold abdominal pain, swallowing difficulty, vomiting, diarrhea.

32. **CHINESE:** Ce-bai-ye 側柏葉 (oriental arborvitae).

BOTANICAL: Biota orientalis (L.) Endl.

PHARMACEUTICAL: Cacumen Biotae Folium et Ramulus Biotae.

PART USED: twig and leaf.

DOSAGES: 9 to 15 g.

FLAVOR: bitter.

ENERGY: slightly cold.

ACTIONS: To cool blood, arrest bleeding, clear heat, expel coagulations.

INDICATIONS: Coughing with blood due to hot lungs, vomiting with blood, nosebleed, urine containing blood, unusual vaginal bleeding.

33. **CHINESE:** Chai-hu 柴胡 (hare's ear).

BOTANICAL: Bupleurum chinense DC./- Bupleurum scorzonerifolium Willd.

PHARMACEUTICAL: Radix Bupleuri.

PART USED: root.

DOSAGES: 3 to 10 g.

FLAVOR: bitter.

ENERGY: slightly cold.

ACTIONS: To elevate yang; disperse heat; relieve congestion; disperse liver energy.

INDICATIONS: Malaria, pain in ribs, irregular menstrual flow, prolapse of rectum and uterus.

34. **CHINESE:** Chang-pu 菖蒲 (Shui-chang-pu 水菖蒲; calamus).

BOTANICAL: Acorus calamus.

PHARMACEUTICAL: Rhizoma Calami.

PART USED: rhizome.

DOSAGES: 2.5 to 5 g.

FLAVOR: pungent.

ENERGY: warm.

ACTIONS: To open up cavities, expel sputum, counteract toxic effects, destroy worms.

INDICATIONS: Mental instability, convulsion, rheumatism.

NOTE: For scabies and carbuncles, apply externally.

35. **CHINESE:** Chen-pi 陳皮 (tangerine peel).

BOTANICAL: Citrus reticulata Blanco/- tangerina Hort. et Tanaka/- erythrosa Tanaka.

PHARMACEUTICAL: Pericarpium Citri reticulatae/Pericarpium Aurantii.

PART USED: ripe fruit peel.

DOSAGES: 3 to 6 g.

FLAVOR: bitter and pungent.

ENERGY: warm.

ACTIONS: To promote energy circulation, strengthen spleen, transform dampness, expel sputum.

INDICATIONS: Excessive dampness, upper abdominal distension, poor appetite, nausea, vomiting, cough.

36. **CHINESE:** Che-qian-zi 車前子 (Asiatic plantain seed).

BOTANICAL: Plantago asiatica L./- depressa Willd.

PHARMACEUTICAL: Semen Plantaginis.

PART USED: ripe seed.

DOSAGES: 6 to 18 g.

FLAVOR: sweet.

ENERGY: cold.

ACTIONS: To clear heat, benefit water, relieve cough, expel sputum.

INDICATIONS: Urination difficulty, edema, diarrhea, jaundice, cough.

37. **CHINESE:** Chi-xiao-dou 赤小豆 (small red bean).

BOTANICAL: Phaseolus calcalatus Roxb./- angularis Wight.

PHARMACEUTICAL: Semen Phaseoli.

PART USED: ripe seed.

DOSAGES: 10 to 15 g.

FLAVOR: sweet and sour.

ENERGY: neutral.

ACTIONS: To promote urination, heal swelling, counteract toxic effects, and drain pus.

INDICATIONS: Edema, beriberi, carbuncle, diarrhea.

NOTE: Chi-xiao-dou is often called azuki bean in the United States, but there is a difference. The Japanese azuki bean is round, whereas the Chinese small red bean is long in shape and has stronger effects as an herb.

38. **CHINESE:** Chuan-bei 川貝 (tendril-leaved fritillary bulb).

BOTANICAL: Fritillaris cirrhosa D. Don.

PHARMACEUTICAL: Bulbus Fritillariae Cirrhosae/- Roylei.

PART USED: bulb.

DOSAGES: 5 to 10 g.

FLAVOR: bitter and sweet.

ENERGY: slightly cold.

ACTIONS: To lubricate lungs, transform dry sputum, disperse accumulations, remove heat.

INDICATIONS: Cough, vomiting of blood, sore throat, goiter.

39. **CHINESE:** Chuan-xiong 川芎 (hemlock parsley).

BOTANICAL: Ligusticum Chuan-xiong (hemlock parsley) Hort./- wallichii Franchet.

PHARMACEUTICAL: Rhizoma Ligustici Chuan- xiong (hemlock parsley).

PART USED: rhizome.

DOSAGES: 3 to 10 g.

FLAVOR: pungent.

ENERGY: warm.

ACTIONS: To activate the blood, disperse coagulations, expel wind, promote energy circulation, relieve pain.

INDICATIONS: Dizziness, headache, suppression of menstruation, abdominal pain, rib pain, carbuncles, irregular periods.

40. **CHINESE:** Cong-bai 葱白 (Welsh onion).

BOTANICAL: Allium fistulosum L.

PHARMACEUTICAL: Allium Fistulosum L.

PART USED: bulb.

DOSAGES: 6 to 15 g.

FLAVOR: pungent.

ENERGY: warm.

ACTIONS: To disperse cold; induce perspiration; connect yang; activate the blood; destroy worms.

INDICATIONS: Common cold, acute diarrhea, cold limbs, biliary ascariasis (infestation of the bile ducts or gallbladder).

41. **CHINESE:** Da-huang 大黃 (rhubarb).

BOTANICAL: Rheum palmatum L./- tanguticum Maxim. ex Balf./- officinale Baill.

PHARMACEUTICAL: Radix et Rhizoma Rhei.

PART USED: root and rhizome.

DOSAGES: 3 to 12 g.

FLAVOR: bitter.

ENERGY: cold.

ACTIONS: To attack accumulations, sedate fire, counteract toxic effects, remove coagulations.

INDICATIONS: Excess heat in stomach and intestines, nosebleed, blood coagulation, vomiting of blood, amenorrhea (suppression of period).

42. **CHINESE:** Da-ji 大薊 (Japanese thistle).

BOTANICAL: Cirsium japonicum DC.

PHARMACEUTICAL: Herba seu Radix Cirsii japonici.

PART USED: whole plant.

DOSAGES: 10 to 15 g.

FLAVOR: sweet.

ENERGY: cool.

ACTIONS: To cool the blood, arrest bleeding, disperse blood coagulations.

INDICATIONS: Vomiting of blood, nosebleed, urine containing blood, vaginal bleeding, carbuncles.

43. **CHINESE:** Dang-gui 當歸 (Chinese angelica).

BOTANICAL: Angelica sinensis (Oliv.) Diels.

PHARMACEUTICAL: Radix Angelicae Sinensis.

PART USED: root.

DOSAGES: 5 to 15 g.

FLAVOR: sweet and pungent.

ENERGY: warm.

ACTIONS: To tone and activate blood, regulate menstruation, moisten the intestines.

INDICATIONS: Blood deficiency and coagulation causing amenorrhea and abdominal pain, rheumatism, constipation.

44. CHINESE: Dang-shen 黨參
(root of pilose asiabell).

BOTANICAL: Codonopsis pilosula (Franch.) Nannf.

PHARMACEUTICAL: Radix Codonopsis Pilosulae.

PART USED: root.

DOSAGES: 10 to 30 g.

FLAVOR: sweet.

ENERGY: neutral.

ACTIONS: To tone middle region, benefit energy, strengthen spleen, produce fluids.

INDICATIONS: Energy deficiency, excessive perspiration, prolapse of rectum and uterus, diarrhea, cough and asthma, diabetes.

45. CHINESE: Dan-pi 丹皮
(Mu-dan-pi 牧丹皮; peony/moutan bark).

BOTANICAL: Paeonia suffruticosa Andr.

PHARMACEUTICAL: Cortex Moutan Radicis.

PART USED: root bark.

DOSAGES: 6 to 15 g.

FLAVOR: sweet and bitter.

ENERGY: cold.

ACTIONS: To clear heat, cool the blood, resolve coagulations.

INDICATIONS: Periodic fever, irregular menstruation, carbuncles, swelling, blood coagulation caused by injuries.

46. CHINESE: Dan-shen 丹參
(purple sage/Salvia root/red sage root).

BOTANICAL: Salvia miltiorrhiza Bge.

PHARMACEUTICAL: Radix Salviae Miltiorrhizae.

PART USED: root.

DOSAGES: 6 to 15 g.

FLAVOR: bitter.

ENERGY: slightly cold.

ACTIONS: To activate the blood, regulate menstruation, clear heat, cool the blood.

INDICATIONS: Irregular periods, vaginal bleeding, abdominal obstructions, amenorrhea (suppression of menstruation), insomnia.

47. CHINESE: Dan-zhu-ye 淡竹葉
(light bamboo leaf).

BOTANICAL: Lophatherum gracile Brongn.

PHARMACEUTICAL: Herba Lophatheri.

PART USED: plant (no tuberous root).

DOSAGES: 6 to 12 g.

FLAVOR: sweet and light.

ENERGY: cool.

ACTIONS: To clear heat, relieve depression, promote urination.

INDICATIONS: Discharge of red urine, mental depression, painful urination, mouth canker, crying at night in children.

48. CHINESE: Da-qing-ye 大青葉
(mayflower glorybower leaf/Isatis leaf).

BOTANICAL: Isatis tinctoria L./- indigotia Fort

PHARMACEUTICAL: Folium Isatidis.

PART USED: leaf.

DOSAGES: 10 to 30 g.

FLAVOR: bitter.

ENERGY: cold.

ACTIONS: To clear heat and counteract toxic effects, cool the blood, heal swelling.

INDICATIONS: Hot disease, spotted fever, erysipelas, sore throat, hepatitis, mumps.

49. **CHINESE:** Da-suan 大蒜 (garlic).

BOTANICAL: Allium sativum L.

PHARMACEUTICAL: Bulbus Allii.

PART USED: bulb.

DOSAGES: 6 to 15 g.

FLAVOR: pungent.

ENERGY: warm.

ACTIONS: To counteract toxic effects, destroy parasites, promote energy circulation, eliminate water, clear heat.

INDICATIONS: Amebic dysentery, tapeworms, trichomonas vaginitis, fish and shellfish poisoning, edema, beriberi.

50. **CHINESE:** Da-zao 大棗 (red date).

BOTANICAL: Ziziphus jujuba Mill.

PHARMACEUTICAL: Fructus Ziziphi Jujubae.

PART USED: ripe fruit.

DOSAGES: 3–12 dates.

FLAVOR: sweet.

ENERGY: warm.

ACTIONS: To strengthen the spleen and stomach, harmonize various herbal ingredients in a formula.

INDICATIONS: Weakness of spleen and stomach.

51. **CHINESE:** Di-fu-zi 地膚子 (summer cypress).

BOTANICAL: Kochia scoparia (L.) Schrad.

PHARMACEUTICAL: Fructus Kochiae.

PART USED: seed and fruit.

DOSAGES: 5 to 10 g.

FLAVOR: sweet and bitter.

ENERGY: cold.

ACTIONS: To clear damp heat, promote urination.

INDICATIONS: Urination difficulty, cystitis, urinary strains, beriberi, edema, urethritis.

52. **CHINESE:** Di-gu-pi 地骨皮 (root bark of Chinese wolfberry).

BOTANICAL: Lycium chinense Mill./- barbarum L.

PHARMACEUTICAL: Cortex Lycii Radicis.

PART USED: root bark.

DOSAGES: 10 to 15 g.

FLAVOR: sweet.

ENERGY: cold.

ACTIONS: To clear deficiency heat, relieve mental depression.

INDICATIONS: Periodic fever, chronic fever.

53. **CHINESE:** Ding-xiang 丁香 (clove).

BOTANICAL: Eugenia caryophyllata Thunberg (Caryophyllus aromaticus L.).

PHARMACEUTICAL: Flos Caryophylli.

PART USED: flower bud.

DOSAGES: 1 to 3 g.

FLAVOR: pungent.

ENERGY: warm.

ACTIONS: To bring down energy, warm spleen and kidneys, relieve pain.

INDICATIONS: Hiccups, vomiting, spleen and kidney cold deficiency, cold abdominal pain.

54. **CHINESE:** Di-yu 地榆 (burnet).

BOTANICAL: Sanguisorba officinalis L.

PHARMACEUTICAL: Radix Sanguisorbae.

PART USED: root and rhizome.

DOSAGES: 6 to 15 g.

FLAVOR: bitter and sour.

ENERGY: slightly cold.

ACTIONS: To cool the blood, arrest bleeding, clear heat, remove dampness.

INDICATIONS: Bloody stool, dysentery, vaginal bleeding due to hot blood, burns, bleeding piles.

55. **CHINESE:** Dong-chong-xia-cao 冬蟲夏草 (Chinese caterpillar fungus).

BOTANICAL: Cordyceps sinensis (Berk.) Sacc.

PHARMACEUTICAL: Cordyceps Sinensis.

PART USED: caterpillar fungus.

DOSAGES: 5 to 10 g.

FLAVOR: sweet.

ENERGY: slightly warm.

ACTIONS: To water and tone lungs and kidneys, benefit semen and marrow, transform sputum, arrest bleeding.

INDICATIONS: Cough due to deficiency fatigue, cough with bloody sputum, spontaneous sweating, impotence, lumbago.

56. **CHINESE:** Dong-gua-ren 冬瓜仁 (wax gourd seed).

BOTANICAL: Benincasa hispida (Thunb.) Cogn.

PHARMACEUTICAL: Semen Benincasae.

PART USED: ripe seed.

DOSAGES: 1 to 30 g.

FLAVOR: sweet and light.

ENERGY: neutral and cool.

ACTIONS: To transform hot sputum, benefit water, suppress cough, drain off pus, promote urination, heal swelling, clear heat, lubricate lungs.

INDICATIONS: Cough, lung abscess, chronic bronchitis, edema, vaginal discharge, diabetes.

57. **CHINESE:** Du-huo 獨活 (downy angelica).

BOTANICAL: Angelica pubescens Maxim.f biserrata Shan et Yuan.

PHARMACEUTICAL: Radix Angelicae Pubescentis.

PART USED: root and rhizome.

DOSAGES: 3 to 10 g.

FLAVOR: pungent and bitter.

ENERGY: slightly warm.

ACTIONS: To remove wind and dampness, induce perspiration, disperse cold.

INDICATIONS: Rheumatism, pain across loins and in legs.

58. **CHINESE:** Du-zhong 杜仲 (eucommia bark).

BOTANICAL: Eucommia ulmoides oliv.

PHARMACEUTICAL: Cortex Eucommiae.

PART USED: bark.

DOSAGES: 3 to 10 g.

FLAVOR: sweet and bitter.

ENERGY: warm.

ACTIONS: To tone liver and kidney, strengthen tendons and bones, secure fetus.

INDICATIONS: Lumbago, fetus motion, headache and dizziness due to kidney deficiency, weak legs.

59. **CHINESE:** E-jiao 阿膠 (donkey-hide gelatin).

ZOOLOGICAL: Colla Corii Asini Equus asinus chinensis.

PHARMACEUTICAL: Colla Corii Asini Gelatina Nigra.

PART USED: prepared glue.

DOSAGES: 3 to 10 g.

FLAVOR: sweet.

ENERGY: neutral.

ACTIONS: To water yin, nourish blood, tone lungs, lubricate dryness, arrest bleeding, secure fetus.

INDICATIONS: Emaciation, irregular periods, insecure fetus, blood deficiency, nosebleed, cough with bloody sputum.

60. **CHINESE:** Fang-feng 防風 (Chinese wind shelter).

BOTANICAL: Ledebouriella divaricata (Turcz.).

PHARMACEUTICAL: Radix Ledebouriellae.

PART USED: root.

DOSAGES: 3 to 9 g.

FLAVOR: pungent.

ENERGY: slightly warm.

ACTIONS: To induce perspiration, disperse cold, relieve pain, overcome dampness.

INDICATIONS: Wind and dampness rheumatism.

61. **CHINESE:** Fan-xie-ye 番瀉葉 (senna leaf).

BOTANICAL: Cassia angustifolia Vahl/-acutifolia Delile (Cassia senna L.).

PHARMACEUTICAL: Folium Sennae.

PART USED: leaf.

DOSAGES: 3 to 10 g.

FLAVOR: sweet and bitter.

ENERGY: cold.

ACTIONS: To induce bowel movements.

INDICATIONS: Constipation, indigestion.

NOTE: Not to be used by pregnant women.

62. **CHINESE:** Fu-ling 茯苓 (tuckahoe/Indian bread).

BOTANICAL: Poria cocos (Schw.) Wolf (Pachyma hoelen Rumph).

PHARMACEUTICAL: Poria.

PART USED: fungus nucleus.

DOSAGES: 10 to 18 g.

FLAVOR: sweet and light.

ENERGY: neutral.

ACTIONS: To transform dampness, strengthen spleen, calm the heart and spirits.

INDICATIONS: Diarrhea due to spleen deficiency, diminished urination, edema, palpitation, insomnia.

63. **CHINESE:** Fu-pen-zi 覆盆子 (wild raspberry).

BOTANICAL: Rubus chingii Hu Rubus palmatus Thunberg.

PHARMACEUTICAL: Fructus Rubi.

PART USED: unripe fruit.

DOSAGES: 6 to 12 g.

FLAVOR: sweet and sour.

ENERGY: warm.

ACTIONS: To tone liver and kidneys, restrain semen, check urination, sharpen vision.

INDICATIONS: Impotence, seminal emission, enuresis, frequent urination, vaginal discharge, blurred vision.

64. **CHINESE:** Fu-shen 茯神 (poria with hostwood).

BOTANICAL: Poria cocos (Schw.) Wolf.

PHARMACEUTICAL: Poria cum Ligno Hospite.

PART USED: mass of fungus with its host wood (usually pine root)

DOSAGES: 10 to 15 g.

FLAVOR: sweet and light.

ENERGY: neutral.

ACTIONS: To calm the heart and spirit, promote urination.

INDICATIONS: Palpitation, forgetfulness, convulsion, urination difficulty.

65. **CHINESE:** Gan-cao 甘草 (licorice).

BOTANICAL: Glycyrrhiza uralensis Fisch./-inflata Bat./- glabra L.

PHARMACEUTICAL: Radix Glycyrrhizae.

PART USED: root and rhizome.

DOSAGES: 2 to 10 g.

FLAVOR: sweet.

ENERGY: neutral.

ACTIONS: To tone spleen, benefit energy, produce fluids, release toxins, harmonize various herbs, slow down symptoms.

INDICATIONS: Spleen and stomach weakness, dry cough, sore throat, acute abdominal pain, carbuncles, swelling, poisoning.

66. **CHINESE:** Gan-jiang 干姜 (dried ginger).

BOTANICAL: Zingiber officinale (Willd.) Rosc.

PHARMACEUTICAL: Rhizoma Zingiberis.

PART USED: rhizome.

DOSAGES: 3 to 10 g.

FLAVOR: pungent.

ENERGY: warm.

ACTIONS: To warm internal region, dispel cold, warm lungs, relieve vomiting.

INDICATIONS: Cold and deficiency of spleen and stomach (spleen-stomach yang deficiency syndrome), cold lungs syndrome with cough.

67. **CHINESE:** Gan-sui 甘遂 (Kansui root).

BOTANICAL: Euphorbia kansui T.N. Liou ex T. P. Wang.

PHARMACEUTICAL: Radix Euphorbiae Kansui.

PART USED: root.

DOSAGES: 2 to 10 g.

FLAVOR: bitter.

ENERGY: cold.

ACTIONS: To expel water, promote urination and bowel movements, expel sputum, counteract toxic effects.

INDICATIONS: Edema, sputum, blood coagulations, schistosomiasis at a late stage, hepatic ascites.

68. **CHINESE:** Gao-liang-jiang 高良姜 (lesser galangal).

BOTANICAL: Alpinia officinarum Hance.

PHARMACEUTICAL: Rhizoma Alpiniae Officinarum.

PART USED: rhizome.

DOSAGES: 3 to 10 g.

FLAVOR: pungent.

ENERGY: warm.

ACTIONS: To warm the internal regions, disperse cold, relieve pain, strengthen the stomach.

INDICATIONS: Stomachache due to cold and deficiency of spleen and stomach (spleen-stomach yang deficiency syndrome), vomiting.

69. **CHINESE:** Ge-gen 葛根 (kudzu vine).

BOTANICAL: Pueraria lobata (Willd.) Ohwi/-thomsanii Benth.

PHARMACEUTICAL: Radix Puerariae.

PART USED: root.

DOSAGES: 10 to 25 g.

FLAVOR: sweet and pungent.

ENERGY: neutral.

ACTIONS: To induce perspiration; clear heat; facilitate measle eruption, elevate clear energy, relieve diarrhea.

INDICATIONS: Measles prior to eruptions, diarrhea (better used in roasted form), headache in forehead area, stiff neck.

70. **CHINESE:** Ge-hua 葛花 (kudzu vine flower).

SCIENTIFIC: Pueraria omeiensis Wang et Tang.

PHARMACEUTICAL: Flos Puerariae.

PART USED: flower.

DOSAGES: 5 to 10 g.

FLAVOR: sweet.

ENERGY: cool.

MERIDIANS: stomach.

ACTIONS: To relieve drunkenness, energize the spleen.

INDICATIONS: Symptoms caused by alcoholism, thirst, poor appetite, vomiting of acid, vomiting of blood, anal bleeding as in hemorrhoids.

71. **CHINESE:** Ge-jie 蛤蚧 (gecko).

ZOOLOGICAL: Gekko gecko L.

PHARMACEUTICAL: Gecko.

PART USED: body.

DOSAGES: 2 to 6 g.

FLAVOR: salty.

ENERGY: neutral.

ACTIONS: To tone lungs and kidneys, benefit semen and kidneys, absorb inspiration.

INDICATIONS: Weakness after chronic illness, cough and asthma due to deficiency, frequent urination, cough with bloody sputum.

72. **CHINESE:** Gou-qi-zi 枸杞子 (matrimony vine fruit).

BOTANICAL: Lycium barbarum L.

PHARMACEUTICAL: Fructus Lycii.

PART USED: ripe fruit.

DOSAGES: 5 to 10 g.

FLAVOR: sweet.

ENERGY: neutral.

ACTIONS: To tone kidneys, nourish liver and blood, sharpen vision.

INDICATIONS: Blood deficiency with dizziness and blurred vision, lumbago, seminal emission, diabetes.

73. **CHINESE:** Gou-teng 鉤藤 (gambir).

BOTANICAL: Uncaria rhynchophylla (Miq.) Jacks./- macrophylla Wall./- hirsuta Havil./- sinensis (Oliv.) Havil./- sessilifructus Roxb.

PHARMACEUTICAL: Ramulus Uncariae Cum Uncis Rhynchophylla.

PART USED: twig.

DOSAGES: 6 to 15 g.

FLAVOR: sweet.

ENERGY: slightly cold.

ACTIONS: To stop wind, remove heat, calm convulsion, stop dizziness.

INDICATIONS: Convulsions in children, dizziness, headache, fever, twitching.

74. **CHINESE:** Gua-lou 瓜蔞子 (snake gourd).

BOTANICAL: Trichosanthes kirilowii Maxim./ - uniflora Hao.

PHARMACEUTICAL: Fructus Trichosanthis.

PART USED: fruit.

DOSAGES: 6 to 15 g.

FLAVOR: sweet and bitter.

ENERGY: cold.

ACTIONS: To clear lungs, transform sputum, expand chest, disperse accumulations, lubricate intestines.

INDICATIONS: Cough, asthma, lungs abscess, chest pain, diabetes, jaundice.

75. **CHINESE:** Gua-lou-ren 瓜蔞仁 (Gua-lou-zi; snake gourd kernel).

BOTANICAL: Trichosanthes kirilowii Maxim./ uniflora Hao.

PHARMACEUTICAL: Semen Trichosanthis.

PART USED: ripe seed.

DOSAGES: 10 to 12 g.

FLAVOR: sweet.

ENERGY: cold.

ACTIONS: To clear heat, expel sputum, lubricate lungs and intestines, heal carbuncles, disperse congestion.

INDICATIONS: Cough with plenty of sputum, constipation, mastitis.

76. **CHINESE:** Gui-zhi 桂枝 (cinnamon stick).

BOTANICAL: Cinnamomum cassia Presl.

PHARMACEUTICAL: Ramulus Cinnamomi.

PART USED: twig.

DOSAGES: 3 to 10 g.

FLAVOR: pungent and sweet.

ENERGY: warm.

ACTIONS: To induce perspiration; disperse cold; warm meridians.

INDICATIONS: Cold rheumatism, decline in heart yang, superficial cold.

77. **CHINESE:** Gu-sui-bu 骨碎補 (rhizome of fortune's drynaria).

BOTANICAL: Drynaria fortunei (Kunze) J.Sm./- baronii (Christ) Diels.

PHARMACEUTICAL: Rhizoma Drynariae.

PART USED: rhizome.

DOSAGES: 5 to 10 g.

FLAVOR: bitter.

ENERGY: warm.

ACTIONS: To tone kidneys, facilitate mending of tendons and bones, activate the blood, relieve pain.

INDICATIONS: Fracture, lumbago, kidney deficiency with ringing in ears.

78. **CHINESE:** Hai-piao-xiao 海螵蛸 (Wuzeigu/Moyugu; cuttlebone).

ZOOLOGICAL: Sepiella maindroni de Rochebrune Sepia esculenta Hoyle.

PHARMACEUTICAL: Os Sepiellae Seu Sepiae Os Sepiae.

PART USED: inner shell.

DOSAGES: 5 to 15 g.

FLAVOR: salty.

ENERGY: slightly warm.

ACTIONS: To solidify semen, check urination, arrest bleeding, relieve pain.

INDICATIONS: Acid indigestion, seminal emission, vaginal discharge, bleeding symptoms.

79. **CHINESE:** Han-lian-cao 旱蓮草 (ink plant).

BOTANICAL: Eclipta prostrata L.

PHARMACEUTICAL: Herba Ecliptae.

PART USED: aerial part.

DOSAGES: 6 to 15 g.

FLAVOR: sweet and sour.

ENERGY: slightly cold.

ACTIONS: To benefit yin, tone kidneys, cool the blood, arrest bleeding, return gray hair to its original color.

INDICATIONS: Periodic fever in yin deficiency, vomiting of blood, coughing with blood, anal bleeding.

80. **CHINESE:** He-huan-pi 合歡皮 (mimosa).

BOTANICAL: Albizia julibrissin Durazz./- kalkora (Roxb.) Prain.

PHARMACEUTICAL: Cortex Albiziae.

PART USED: bark.

DOSAGES: 6 to 12 g.

FLAVOR: sweet.

ENERGY: neutral.

ACTIONS: To calm the spirits, disperse energy congestion, harmonize the blood, relieve pain, facilitate mending of bones.

INDICATIONS: Nervousness, insomnia, lung disease, bone fracture.

81. **CHINESE:** He-shou-wu 何首烏 (tuber of multiflower knotweed/ Fleeceflower root).

BOTANICAL: Polygonum multiflorum Thunb.

PHARMACEUTICAL: Radix Polygoni Multiflori.

PART USED: tuberous root.

DOSAGES: 10 to 25 g.

FLAVOR: bitter and sweet.

ENERGY: slightly warm.

ACTIONS: To tone up liver and kidneys, nourish semen and blood.

INDICATIONS: Seminal emission, vaginal discharge, lumbago, premature gray hair.

82. **CHINESE:** He-ye 荷葉 (lotus leaf).

BOTANICAL: Nelumbo nucifera Gaertn.

PHARMACEUTICAL: Folium Nelumbinis.

PART USED: leaf.

DOSAGES: 3 to 10 g.

FLAVOR: bitter.

ENERGY: neutral.

ACTIONS: To relieve summer heat, elevate yang, arrest bleeding.

INDICATIONS: Summer heat injuries, common colds, nosebleed, diarrhea.

83. **CHINESE:** Hong-hua 紅花 (safflower).

BOTANICAL: Carthamus tinctorius L.

PHARMACEUTICAL: Flos Carthami.

PART USED: corolla.

DOSAGES: 3 to 10 g.

FLAVOR: pungent.

ENERGY: warm.

ACTIONS: To activate the blood, facilitate menstrual flow, disperse blood coagulations, relieve pain.

INDICATIONS: Period pain, amenorrhea (suppression of menstruation), stillbirth, swelling, lochiostasis (retention of blood or mucus from the uterus during the period immediately following childbirth).

84. **CHINESE:** Hou-pu 厚朴 (official magnolia).

BOTANICAL: Magnolia officinalis Rehd.et. Wils./- officinalis Rehd. et. Wils. var. biloba Rehd. et Wils.

PHARMACEUTICAL: Cortex Magnoliae Officinalis.

PART USED: bark.

DOSAGES: 3 to 12 g.

FLAVOR: bitter and pungent.

ENERGY: warm.

ACTIONS: To promote energy circulation, resolve retention of food, warm middle region, bring down energy.

INDICATIONS: Abdominal distention with pain, vomiting, abdominal pain, diarrhea, asthma.

85. **CHINESE:** Huai-hua 槐花 (Japanese pagoda tree flower).

BOTANICAL: Sophora japonica L.

PHARMACEUTICAL: Flos Sophorae.

PART USED: flower.

DOSAGES: 6 to 15 g.

FLAVOR: bitter.

ENERGY: slightly cold.

ACTIONS: To sedate heat, cool the blood, arrest bleeding.

INDICATIONS: Hemorrhoids, bloody stools, urination with blood, nosebleed, dysentery.

86. **CHINESE:** Huai-mi 槐米 (Japanese pagoda tree flower bud).

BOTANICAL: Sophora japonica L.

PHARMACEUTICAL: Flos Sophorae Immaturus.

PART USED: flower bud.

DOSAGES: 5 to 10 g.

FLAVOR: bitter.

ENERGY: neutral.

ACTIONS: To cool the blood, clear heat, arrest bleeding.

INDICATIONS: Dysentery, anal bleeding, vomiting of blood, nosebleed, unusual vaginal bleeding.

87. **CHINESE:** Hua-jiao 椒角 (Chinese prickly ash).

BOTANICAL: Zanthoxylum schinifolium Sieb. et Zucc./- bungeanum Maxim.

PHARMACEUTICAL: Pericarpium Zanthoxyli.

PART USED: peel.

DOSAGES: 3 to 10 g.

FLAVOR: pungent.

ENERGY: warm.

ACTIONS: To warm internal regions, disperse cold, relieve pain, destroy parasites.

INDICATIONS: Cold abdominal pain, roundworm disease.

88. **CHINESE:** Huang-bai 黄柏
(cork tree).

BOTANICAL: Phellodendron chinense Schneid./- amurense Rupr.

PHARMACEUTICAL: Cortex Phellodendri.

PART USED: bark.

DOSAGES: 3 to 10 g.

FLAVOR: bitter.

ENERGY: cold.

ACTIONS: To clear heat, dry dampness, sedate fire, counteract toxic effects, promote urination.

INDICATIONS: Diarrhea due to damp heat, dysentery, jaundice, urinary problems, leukorrhea, eczema, many dreams.

89. **CHINESE:** Huang-jing 黄精
(sealwort).

BOTANICAL: Polygonatum kingianum Coll. et Hemsl./- sibiricum Red./- cyrtonema Hua.

PHARMACEUTICAL: Rhizoma Polygonati.

PART USED: rhizome.

DOSAGES: 10 to 18 g.

FLAVOR: sweet.

ENERGY: neutral.

ACTIONS: To water and lubricate heart and lungs, tone middle region, promote energy, nourish semen and marrow.

INDICATIONS: Yin deficiency, blood deficiency, gray hair, dry throat, thirst, diabetes.

90. **CHINESE:** Huang-lian 黄蓮
(goldthread).

BOTANICAL: Coptis chinensis Franch./- deltoidea C. Y. Cheng et Hsiao/- teetoides C. Y. Cheng.

PHARMACEUTICAL: Rhizoma Coptidis.

PART USED: root.

DOSAGES: 3 to 10 g.

FLAVOR: bitter.

ENERGY: cold.

ACTIONS: To clear heat, sedate fire, counteract toxic effects, dry dampness.

INDICATIONS: Mouth canker, vomiting, dysentery, diarrhea, pink eyes with pain and swelling, carbuncles and eczema.

91. **CHINESE:** Huang-qi 黄耆
(membranous milk vetch).

BOTANICAL: Astragalus membranaceus (Fisch.). Bge./- membranaceus Bge. var. mongholicus. (Bge.) Hsiao.

PHARMACEUTICAL: Radix Astragali.

PART USED: root.

DOSAGES: 5 to 25 g.

FLAVOR: sweet.

ENERGY: slightly warm.

ACTIONS: To tone energy, elevate yang, solidify superficial region, check perspiration, benefit water.

INDICATIONS: Excessive perspiration due to yang deficiency, fatigue, edema, gastroptosis, prolapse of rectum and uterus.

92. **CHINESE:** Huang-qin 黄芩
(skullcap).

BOTANICAL: Scutellaria baicalensis Georgi.

PHARMACEUTICAL: Radix Scutellariae.

PART USED: root.

DOSAGES: 10 to 15 g.

FLAVOR: bitter.

ENERGY: cold.

ACTIONS: To clear heat, dry dampness, arrest bleeding, secure fetus.

INDICATIONS: Cough, insecure fetus, infections of upper respiratory tract, diarrhea, bleeding of various kinds.

93. **CHINESE:** Huang-yao-zi 黄藥子
(Ceylon white yam).

BOTANICAL: Dioscorea bulbifera Linne.

PHARMACEUTICAL: Rhizoma Dioscoreae.

PART USED: rhizome.

DOSAGES: 5 to 10 g.

FLAVOR: bitter.

ENERGY: neutral.

ACTIONS: To cool blood, bring down fire, counteract toxic effects.

INDICATIONS: Swelling of various kinds, sore throat, snake bites, dog bites, nosebleed, vomiting of blood.

94. CHINESE: Hua-shi 滑石 (talc).

MINERAL: Talcum.

PHARMACEUTICAL: Talcum.

PART USED: mineral.

DOSAGES: 10 to 30 g.

FLAVOR: sweet.

ENERGY: cold.

ACTIONS: To promote urination, transform dampness, clear summer heat.

INDICATIONS: Summer heat, diarrhea, diminished or blocked urination, painful urination, urinary stones.

95. CHINESE: Huo-ma-ren 火痲仁 (hemp).

BOTANICAL: Cannabis sativa L.

PHARMACEUTICAL: Fructus Cannabis.

PART USED: fruit.

DOSAGES: 10 to 15 g.

FLAVOR: sweet.

ENERGY: neutral.

ACTIONS: To lubricate dryness and dry intestines.

INDICATIONS: Constipation with dryness, senile constipation, chronic constipation, constipation after childbirth.

96. CHINESE: Huo-xiang 藿香 (Korean mint).

BOTANICAL: Agastache rugosus. (Fisch. et Mey) O. Ktze./Pogostemon cablin (Blanco) Benth.

PHARMACEUTICAL: Herba Agastachis.

PART USED: stalk and leaf.

DOSAGES: 3 to 10 g.

FLAVOR: pungent.

ENERGY: slightly warm.

ACTIONS: To transform dampness, harmonize the stomach, relieve vomiting.

INDICATIONS: Nausea, vomiting.

97. CHINESE: Jie-geng 桔梗 (kikio root).

BOTANICAL: Platycodon grandiflorum (Jacq.) A. DC.

PHARMACEUTICAL: Radix Platycodi.

PART USED: root.

DOSAGES: 3 to 10 g.

FLAVOR: pungent and bitter.

ENERGY: slightly warm.

ACTIONS: To expand lung energy, expel sputum, suppress cough, drain pus.

INDICATIONS: Sore throat, hoarseness, cough and copious sputum, lung abscess, pneumonia, pulmonary gangrene.

98. CHINESE: Ji-nei-jin 雞内金 (membrane of chicken gizzard).

ZOOLOGICAL: Gallus gallus domesticus Briss.

PHARMACEUTICAL: Endothelium Corneum Gigeriae Galli.

PART USED: inner membrane of chicken gizzard.

DOSAGES: 3 to 10 g.

FLAVOR: sweet.

ENERGY: neutral.

ACTIONS: To eliminate accumulation, strengthen the spleen, dissolve stones.

INDICATIONS: Indigestion, poor appetite due to spleen deficiency, abdominal lump, urinary stones.

99. CHINESE: Jing-jie 荊芥 (Japanese ground-ivy).

BOTANICAL: Schizonepeta tenuifolia Briq.

PHARMACEUTICAL: Herba Seu Flos Schizonepetae.

PART USED: aerial part.

DOSAGES: 3 to 10 g.

FLAVOR: pungent.

ENERGY: warm.

ACTIONS: To induce perspiration, disperse cold, expel wind, relieve pain, arrest bleeding (pan fry until charred black and consume).

INDICATIONS: Carbuncles, swelling, unusual vaginal bleeding, bloody stools as in hemorrhoids.

100. **CHINESE:** Jin-qian-cao 金錢草 (coin grass).

BOTANICAL: Glechoma longituba (Nakai) Kupr.

PHARMACEUTICAL: Herba Glechoma.

PART USED: whole plant.

DOSAGES: 10 to 15 g.

FLAVOR: bitter and pungent.

ENERGY: cool.

ACTIONS: To clear heat, promote urination, suppress cough, heal swelling, counteract toxic effects.

INDICATIONS: Jaundice, edema, bladder stones, malaria, lung disease, cough, vomiting of blood, rheumatism.

101. **CHINESE:** Jin-ying-zi 金櫻子 (Cherokee rose hips).

BOTANICAL: Rosa laevigata Michx.

PHARMACEUTICAL: Fructus Rosae Laevigatae.

PART USED: ripe fruit.

DOSAGES: 6 to 12 g.

FLAVOR: sweet and sour.

ENERGY: neutral.

ACTIONS: To benefit kidneys, restrain semen, relieve diarrhea.

INDICATIONS: Frequent urination, enuresis, chronic diarrhea, seminal emission, excessive vaginal bleeding and discharge.

102. **CHINESE:** Jin-yin-hua 金銀花 (Japanese honeysuckle).

BOTANICAL: Lonicera japonica Thunb./- hypoglauca Miq./- confusa DC./- dasystyla Rehd.

PHARMACEUTICAL: Flos Lonicerae.

PART USED: flower bud.

DOSAGES: 10 to 15 g.

FLAVOR: sweet.

ENERGY: cold.

ACTIONS: To clear heat, counteract toxic effects, cool the blood, disperse wind and heat.

INDICATIONS: Carbuncles, dysentery, sore throat with swelling.

103. **CHINESE:** Ji-xing-zi 急性子 (Fengxianhua; seed of garden balsam).

BOTANICAL: Impatiens balsamina L.

PHARMACEUTICAL: Semen Impatientis.

PART USED: seed.

DOSAGES: 3 to 10 g.

FLAVOR: bitter.

ENERGY: warm.

ACTIONS: To bring down energy, remove coagulations, disperse accumulations.

INDICATIONS: Fish bone stuck in the throat (chew the seed slowly and wash down with warm water to induce the bone to move downward), amenorrhea, cancer of esophagus.

104. **CHINESE:** Jiu-cai-zi 韭菜子 (Jiuzi; Chinese chive seed).

BOTANICAL: Allium tuberosum Rottl.

PHARMACEUTICAL: Semen Allii Tuberosi.

PART USED: seed.

DOSAGES: 3 to 10 g.

FLAVOR: pungent, salty, and sweet.

ENERGY: warm.

ACTIONS: To tone the liver and kidneys,

warm the loins, strengthen yang, and solidify semen.

INDICATIONS: Impotence, seminal ejaculation with erotic dreams, frequent urination, enuresis, cold pain in the lower back and feet, diarrhea, unusual vaginal discharge.

105. **CHINESE:** Jue-ming-zi 决明子 (coffee weed/cassia seed).

BOTANICAL: Cassia obtusifolia L./- tora L.

PHARMACEUTICAL: Semen Cassiae.

PART USED: ripe seed.

DOSAGES: 6 to 12 g.

FLAVOR: salty.

ENERGY: neutral.

ACTIONS: To clear liver, benefit kidneys, expel wind, sharpen vision, lubricate intestines for constipation.

INDICATIONS: Headache due to hot liver, amaurosis (complete loss of vision with no apparent cause), pink eyes with swelling, discharge of dry stools and constipation.

106. **CHINESE:** Ju-he 橘核 (tangerine seed).

BOTANICAL: Citrus Reticulata Blanco.

PHARMACEUTICAL: Semen reticulata Blanco.

PART USED: seed.

DOSAGES: 6 to12 g.

FLAVOR: bitter.

ENERGY: slightly warm.

ACTIONS: To bring down energy, disperse accumulations, expand the middle region.

INDICATIONS: Chest and abdominal congestion and pain, hernial pain, mastitis, excessive milk secretion.

107. **CHINESE:** Ju-hong 橘紅 (red outer layer of tangerine peel).

BOTANICAL: Citrus grandis Osbeck var. tomentosa Hort./- grandis Osbeck.

PHARMACEUTICAL: Exocarpium Citri Grandis/- Citri Rubrum.

PART USED: red part of outer layer.

DOSAGES: 30 to 45 g.

FLAVOR: pungent and bitter.

ENERGY: warm.

ACTIONS: To bring down energy, transform sputum, warm lungs, dry dampness.

INDICATIONS: Stomachache, vomiting, belching, hernial pain, chest congestion, cough with copious sputum.

108. **CHINESE:** Ju-hua 菊花 (mulberry-leaved chrysanthemum).

BOTANICAL: Chrysanthemum morifolium Ramat.

PHARMACEUTICAL: Flos Chrysanthemi.

PART USED: inflorescence (a flower cluster).

DOSAGES: 3 to 10 g.

FLAVOR: sweet and bitter.

ENERGY: cool.

ACTIONS: To induce perspiration; clear heat; clear liver; detoxicate.

INDICATIONS: Eye disease, pain in ears, dizziness, headache due to wind heat, carbuncles, and swelling.

109. **CHINESE:** Kuan-dong-hua 款冬花 (coltsfoot).

BOTANICAL: Tussilago farfara L.

PHARMACEUTICAL: Flos Farfarae.

PART USED: flower bud.

DOSAGES: 3 to 10 g.

FLAVOR: pungent and sweet.

ENERGY: warm.

ACTIONS: To expel sputum, suppress cough, calm asthma.

INDICATIONS: Chronic cough and asthma

due to lung deficiency, pulmonary tuberculosis, chronic bronchitis, bronchiectasis.

110. **CHINESE:** Ku-shen 苦參 (bitter sophora).

BOTANICAL: Sophora flavescens Ait.

PHARMACEUTICAL: Radix Sophorae Flavescentis.

PART USED: root.

DOSAGES: 6 to 12 g.

FLAVOR: bitter.

ENERGY: cold.

ACTIONS: To clear heat, dry dampness, benefit water, destroy worms, relieve itch.

INDICATIONS: Diarrhea, dysentery, urination difficulty, scabies, trichomonas vaginitis.

111. **CHINESE:** Lai-fu-zi 萊菔子 (radish seed).

BOTANICAL: Raphanus sativus L.

PHARMACEUTICAL: Semen Raphani.

PART USED: seed.

DOSAGES: 3 to 10 g.

FLAVOR: pungent and sweet.

ENERGY: neutral.

ACTIONS: To eliminate accumulation, bring down energy, expel sputum, suppress cough.

INDICATIONS: Indigestion, cough, asthma.

112. **CHINESE:** Lian-xu 蓮須 (lotus stamen).

BOTANICAL: Nelumbo nucifera Gaertn.

PHARMACEUTICAL: Stamen Nelumbinis.

PART USED: stamen.

DOSAGES: 5 to 10 g.

FLAVOR: sweet.

ENERGY: warm.

ACTIONS: To restrain semen, arrest bleeding.

INDICATIONS: Seminal emission, vomiting of blood, excessive vaginal bleeding and discharge.

113. **CHINESE:** Lian-zi 蓮子 (Lianzirou; East Indian lotus).

BOTANICAL: Nelumbo nucifera Gaertn.

PHARMACEUTICAL: Semen Nelumbinis Semen Loti.

PART USED: seed.

DOSAGES: 6 to 15 g.

FLAVOR: sweet.

ENERGY: neutral.

ACTIONS: To strengthen spleen, relieve diarrhea, restrain semen.

INDICATIONS: Spleen deficiency causing chronic diarrhea, seminal emission, excessive vaginal bleeding.

114. **CHINESE:** Lian-zi-xin 蓮子心 (lotus plumule).

BOTANICAL: Nelumbo nucifera Gaertn.

PHARMACEUTICAL: Plumula Nelumbinis.

PART USED: ripe seed radicle.

DOSAGES: 2 to 3 g.

FLAVOR: bitter.

ENERGY: cold.

ACTIONS: To calm the heart, remove heat.

INDICATIONS: Delirium, depression, vomiting of blood.

115. **CHINESE:** Ling-zhi 靈芝 (Ling-zhi-cao 靈芝草; lucid ganoderma).

BOTANICAL: Ganoderma lucidum (Leyss. ex Fr.) Karst./Ganoderma japonicum (Fr.) Lloyd.

PHARMACEUTICAL: Ganoderma Lucidum Seu Japonicum.

PART USED: whole plant.

DOSAGES: 2 to 4 g in powder.

FLAVOR: sweet.

ENERGY: neutral.

ACTIONS: To benefit joints, calm the nervous system, increase energy, strengthen tendons and bones, improve complexion.

INDICATIONS: Deficiency fatigue, cough, asthma, insomnia, indigestion, deafness, chronic tracheitis, bronchial asthma, leukocytopenia, coronary heart disease, irregular heartbeat.

116. CHINESE: Long-dan-cao 龍膽草 (gentian).

BOTANICAL: Gentiana manshurica Kitag./ - scabra Bge./- triflora Pall./- regescens Franch.

PHARMACEUTICAL: Radix Gentianae.

PART USED: root.

DOSAGES: 3 to 10 g.

FLAVOR: bitter.

ENERGY: cold.

ACTIONS: To sedate excess fire in liver and gallbladder, clear damp heat in lower burning space.

INDICATIONS: Excess heat in liver and gallbladder, twitching due to high fever, pain on urination, itch and eczema around genital area.

117. CHINESE: Lou-lu 漏蘆 (rhaponticum root).

BOTANICAL: Rhaponticum uniflorum (L.) DC.

PHARMACEUTICAL: Radix Rhapontici Seu Echinopsis.

PART USED: root.

DOSAGES: 3 to 6 g.

FLAVOR: salty.

ENERGY: cold.

ACTIONS: To clear heat, counteract toxic effects, heal swelling, promote milk secretion.

INDICATIONS: Carbuncles, tuberculosis of lymph node, mastitis, shortage of milk secretion, tumors of various kinds.

118. CHINESE: Lu-gen 蘆根 (reed rhizome).

BOTANICAL: Phragmites communis (L.) Trin.

PHARMACEUTICAL: Rhizoma Phragmitis.

PART USED: rhizome.

DOSAGES: 15 to 30 g.

FLAVOR: sweet.

ENERGY: cold.

ACTIONS: To clear heat, produce fluids, promote urination.

INDICATIONS: Unusual thirst, short streams of urine, vomiting due to hot stomach, dry cough due to hot lungs, lung disease.

119. CHINESE: Lu-hui 蘆薈 (aloe).

BOTANICAL: Aloe vera L. var. chinensis. (Haw.) Berger.

PHARMACEUTICAL: Aloe.

PART USED: residue of juice from the leaf.

DOSAGES: 2 to 3 g.

FLAVOR: bitter.

ENERGY: cold.

ACTIONS: To induce bowel movements, destroy worms, clear heat, cool the blood.

INDICATIONS: Constipation, indigestion, convulsion; not to be consumed by pregnant women.

120. CHINESE: Lu-jiao-jiao 鹿角膠 (antler glue).

ZOOLOGICAL: Cervus elaphus L.

PHARMACEUTICAL: Colla Cornus Cervi.

PART USED: antler.

DOSAGES: 6 to 12 g.

FLAVOR: sweet and salty.

ENERGY: warm.

ACTIONS: To tone blood, benefit semen, strengthen tendons and bones, heal sores and nourish muscles.

INDICATIONS: Deficiency fatigue, excessive perspiration, lumbago, impotence, cold uterus, seminal emission, vaginal bleeding and discharge.

121. **CHINESE:** Lu-rong 鹿茸 (pilose antler of a young stag).

ZOOLOGICAL: Cervus nippon Temminck/- elephus L.

PHARMACEUTICAL: Cornu Cervi Pantotrichum/- Cornu Cervi Parvum.

PART USED: hairy young horn.

DOSAGES: 2 to 5 g.

FLAVOR: sweet and salty.

ENERGY: warm.

ACTIONS: To produce semen and marrow, strengthen tendons and bones.

INDICATIONS: Infantile maldevelopment, impotence, frigidity, infertility, seminal emission, enuresis, lumbago, dizziness, pain in legs, loss of hearing.

122. **CHINESE:** Ma-bo 馬勃 (puff ball).

BOTANICAL: Lasiosphaera fenzlii Reich. Calvatia gigantea (Batsch ex Pers.).

PHARMACEUTICAL: Lasiosphaera Seu Calvatia.

PART USED: sporophore.

DOSAGES: 3 to 6 g.

FLAVOR: pungent.

ENERGY: neutral.

ACTIONS: To clear heat, detoxify, benefit throat, heal swelling, arrest bleeding.

INDICATIONS: Sore throat, mumps, cough due to hot lungs, external application to arrest bleeding.

123. **CHINESE:** Ma-huang 麻黃 (Chinese ephedra).

BOTANICAL: Ephedra sinica Stapf/- intermedia Schrenk et C.A.May/- equisetina Bge.

PHARMACEUTICAL: Herba Ephedrae.

PART USED: stalk.

DOSAGES: 3 to 10 g.

FLAVOR: pungent and bitter.

ENERGY: warm.

ACTIONS: To induce perspiration; disperse cold (when consumed raw), overcome asthma (when consumed fried), promote urination.

INDICATIONS: Asthma, edema, hypertension (used with great care).

124. **CHINESE:** Mai-dong 麥冬 (lilyturf).

BOTANICAL: Ophiopogon japonicus (Thunb.). Ker-Gawl.

PHARMACEUTICAL: Radix Ophiopogonis.

PART USED: tuberous root.

DOSAGES: 5 to 10 g.

FLAVOR: sweet and bitter.

ENERGY: slightly cold.

ACTIONS: To lubricate lungs, calm the heart, nourish stomach, produce fluids.

INDICATIONS: Deficiency fatigue, cough, cough with blood, dry throat, skin itch.

125. **CHINESE:** Mai-ya 麥芽 (barley malt).

BOTANICAL: Hordeum vulgare L.

PHARMACEUTICAL: Fructus Hordei Germinatus.

PART USED: germinated barley.

DOSAGES: 10 to 25 g.

FLAVOR: salty.

ENERGY: warm.

ACTIONS: To eliminate accumulation,

harmonize stomach, relax the liver, relieve excessive milk secretion.

INDICATIONS: Excessive milk secretion (lactifuge), indigestion, pain in ribs, swelling of breast due to excessive milk.

126. **CHINESE:** Mo-yao 沒藥 (myrrh).

BOTANICAL: Commiphor myrrha Engler. (C. myrrha Holmes)/- abyssinica (Berg) Engler.

PHARMACEUTICAL: Myrrha.

PART USED: resin.

DOSAGES: 3 to 10 g.

FLAVOR: bitter.

ENERGY: neutral.

ACTIONS: To promote energy circulation, activate the blood, heal swelling, relieve pain.

INDICATIONS: Carbuncles, swelling, chest and abdominal pain, amenorrhea, abdominal obstructions.

127. **CHINESE:** Mu-gua 木瓜 (Chinese flowering quince).

BOTANICAL: Chaenomeles speciosa (Sweet). Nakai/- sinensis (thouin) Koehne.

PHARMACEUTICAL: Fructus Chaenomelis.

PART USED: ripe fruit.

DOSAGES: 6 to 12 g.

FLAVOR: sour.

ENERGY: warm.

ACTIONS: To remove dampness, relax tendons, relieve vomiting and diarrhea.

INDICATIONS: Beriberi, damp rheumatism, inflexible joints, vomiting, diarrhea, spasms.

128. **CHINESE:** Mu-li 牧蠣 (oyster shell).

ZOOLOGICAL: Ostrea gigas Thunb./- talienwhanensis Crosse/- rivularis Gould.

PHARMACEUTICAL: Concha Ostreae.

PART USED: shell.

DOSAGES: 15 to 30 g.

FLAVOR: salty.

ENERGY: slightly cold.

ACTIONS: To suppress yang, stabilize and obstruct, transform sputum, soften hardness.

INDICATIONS: Excessive perspiration, night sweats, seminal emission, unusual vaginal bleeding and discharge, scrofula.

129. **CHINESE:** Mu-tong 木通 (akebi).

BOTANICAL: Aristolochia manshuriensis Kom. Akebia quinata (Thunb.) Decne).

PHARMACEUTICAL: Caulis Aristolochiae. Manshuriensis (Caulis Akebiae).

PART USED: vine.

DOSAGES: 3 to 10 g.

FLAVOR: bitter.

ENERGY: cold.

ACTIONS: To clear the heart, benefit water, and promote milk secretion.

INDICATIONS: Urination difficulty, shortage of milk secretion.

NOTE: Not to be used by pregnant women.

130. **CHINESE:** Mu-xiang 木香 (costus root).

BOTANICAL: Aucklandia lappa Decne./ Saussurae lappa Clarke.

PHARMACEUTICAL: Radix Aucklandiae/ Radix Saussureae.

PART USED: root.

DOSAGES: 2 to 10 g.

FLAVOR: pungent.

ENERGY: warm.

ACTIONS: To promote energy circulation, relieve pain, disperse accumulations.

INDICATIONS: Abdominal swelling and pain, diarrhea, dysentery.

131. **CHINESE:** Niu-bang-zi 牛蒡子 (burdock fruit).

BOTANICAL: Arctium lappa L.

PHARMACEUTICAL: Fructus Arctii.

PART USED: ripe fruit.

DOSAGES: 5 to 10 g.

FLAVOR: pungent and bitter.

ENERGY: cold.

ACTIONS: To disperse wind heat, heal swelling, release toxins, expand lungs, facilitate measle eruption.

INDICATIONS: Common cold, sore throat, measles, carbuncles, swelling.

132. **CHINESE:** Niu-xi 牛膝 (two-toothed amaranthus).

BOTANICAL: Achyranthes bidentata Bl.

PHARMACEUTICAL: Radix Achyranthis Bidentatae.

PART USED: root.

DOSAGES: 6 to 12 g.

FLAVOR: bitter and sour.

ENERGY: neutral.

ACTIONS: To activate blood and faciliate menstrual flow (consume fresh), tone liver and kidneys (consume cooked).

INDICATIONS: Amenorrhea, abdominal obstructions, headache due to liver fire, pain in bones.

133. **CHINESE:** Nu-zhen-zi 女貞子 (wax tree).

BOTANICAL: Ligustrum lucidum Ait.

PHARMACEUTICAL: Fructus Ligustri Lucidi.

PART USED: ripe fruit.

DOSAGES: 10 to 15 g.

FLAVOR: sweet and bitter.

ENERGY: neutral.

ACTIONS: To nourish yin, tone liver and kidneys.

INDICATIONS: Liver-kidney yin deficiency, dizziness, seminal emission, palpitation.

134. **CHINESE:** Pei-lan 佩蘭 (boneset).

BOTANICAL: Eupatorium fortunei Turcz./-japonicum Thunberg.

PHARMACEUTICAL: Herba Eupatorii.

PART USED: stalk and leaf.

DOSAGES: 3 to 10 g.

FLAVOR: pungent.

ENERGY: neutral.

ACTIONS: To transform dampness by aromatic flavor, relieve summer heat.

INDICATIONS: Headache due to summer heat.

135. **CHINESE:** Pi-pa-ye 枇杷葉 (loquat leaf).

BOTANICAL: Eriobotrya japonica (Thunb.) Lindl.

PHARMACEUTICAL: Folium Eriobotryae.

PART USED: leaf.

DOSAGES: 3 to 10 g.

FLAVOR: bitter.

ENERGY: neutral.

ACTIONS: To clear lungs, bring down energy, suppress cough, harmonize stomach.

INDICATIONS: Cough due to hot lungs, vomiting, hiccups.

136. **CHINESE:** Pu-gong-ying 蒲公英 (Asian dandelion).

BOTANICAL: Taraxacum mongolicum Hand. -Mazz./- sinicum Kitag./- heterolepis. Nakai et H. Koidz.

PHARMACEUTICAL: Herba Taraxaci.

PART USED: whole plant.

DOSAGES: 10 to 30 g.

FLAVOR: bitter and sweet.

ENERGY: cold.

ACTIONS: To clear up heat, counteract toxic effects, disperse swelling, and heal carbuncles.

INDICATIONS: Carbuncles, swelling, mastitis, urinary infections, acute tonsillitis.

137. **CHINESE:** Pu-huang 蒲黃 (cattail pollen).

BOTANICAL: Typha angustifolia L./- orientalis Presl.

PHARMACEUTICAL: Pollen Typhae.

PART USED: pollen.

DOSAGES: 3 to 10 g.

FLAVOR: sweet.

ENERGY: neutral.

ACTIONS: To disperse blood coagulation (consume fresh), arrest bleeding (consume fried).

INDICATIONS: Menstrual pain due to blood coagulation, pain due to blood coagulation from injuries, sore throat, unusual bleeding.

138. **CHINESE:** Qian-hu 前胡 (purple-flowered peucedanum).

BOTANICAL: Peucedanum praeruptorum Dunn./- decursivum Maxim.

PHARMACEUTICAL: Radix Peucedani.

PART USED: root.

DOSAGES: 6 to 12 g.

FLAVOR: bitter and pungent.

ENERGY: slightly cold.

ACTIONS: To disperse wind, expand lungs, remove sputum, suppress cough.

INDICATIONS: Cough due to wind heat, sticky sputum with asthma.

139. **CHINESE:** Qian-shi 芡實 (water lily).

BOTANICAL: Euryale ferox Salisb.

PHARMACEUTICAL: Semen Euryales.

PART USED: kernel.

DOSAGES: 3 to 10 g.

FLAVOR: sweet.

ENERGY: neutral.

ACTIONS: To strengthen spleen, benefit kidneys, solidify semen, relieve diarrhea.

INDICATIONS: Diarrhea due to spleen deficiency, seminal emission, leukorrhea.

140. **CHINESE:** Qing-dai 青黛 (blue indigo).

BOTANICAL: Baphicacanthus cusia (Nees) Bremek./Indigofera suffruticosa Mill./ Polygonum tinctorium Ait./Isatis tinctoria L.

PHARMACEUTICAL: Indigo Naturalis.

PART USED: indigo prepared from the leaf.

DOSAGES: 2 to 3 g.

FLAVOR: salty.

ENERGY: cold.

ACTIONS: To clear heat, counteract toxic effects, cool the blood, heal swelling.

INDICATIONS: Erysipelas, hepatitis, mumps, sore throat.

141. **CHINESE:** Qing-pi 青皮 (green tangerine peel).

BOTANICAL: Cirtrus reticulata Blanco/- tangerina Hortorum et Tanaka/- sinensis (L.) Osbeck/- unshiu Marcovitch/- wilsonii Tanaka.

PHARMACEUTICAL: Pericarpium Citri Reticulatae Viride/Fructus Aurantii Immaturus.

PART USED: unripe fruit peel/fruit.

DOSAGES: 3 to 6 g.

FLAVOR: bitter and pungent.

ENERGY: warm.

ACTIONS: To disperse energy congestion, disperse accumulations, promote energy flow, relieve pain.

INDICATIONS: Chest swelling and pain, hernial pain in the lower abdomen.

142. **CHINESE:** Qin-jiao 秦艽 (large-leaved gentian).

BOTANICAL: Gentiana macrophylla Pall./ Gentiana straminea Maxim./Gentiana crassicaulis Duthie. ex Burk./Gentiana dahurica Fisch.

PHARMACEUTICAL: Radix Gentianae Macrophyllae.

PART USED: root.

DOSAGES: 3 to 10 g.

FLAVOR: bitter.

ENERGY: neutral.

ACTIONS: To remove wind and dampness, relax tendons, relieve pain, clear heat arising from yin deficiency, promote urination.

INDICATIONS: Rheumatism, gout, jaundice, constipation.

143. **CHINESE:** Qu-mai 瞿麥 (rainbow pink).

BOTANICAL: Dianthus superbus L./- chinensis L.

PHARMACEUTICAL: Herba Dianthi.

PART USED: whole plant.

DOSAGES: 3 to 10 g.

FLAVOR: bitter.

ENERGY: cold.

ACTIONS: To clear heat, benefit water, relieve urinary problems, cool the blood.

INDICATIONS: Urinary problems (particularly discharge of bloody urine), amenorrhea.

144. **CHINESE:** Ren-shen 人參 (Chinese ginseng).

BOTANICAL: Panax ginseng C. A. Mey.

PHARMACEUTICAL: Radix Ginseng.

PART USED: root.

DOSAGES: 3 to 10 g.

FLAVOR: sweet and slightly bitter.

ENERGY: warm.

ACTIONS: To replenish energy, fix prolapse, produce fluids, calm spirits, benefit the brain.

INDICATIONS: Weakness after chronic illness, abnormal vaginal bleeding, diabetes, prolapse, palpitation, forgetfulness.

145. **CHINESE:** Rou-cong-rong 肉蓯蓉 (saline cistanche).

BOTANICAL: Cistanche deserticola Y. C. Ma/Cistanchis salsa Bentham et Hooker f.

PHARMACEUTICAL: Herba Cistanchis Caulis Cistanchis.

PART USED: fleshy stalk.

DOSAGES: 6 to 12 g.

FLAVOR: sweet.

ENERGY: slightly warm.

ACTIONS: To benefit semen, strengthen yang, lubricate intestines.

INDICATIONS: Impotence, seminal emission, lumbago with cold pain, blood deficiency constipation.

146. **CHINESE:** Rou-gui 肉桂 (Chinese cassia bark).

BOTANICAL: Cinnamomum cassia Presl.

PHARMACEUTICAL: Cortex Cinnamomi.

PART USED: bark.

DOSAGES: 1 to 3 g.

FLAVOR: pungent and sweet.

ENERGY: warm.

ACTIONS: To warm and tone kidney fire, disperse cold, relieve pain.

INDICATIONS: Kidney yang deficiency, cold abdominal pain.

147. **CHINESE:** Ru-xiang 乳香 (frankincense).

BOTANICAL: Pistacia lentisus Linne./Boswellia carterri Birdw.

PHARMACEUTICAL: Mastix/Resina olibani/olibanum.

PART USED: resin.

DOSAGES: 3 to 10 g.

FLAVOR: bitter and pungent.

ENERGY: warm.

ACTIONS: To promote energy circulation, activate the blood, relax tendons, relieve pain, heal swelling.

INDICATIONS: Chest pain, abdominal pain, tendon spasms, amenorrhea, period pain.

148. **CHINESE:** Sang-bai-pi 桑白皮 (root bark of white mulberry).

BOTANICAL: Morus alba L.

PHARMACEUTICAL: Cortex Mori Radicis.

PART USED: root bark.

DOSAGES: 6 to 12 g.

FLAVOR: sweet.

ENERGY: cold.

ACTIONS: To clear lungs, reduce water in the body, suppress cough, calm asthma.

INDICATIONS: Cough and asthma due to hot lungs, edema, diminished urination.

149. **CHINESE:** Sang-ji-sheng 桑寄生 (mistletoe).

BOTANICAL: Loranthus parasiticus (L.) Merr./Taxillus chinensis (D.C.) Danser

PHARMACEUTICAL: Ramulus Loranthi Ramulus Taxilli.

PART USED: stalk.

DOSAGES: 10 to 15 g.

FLAVOR: bitter.

ENERGY: neutral.

ACTIONS: To nourish blood, expel wind, strengthen tendons and bones, secure fetus, promote milk secretion.

INDICATIONS: Blood deficiency, lumbago, weak legs, insecure fetus, shortage of milk secretion.

150. **CHINESE:** Sang-shen 桑椹 (mulberry).

BOTANICAL: Morus alba L.

PHARMACEUTICAL: Fructus Mori.

PART USED: fruit.

DOSAGES: 10 to 15 g.

FLAVOR: sweet and sour.

ENERGY: neutral.

MERIDIANS: liver, kidney.

ACTIONS: To moisten and tone liver and kidneys, nourish blood, sharpen vision, produce fluids, quench thirst.

INDICATIONS: Liver-kidney yin deficiency, ringing in ears, dizziness, premature gray hair, constipation, diabetes.

151. **CHINESE:** Sang-ye 桑葉 (mulberry leaf).

BOTANICAL: Morus alba L.

PHARMACEUTICAL: Folium Mori.

PART USED: leaf.

DOSAGES: 3 to 10 g.

FLAVOR: bitter and sweet.

ENERGY: cold.

ACTIONS: To induce perspiration, clear the liver, expel wind, and clear heat in the lungs.

INDICATIONS: Cough, eye disease, or dizziness and headache due to wind heat.

152. **CHINESE:** Sang-zhi 桑枝 (mulberry twig).

BOTANICAL: Morus alba L.

PHARMACEUTICAL: Ramulus Mori.

PART USED: twig.

DOSAGES: 15 to 25 g.

FLAVOR: bitter.

ENERGY: neutral.

ACTIONS: To remove wind and dampness, improve joint functions.

INDICATIONS: Rheumatism, pain in limbs.

153. **CHINESE:** San-leng 三稜 (triangular rhizome).

BOTANICAL: Sparganium stoloniferum

Buch.-Ham./Sparganium ramosum Huds./Sparganium simplex Huds.

PHARMACEUTICAL: Rhizoma Sparganii.

PART USED: rhizome.

DOSAGES: 5 to 10 g.

FLAVOR: bitter.

ENERGY: neutral.

ACTIONS: To disperse blood coagulations, promote energy circulation, relieve pain, faciliate menstruation.

INDICATIONS: Period pain due to blood stagnation, amenorrhea, shortage of milk secretion, rib pain.

154. **CHINESE:** San-qi 三七 (pseudo-ginseng).

BOTANICAL: Panax pseudo-ginseng Wallich.

PHARMACEUTICAL: Radix Pseudoginseng.

PART USED: root.

DOSAGES: 2 to 3 g.

FLAVOR: sweet and slightly bitter.

ENERGY: warm.

ACTIONS: To arrest bleeding, relieve pain, disperse blood coagulations, heal swelling.

INDICATIONS: Vomiting of blood, nosebleed, bleeding from external injuries, abnormal vaginal bleeding, abdominal pain, carbuncles.

155. **CHINESE:** Shang-lu 商陸 (pokeberry).

BOTANICAL: xhytolacca acinosa Roxb./-americana L.

PHARMACEUTICAL: Radix Phytolaccae.

PART USED: root.

DOSAGES: 3 to 6 g.

FLAVOR: bitter.

ENERGY: cold.

ACTIONS: To promote bowel movements and urination, expel water, counteract toxic effects.

INDICATIONS: Edema, abdominal swelling, constipation.

156. **CHINESE:** Shan-yao 山葯 (Chinese yam).

BOTANICAL: Dioscorea opposita Thunb. Dioscorea batatas Decaisne.

PHARMACEUTICAL: Rhizoma Dioscoreae Rhizoma Batatatis.

PART USED: tuberous root.

DOSAGES: 10 to 30 g.

FLAVOR: sweet.

ENERGY: neutral.

ACTIONS: To strengthen spleen and stomach, relieve diarrhea, tone lungs and kidneys.

INDICATIONS: Spleen deficiency with poor appetite, chronic diarrhea, seminal emission, unusual vaginal discharge, diabetes.

157. **CHINESE:** Shan-zha 山楂 (Chinese hawthorn).

BOTANICAL: Crataegus pinnatifida Bge. var. major N.E.Br.

PHARMACEUTICAL: Fructus Crataegi.

PART USED: fruit.

DOSAGES: 6 to 25 g.

FLAVOR: sour.

ENERGY: slightly warm.

ACTIONS: To eliminate accumulations, promote energy flow, disperse blood coagulations.

INDICATIONS: Indigestion, dysentery, hernia, blood coagulations, suppression of menses.

158. **CHINESE:** Shan-zhu-yu 山茱萸 (fruit of medicinal cornel).

BOTANICAL: Cornus officinalis Sieb et Zucc.

PHARMACEUTICAL: Fructus Corni.

PART USED: fruit.

DOSAGES: 5 to 10 g.

FLAVOR: sour.

ENERGY: slightly warm.

ACTIONS: To tone liver and kidneys, restrain semen, check perspiration.

INDICATIONS: Seminal emission, excessive perspiration, lumbago, dizziness, ringing in ears.

159. **CHINESE:** Sha-ren 砂仁 (grains of paradise).

BOTANICAL: Amomum villosum Lour./- longiligulare T. L. Wu/- xanthioides Wallich.

PHARMACEUTICAL: Fructus Amomi.

PART USED: ripe fruit.

DOSAGES: 3 to 6 g.

FLAVOR: pungent.

ENERGY: warm.

ACTIONS: To promote energy circulation, expand middle region, relieve vomiting, secure fetus.

INDICATIONS: Stomach and abdominal swelling with pain, belching, vomiting, indigestion, cold diarrhea, insecure fetus.

160. **CHINESE:** She-chuang-zi 蛇床子 (snake bed seed).

BOTANICAL: Cnidium monnieri (L.) Cuss.

PHARMACEUTICAL: Fructus Cnidii.

PART USED: ripe fruit.

DOSAGES: 3 to 10 g.

FLAVOR: pungent and bitter.

ENERGY: warm.

ACTIONS: To destroy worms, transform dampness, strengthen yang.

INDICATIONS: Chronic tinea and scabies, eczema involving scrotum, vaginal trichomoniasis, infertility.

161. **CHINESE:** Sheng-di 生地 (dried glutinous rehmannia).

BOTANICAL: Rehmannia glutinosa Libosch.

PHARMACEUTICAL: Radix Rehmanniae.

PART USED: tuberous root.

DOSAGES: 10 to 30 g.

FLAVOR: sweet and bitter.

ENERGY: cold.

ACTIONS: To water yin, bring down fire, cool the blood, lubricate intestines, produce fluids.

INDICATIONS: Sore throat, vomiting of blood, coughing with blood, nosebleed, discharge of urine containing blood, diabetes.

162. **CHINESE:** Sheng-ma 升麻 (skunk bugbane).

BOTANICAL: Cimicifuga heracleifolia Kom/- dahurica (Turcz.) Maxim./- foetida L.

PHARMACEUTICAL: Rhizoma Cimicifugae.

PART USED: rhizome.

DOSAGES: 3 to 10 g.

FLAVOR: pungent, sweet, and bitter.

ENERGY: cool.

ACTIONS: To elevate yang, facilitate measle eruption, to detoxify, arrest bleeding.

INDICATIONS: Chronic diarrhea, prolapse of rectum and uterus, measles that fail to erupt, sore throat, mouth canker, abormal vaginal bleeding.

163. **CHINESE:** Shen-qu 神麯 (digestive tea).

BOTANICAL: Massa Medicata Fermentata.

PHARMACEUTICAL: Massa Medicata Fermentata.

PART USED: blend of fermented tea leaves.

DOSAGES: 6 to 12 g.

FLAVOR: pungent and sweet.

ENERGY: warm.

ACTIONS: To eliminate congestion in

the abdomen, induce perspiration, disperse cold.

INDICATIONS: Indigestion, gastro-intestinal type of common cold.

164. **CHINESE:** Shi-chang-pu 石菖蒲 (grass-leaved sweetflag).

BOTANICAL: Acorus gramineus Soland.

PHARMACEUTICAL: Rhizoma Acori Graminei.

PART USED: rhizome.

DOSAGES: 2 to 10 g.

FLAVOR: pungent.

ENERGY: warm.

ACTIONS: To expel sputum, open cavities, transform dampness, harmonize the middle region.

INDICATIONS: Convulsions, fainting, congested chest, abdominal swelling, poor appetite.

165. **CHINESE:** Shi-di 柿蒂 (Japanese persimmon).

BOTANICAL: Diospyros kaki L.f.

PHARMACEUTICAL: Calyx Kaki.

PART USED: calyx.

DOSAGES: 2 to 5 g.

FLAVOR: bitter.

ENERGY: slightly warm.

ACTIONS: To bring down energy, stop hiccups.

INDICATIONS: Hiccups, vomiting.

166. **CHINESE:** Shi-gao 石膏 (gypsum).

MINERAL: Calcium sulfate ($CaSO_4$)

PHARMACEUTICAL: Gypsum Fibrosum.

PART USED: mineral.

DOSAGES: 15 to 60 g.

FLAVOR: pungent and sweet.

ENERGY: cold.

ACTIONS: To clear heat, sedate fire, relieve thirst and mental depression.

INDICATIONS: Asthma and cough due to hot lungs, carbuncles, and eczema.

167. **CHINESE:** Shi-hu 石斛 (orchid).

BOTANICAL: Dendrobium loddigesii Rolfe/- chrysanthum Wall./- fimbriatum Hook. var. oculatum Hook/- nobile Lindl./- candidum Wall. ex Lindl.

PHARMACEUTICAL: Herba Dendrobii.

PART USED: stalk.

DOSAGES: 6 to 12 g.

FLAVOR: sweet, bland, and slightly salty.

ENERGY: cold.

ACTIONS: To water yin, benefit stomach, produce fluids.

INDICATIONS: Unusual thirst, dehydration in a hot disease.

168. **CHINESE:** Shi-wei 石葦 (stony reed).

BOTANICAL: Pyrrosia sheareri (Bak.) Ching/- lingua (Thunb.) Farwell./- petiolosa (Christ) Ching.

PHARMACEUTICAL: Folium Pyrrosiae.

PART USED: leaf.

DOSAGES: 3 to 10 g.

FLAVOR: sweet and bitter.

ENERGY: cool.

ACTIONS: To clear heat, benefit water (promote water metabolism), relieve urinary problems, arrest bleeding.

INDICATIONS: Urinary problems (particularly discharge of muddy urine), diarrhea.

169. **CHINESE:** Shu-di 熟地 (processed glutinous rehmannia).

BOTANICAL: Rehmannia glutinosa Libosch.

PHARMACEUTICAL: Radix Rehmanniae (steamed).

PART USED: tuberous root.

DOSAGES: 10 to 25 g.

FLAVOR: sweet.

ENERGY: slightly warm.

ACTIONS: To tone blood, water kidneys, nourish yin, return gray hair to its original color.

INDICATIONS: Blood deficiency, gray hair, ringing in ears, night sweats, excessive vaginal bleeding, diabetes, seminal emission.

170. **CHINESE:** Suan-zao-ren 酸棗仁 (jujube).

BOTANICAL: Ziziphus spinosa Hu.

PHARMACEUTICAL: Semen Ziziphi Spinosae.

PART USED: kernel.

DOSAGES: 6 to 15 g.

FLAVOR: sweet.

ENERGY: neutral.

ACTIONS: To calm the heart and spirits, check perspiration, produce fluids.

INDICATIONS: Insomnia, palpitation, forgetfulness, deficiency perspiration.

171. **CHINESE:** Tao-ren 桃仁 (peach kernel).

BOTANICAL: Prunus persica (L.) Batsch./- davidiana (Carr.) Franch.

PHARMACEUTICAL: Semen Persicae.

PART USED: kernel.

DOSAGES: 3 to 10 g.

FLAVOR: bitter and sweet.

ENERGY: neutral.

ACTIONS: To remove blood stagnation, lubricate dryness in the intestines.

INDICATIONS: Period pain due to blood coagulation, suppression of menstruation, abdominal obstructions, constipation.

172. **CHINESE:** Tian-dong 天冬 (lucid asparagus).

BOTANICAL: Asparagus cochinchinensis. (Lour.) Merr.

PHARMACEUTICAL: Radix Asparagi.

PART USED: tuberous root.

DOSAGES: 2 to 10 g.

FLAVOR: sweet and bitter.

ENERGY: extremely cold.

ACTIONS: To water yin, lubricate dryness, clear heat, transform sputum.

INDICATIONS: Cough, vomiting of blood, coughing of blood, diabetes, constipation, hot diseases.

173. **CHINESE:** Tian-hua-fen 天花粉 (Chinese trichosanthes).

BOTANICAL: Trichosanthes kirilowii Maxim./- japonica Regel.

PHARMACEUTICAL: Radix Trichosanthis.

PART USED: tuberous root.

DOSAGES: 10 to 15 g.

FLAVOR: sweet and bitter.

ENERGY: cool.

ACTIONS: To clear heat, produce fluids, lubricate lungs, suppress cough, detoxify, heal swelling.

INDICATIONS: Thirst in hot diseases, dry cough due to hot lungs, carbuncles, swelling, diabetes.

174. **CHINESE:** Tian-nan-xing 天南星 (serrated arum).

BOTANICAL: Trichosanthes kirilowii maxim./- beterophyllum Bl./- amurense Maxim.

PHARMACEUTICAL: Rhizoma Arisaematis.

PART USED: rhizome.

DOSAGES: 3 to 10 g.

FLAVOR: bitter and pungent.

ENERGY: warm.

ACTIONS: To expel sputum, calm convulsions, relieve spasms.

INDICATIONS: Cough and asthma with cold sputum (sputum caused by cold), apoplexy and aftereffects, facial paralysis, tetanus.

175. **CHINESE:** Tian-xing-ren 甜杏仁 (sweet apricot seed).

BOTANICAL: Prunus armeniaca Linne.

PHARMACEUTICAL: Semen Armeniacae Dulcis.

PART USED: ripe seed.

DOSAGES: 6 to 15 g.

FLAVOR: sweet.

ENERGY: neutral.

ACTIONS: To lubricate lungs, expel sputum, suppress cough, relieve asthma.

INDICATIONS: Dry cough, asthma, constipation.

176. **CHINESE:** Ting-li-zi 葶藶子 (seed of pepperweed).

BOTANICAL: Lepidium apetalum Willd. Descurainia sophia (L.) Webb ex. Prantl/- Draba nemorosa Linne.

PHARMACEUTICAL: Semen Lepidii seu Descurainiae/Semen Drabae.

PART USED: ripe seed.

DOSAGES: 3 to 10 g.

FLAVOR: pungent and bitter.

ENERGY: extremely cold.

ACTIONS: To expel sputum, calm asthma, sedate lungs, promote water flow.

INDICATIONS: Asthma and cough with copious sputum, edema, diminished urination, accumulation of fluids in chest and abdomen.

177. **CHINESE:** Tong-cao 通草 (rice-paper plant).

BOTANICAL: Tetrapanax papyriferus. (Hook.) K. Koch.

PHARMACEUTICAL: Medulla Tetrapanacis.

PART USED: pith of stalk.

DOSAGES: 2 to 5 g.

FLAVOR: sweet and light.

ENERGY: cold.

ACTIONS: To promote water metabolism, transform dampness, clear heat, promote milk secretion.

INDICATIONS: Diminished urination, urinary strains, edema, shortage of milk secretion

NOTE: Not to be used during pregnancy.

178. **CHINESE:** Tu-fu-ling 土茯苓 (wild tuckahoe, wild Indian bread).

BOTANICAL: Smilax glabra Roxb.

PHARMACEUTICAL: Rhizoma Smilacis Glabrae.

PART USED: tuberous root.

DOSAGES: 3 to 6 g.

FLAVOR: sweet and light.

ENERGY: neutral.

ACTIONS: To expel dampness, detoxify.

INDICATIONS: Eczema, syphilis, toxic dampness, gonorrhea, leukorrhea, bone pain in rheumatism.

179. **CHINESE:** Tu-si-zi 菟絲子 (dodder seed).

BOTANICAL: Cuscuta chinensis Lam./-japonica Choisy.

PHARMACEUTICAL: Semen Cuscutae.

PART USED: ripe seed.

DOSAGES: 5 to 10 g.

FLAVOR: pungent and sweet.

ENERGY: neutral.

ACTIONS: To tone liver and kidneys, strengthen yang, relieve diarrhea.

INDICATIONS: Impotence, seminal emission, diarrhea, lumbago, insecure fetus.

180. **CHINESE:** Wa-leng-zi 瓦楞子 (arca shell).

ZOOLOGICAL: Arca subcrenata Lischke./- granosa L./- inflata Reeve.

PHARMACEUTICAL: Concha Arcae.

PART USED: shell.

DOSAGES: 6 to 12 g.

FLAVOR: sweet and salty.

ENERGY: neutral.

ACTIONS: To arrest bleeding, disperse coagulations, relieve pain, eliminate sputum, soften hardness.

INDICATIONS: Stomachache, belching, abdominal obstructions.

181. **CHINESE:** Wang-bu-liu-xing 王不留行 (Wangbuliu; seed of cow-basil).

BOTANICAL: Vaccaria segetalis (Neck.) Garcke.

PHARMACEUTICAL: Semen Vaccariae.

PART USED: ripe seed.

DOSAGES: 6 to 15 g.

FLAVOR: sweet and bitter.

ENERGY: neutral.

ACTIONS: To activate the blood, disperse blood coagulation, heal swelling, relieve pain.

INDICATIONS: Amenorrhea, shortage of milk secretion, abdominal obstructions, difficulty urinating.

182. **CHINESE:** Wei-ling-xian 威靈仙 (Chinese clematis).

BOTANICAL: Clematis chinensis Osbeck/- hexapetala Pall./- manshurica Rupr.

PHARMACEUTICAL: Radix Clematidis.

PART USED: root.

DOSAGES: 3 to 10 g.

FLAVOR: pungent.

ENERGY: warm.

ACTIONS: To remove wind and dampness, facilitate passage of meridians, relieve pain.

INDICATIONS: Rheumatism, jaundice, edema.

183. **CHINESE:** Wu-bei-zi 五倍子 (Chinese nutgall).

ZOOLOGICAL: Rhus chinensis Mill./- potaninii Maxim.

PHARMACEUTICAL: Galla Chinensis.

PART USED: insect gall.

DOSAGES: 2 to 6 g.

FLAVOR: sour.

ENERGY: neutral.

ACTIONS: To act as an intestinal astringent, arrest bleeding, check perspiration.

INDICATIONS: Chronic dysentery, prolapse of rectum and uterus, anal bleeding, excessive perspiration, unusual vaginal bleeding.

184. **CHINESE:** Wu-jia-pi 五加皮 (slender acanthopanax root bark).

BOTANICAL: Acanthopanax gracilistylus. W.W. Smith.

PHARMACEUTICAL: Cortex Acanthopanacis Radicis.

PART USED: root bark.

DOSAGES: 6 to 12 g.

FLAVOR: pungent.

ENERGY: warm.

ACTIONS: To remove wind and dampness, strengthen bones and tendons.

INDICATIONS: Rheumatism, beriberi, weak limbs.

185. **CHINESE:** Wu-mei 烏梅 (black plum).

BOTANICAL: Prunus mume (Sieb.) Sieb. et Zucc.

PHARMACEUTICAL: Fructus Mume/Fructus Mume Praeparatus.

PART USED: prepared unripe fruit.

DOSAGES: 3 to 10 g.

FLAVOR: sour.

ENERGY: warm.

ACTIONS: To act as an intestinal astringent, constrict lungs, produce fluids, destroy worms.

INDICATIONS: Chronic cough, diarrhea and dysentery due to spleen deficiency, unusual thirst, roundworm.

186. **CHINESE:** Wu-wei-zi 五味子 (magnolia vine fruit).

BOTANICAL: Schisandra chinensis (Turcz.). Baill./- sphenanthera Rehd. et Wils.

PHARMACEUTICAL: Fructus Schisandrae.

PART USED: ripe fruit.

DOSAGES: 2 to 6 g.

FLAVOR: sour.

ENERGY: warm.

ACTIONS: To water kidneys, constrict lungs, produce fluids, check perspiration and diarrhea, restrain semen.

INDICATIONS: Asthma and cough, excessive perspiration, night sweats, diarrhea, seminal emission, abnormal vaginal bleeding.

187. **CHINESE:** Wu-zhu-yu 吳茱萸 (evodia).

BOTANICAL: Euodia rutaecarpa (Juss.) Benth./- var. officinalis (Dode) Huang/- var. bodinieri (Dode) Huang.

PHARMACEUTICAL: Fructus Evodiae.

PART USED: unripe fruit.

DOSAGES: 3 to 10 g.

FLAVOR: pungent.

ENERGY: warm.

ACTIONS: To warm the internal regions, disperse cold, relieve vomiting, relieve pain due to cold.

INDICATIONS: Cold abdominal pain, vomiting, diarrhea, headache.

188. **CHINESE:** Xia-ku-cao 夏枯草 (self-heal).

BOTANICAL: Prunella vulgaris L.

PHARMACEUTICAL: Spica Prunellae.

PART USED: ear of fruit.

DOSAGES: 10 to 30 g.

FLAVOR: slightly bitter.

ENERGY: cool.

ACTIONS: To calm the liver, clear heat, soften hardness, disperse congestion.

INDICATIONS: Headache, pink eye, carbuncles of the head, scrofula.

189. **CHINESE:** Xiang-fu 香附 (nutgrass flatsedge rhizome).

BOTANICAL: Cyperus rotundus L.

PHARMACEUTICAL: Rhizoma Cyperi.

PART USED: rhizome.

DOSAGES: 6 to 15 g.

FLAVOR: pungent and sweet.

ENERGY: slightly warm.

ACTIONS: To promote energy flow, disperse energy congestion, relieve pain, regulate menstruation.

INDICATIONS: Discomfort with energy congestion, chest pain, irregular menstruation, period pain.

190. **CHINESE:** Xian-he-cao 仙鶴草 (Longyacao; agrimony).

BOTANICAL: Agrimonia pilosa Ledeb.

PHARMACEUTICAL: Herba Agrimoniae.

PART USED: whole plant.

DOSAGES: 10 to 25 g.

FLAVOR: bitter.

ENERGY: neutral.

ACTIONS: To check and arrest bleeding.

INDICATIONS: Vomiting of blood, coughing with blood, nosebleed, uterine bleeding.

191. **CHINESE:** Xiao-hui-xiang 小茴香 (fennel fruit).

BOTANICAL: Foeniculum vulgare Mill.

PHARMACEUTICAL: Fructus Foeniculi.

PART USED: ripe fruit.

DOSAGES: 2 to 5 g.

FLAVOR: pungent.

ENERGY: warm.

ACTIONS: To promote energy flow, disperse congestion, warm the internal regions and relieve pain.

INDICATIONS: Hernia, pain in the lower abdomen, intestinal rumbling.

192. **CHINESE:** Xiao-ji 小薊 (cornfield thistle).

BOTANICAL: Cephalanoplos segetum (Bge.) Kitam./- setosum (Willd.) Kitam. Phalanoplos segetum (Bunge). Kitamura.

PHARMACEUTICAL: Herba Cephalanoploris, Herba Cephalanopli.

PART USED: whole plant.

DOSAGES: 10 to 18 g.

FLAVOR: sweet.

ENERGY: cool.

ACTIONS: To disperse blood coagulations, arrest bleeding, clear heat, promote urination.

INDICATIONS: Vomiting of blood, nosebleed, bloody urine, hypertension, abnormal vaginal discharge, nephritis, edema.

193. **CHINESE:** Xing-ren 杏仁 (Ku-xing-ren 苦杏仁; apricot kernel).

BOTANICAL: Prunus armeniaca L. var. ansu. Maxim/- sibirica L./- mandshurica. (Maxim) Koehne/- armeniaca L.

PHARMACEUTICAL: Semen Armeniacae Amarum.

PART USED: ripe kernel.

DOSAGES: 5 to 10 g.

FLAVOR: bitter.

ENERGY: warm.

ACTIONS: To suppress cough, expel sputum, expand lungs, calm asthma.

INDICATIONS: Cough in common cold, asthma with copious sputum, constipation due to exhaustion of fluids.

194. **CHINESE:** Xuan-fu-hua 旋覆花 (elecampane).

BOTANICAL: Inula japonica Thunb.

PHARMACEUTICAL: Flos Inulae.

PART USED: flower.

DOSAGES: 3 to 10 g.

FLAVOR: salty.

ENERGY: warm.

ACTIONS: To expel sputum, suppress cough, bring down energy, calm asthma.

INDICATIONS: Cough, asthma, hiccups.

195. **CHINESE:** Xu-duan 續斷 (Chunduan; teasel).

BOTANICAL: Dipsacus asper Wall.

PHARMACEUTICAL: Radix Dipsaci.

PART USED: root.

DOSAGES: 5 to 10 g.

FLAVOR: bitter and pungent.

ENERGY: slightly warm.

ACTIONS: To tone liver and kidneys, strengthen loins and knees, strengthen tendons and bones, secure fetus.

INDICATIONS: Lumbago, weak legs, disconnected tendons and fracture, insecure fetus, profuse menstrual flow.

196. **CHINESE:** Ya-dan-zi 鴉膽子 (brucea fruit/duck gall).

BOTANICAL: Brucea javanica (L.) Merr.

PHARMACEUTICAL: Fructus Bruceae.

PART USED: fruit.

DOSAGES: 10-20 fruits.

FLAVOR: bitter.

ENERGY: cold.

ACTIONS: To destroy worms, dry dampness, relieve dysentery.

INDICATIONS: Dysentery, hemorrhoids, warts (applied externally).

197. **CHINESE:** Yan-hu-suo 延胡索 (Yuanhu; Chinese yanhusuo).

BOTANICAL: Corydalis yanhusuo W. T. Wang/- ambigua Cham. Et Schlecht. var. amurensis Maxim.

PHARMACEUTICAL: Rhizoma Corydalis/ Tuber Corydalis.

PART USED: rhizome.

DOSAGES: 3 to 10 g.

FLAVOR: pungent.

ENERGY: slightly warm.

ACTIONS: To activate the blood, disperse blood coagulations, benefit energy, relieve pain.

INDICATIONS: Abdominal pain, hernial pain in the lower abdomen, heart pain in coronary heart disease, period pain.

198. **CHINESE:** Ye-ju-hua 野菊花 (wild chrysanthemum).

BOTANICAL: Chrysanthemum indicum L.

PHARMACEUTICAL: Flos Chrysanthemi Indici.

PART USED: whole flower.

DOSAGES: 9 to 15 g.

FLAVOR: bitter and pungent.

ENERGY: cool.

ACTIONS: To detoxify, cool the blood, lower blood pressure.

INDICATIONS: Carbuncles, erysipelas, acute lymphadenitis, mastitis, hypertension, tonsillitis, laryngopharygitis.

199. **CHINESE:** Yi-mu-cao 益母草 (Chongwei; Siberian motherwort).

BOTANICAL: Leonurus heterophyllus Sweet.

PHARMACEUTICAL: Herba Leonuri.

PART USED: whole plant.

DOSAGES: 6 to 15 g.

FLAVOR: bitter and pungent.

ENERGY: neutral.

ACTIONS: To activate the blood, regulate menstruation, move blood coagulations, heal edema.

INDICATIONS: Abdominal pain due to blood coagulations after childbirth, irregular period, excessive vaginal bleeding.

200. **CHINESE:** Yin-chen 茵陳 (capillary artemisia).

BOTANICAL: Artemisia capillaris Thunberg.

PHARMACEUTICAL: Herba Artemisiae Capillaris.

PART USED: seedling.

DOSAGES: 15 to 30 g.

FLAVOR: bitter and pungent.

ENERGY: slightly cold.

ACTIONS: To clear damp heat, treat jaundice.

INDICATIONS: Jaundice due to damp heat, acute jaundice, infectious hepatitis.

201. **CHINESE:** Yin-yang-huo 淫羊藿 (longspur epimendium).

BOTANICAL: Epimedium brevicornum Maxim./- koreanum Nakai/- sagittatum. (Sieb. et Zucc.) Maxim.

PHARMACEUTICAL: Herba Epimedii.

PART USED: aerial part.

DOSAGES: 3 to 10 g.

FLAVOR: pungent.

ENERGY: warm.

ACTIONS: To tone the kidneys, strengthen tendons and bones.

INDICATIONS: Impotence, rheumatism.

202. **CHINESE:** Yi-tang 飴糖 (maltose).

PHARMACEUTICAL: Saccharum Granorum.

PART USED: maltose (a sugar formed by the action of an enzyme or starch of rice, barley, wheat, corn, or millet).

DOSAGES: 10 to 30 g.

FLAVOR: sweet.

ENERGY: warm.

ACTIONS: To strengthen the spleen, lubricate dryness, slow down acute symptoms, relieve pain.

INDICATIONS: Weak stomach, abdominal pain due to deficiency cold, dry lungs and dry throat, constipation due to deficiency.

203. **CHINESE:** Yi-yi-ren 薏苡仁 (Job's tears).

BOTANICAL: Coix lacryma-jobi L. var. ma-yuen (Roman.) Stapf.

PHARMACEUTICAL: Semen Coicis.

PART USED: kernel.

DOSAGES: 10 to 30 g.

FLAVOR: sweet.

ENERGY: neutral.

ACTIONS: To transform dampness and promote water metabolism, strengthen spleen, relieve diarrhea, relax tendons, drain pus.

INDICATIONS: Diminished urination, edema, diarrhea, twitching, beriberi, rheumatism, lung disease.

204. **CHINESE:** Yuan-zhi 遠志 (slender-leaved milkwort).

BOTANICAL: Polygala tenuifolia Willd./-sibirica L.

PHARMACEUTICAL: Radix Polygalae.

PART USED: root.

DOSAGES: 3 to 10 g.

FLAVOR: bitter and pungent.

ENERGY: warm.

ACTIONS: To calm the spirits, transform sputum, open cavities, disperse and eliminate.

INDICATIONS: Insomnia, palpitation, forgetfulness, cough with copious sputum, carbuncles, sore throat.

205. **CHINESE:** Yu-jin 郁金 (aromatic turmeric root-tuber).

BOTANICAL: Curcuma aromatica Salisb./- kwangsiensis S. Lee et C. F. Liang/-longa L./- zedoaria Rosc.

PHARMACEUTICAL: Radix Curcumae/Tuber Curcumae.

PART USED: tuberous root.

DOSAGES: 3 to 10 g.

FLAVOR: bitter and pungent.

ENERGY: slightly cold.

ACTIONS: To promote energy circulation, disperse energy congestion, activate blood, break up coagulations.

INDICATIONS: Abdominal swelling, chest and rib pain, period pain, vomiting of blood, nosebleed, bloody urine.

206. **CHINESE:** Yu-li-ren 郁李仁 (dwarf flowering cherry).

BOTANICAL: Prunus humilis Bge./- japonica Thunb.

PHARMACEUTICAL: Semen Pruni/Semen Pruni Japonicae.

PART USED: kernel.

DOSAGES: 3 to 10 g.

FLAVOR: pungent, sweet, and bitter.

ENERGY: neutral.

ACTIONS: To induce bowel movements, promote urination, heal swelling.

INDICATIONS: Discharge of dry stools, edema, ascites.

NOTE: Not for pregnant women or those with diarrhea due to spleen deficiency.

207. **CHINESE:** Yu-mi-xu 玉米須 (corn silk).

BOTANICAL: Zea mays L.

PHARMACEUTICAL: Stigma Maydis.

PART USED: stigma.

DOSAGES: 30 to 60 g.

FLAVOR: sweet.

ENERGY: neutral.

ACTIONS: To promote urination, sedate heat, calm liver, benefit gallbladder.

INDICATIONS: Nephritis, edema, beriberi, jaundice-type hepatitis, hypertension, cholecystitis, gallstones, diabetes, vomiting blood, nosebleed, sinusitis, mastitis.

208. **CHINESE:** Yu-xing-cao 魚腥草 (Ji-cai; cordate houttuynia).

BOTANICAL: Houttuynia cordata Thunb.

PHARMACEUTICAL: Herba Houttuyniae.

PART USED: whole plant.

DOSAGES: 10 to 15 g, 30 to 60 g (fresh).

FLAVOR: pungent.

ENERGY: cold.

ACTIONS: To clear heat and detoxify, promote urination and reduce swelling.

INDICATIONS: Pneumonia, hot diarrhea, edema, muddy urine with urinary problems, leukorrhea, carbuncles, hemorrhoids, prolapse of rectum and uterus, eczema.

209. **CHINESE:** Yu-zhu 玉竹 (Solomon's seal).

BOTANICAL: Polygonatum odoratum (Mill.) Druce.

PHARMACEUTICAL: Rhizoma Polygonati Odorati.

PART USED: rhizome.

DOSAGES: 5 to 10 g.

FLAVOR: sweet.

ENERGY: slightly cold.

ACTIONS: To nourish yin, lubricate dryness, produce fluids, quench thirst.

INDICATIONS: Chronic thirst, diabetes, cough, excessive perspiration.

210. **CHINESE:** Ze-lan 澤蘭 (water-horehound).

BOTANICAL: Lycopus lucidus Turczaninow. var. hirtus Regel.

PHARMACEUTICAL: Herba Lycopi.

PART USED: whole plant.

DOSAGES: 3 to 10 g.

FLAVOR: bitter.

ENERGY: slightly warm.

ACTIONS: To activate the blood, disperse blood coagulations, facilitate passages of meridians, promote water flow.

INDICATIONS: Period pain due to blood coagulation, irregular periods, suppression of period, rib pain.

211. **CHINESE:** Ze-xie 澤瀉 (water plantain).

BOTANICAL: Alisma orientalis (Sam.) Juzep.

PHARMACEUTICAL: Rhizoma Alismatis.

PART USED: rhizome.

DOSAGES: 6 to 15 g.

FLAVOR: sweet.

ENERGY: neutral.

ACTIONS: To transform dampness, benefit water, sedate deficiency fire.

INDICATIONS: Diminished urination, edema, urinary strains, diarrhea and dysentery, seminal emission.

212. **CHINESE:** Zhe-bei 浙貝 (Zhebeimu; Zhe fritillary bulb).

BOTANICAL: Fritillaria thunbergii Miq./ Fritillaria verticillata Willdenow var. thunbergii Baker.

PHARMACEUTICAL: Bulbus Fritillariae. Thunbergii.

PART USED: bulb.

DOSAGES: 3 to 10 g.

DOSAGES: 3 to 10 g.

FLAVOR: bitter and sweet.

ENERGY: slightly cold.

ACTIONS: To expel sputum, stop cough, lubricate lungs, disperse accumulations.

INDICATIONS: Cough with hot sputum, dry lungs, dry cough, lipoma, fibroma, tuberculosis of lymph nodes, carbuncles.

213. CHINESE: Zhi-ju-zi 枳椇子 (Japanese raisin tree).

BOTANICAL: Hovenia dulcis Thunberg.

PHARMACEUTICAL: Semen Hoveniae.

PART USED: ripe seed.

DOSAGES: 10 to 15 g.

FLAVOR: sweet and sour.

ENERGY: neutral.

INDICATIONS: Intoxication, mental depression and heat, chronic thirst, vomiting, urination difficulty, constipation.

214. CHINESE: Zhi-ma 芝麻 (Hu-ma-ren 胡麻仁; sesame seed).

BOTANICAL: Linum usitatissimum L.

PHARMACEUTICAL: Semen Lini.

PART USED: ripe seed.

DOSAGES: 3 to 10 g.

FLAVOR: sweet.

ENERGY: neutral.

ACTIONS: To tone liver and kidneys, nourish blood, expel wind, lubricate dryness.

INDICATIONS: Weakness after illness, constipation due to dryness, rheumatism, paralysis.

215. CHINESE: Zhi-mu 知母 (wind weed).

BOTANICAL: Anemarrhena asphodeloides Bge.

PHARMACEUTICAL: Rhizoma Anemarrhenae.

FLAVOR: bitter and sweet.

PART USED: rhizome.

DOSAGES: 6 to 12 g.

FLAVOR: bitter.

ENERGY: cold.

ACTIONS: To clear heat, sedate fire, tra form dryness, and moisten intestines.

INDICATIONS: Periodic fever in pulmon tuberculosis, chronic thirst, constipatio

216. CHINESE: Zhi-qiao 枳殼 (unripe citron).

BOTANICAL: Citrus aurantium L./Po cirus trifoliata (L.) Raf./Citrus Wilso Tanaka.

PHARMACEUTICAL: Fructus Aurantii Citri Immaturus Exsiccatus.

PART USED: fruit.

DOSAGES: 3 to 10 g.

FLAVOR: bitter.

ENERGY: slightly cold.

ACTIONS: To promote energy fl relieve pain, with similar actions China orange (Zhi-shi) but weaker.

INDICATIONS: Difficult bowel moveme indigestion, copious sputum, chest co gestion.

217. CHINESE: Zhi-shi 枳實 (China orange).

BOTANICAL: Citrus aurantium L. Pc cirus trifoliata Rafinesque Raf. Citr wilsonii Tanaka.

PHARMACEUTICAL: Fructus Aurantii Immaturus.

PART USED: ripe fruit.

DOSAGES: 3 to 10 g.

FLAVOR: pungent and bitter.

ENERGY: neutral.

ACTIONS: To promote flow of energy a relieve pain, disperse accumulations.

INDICATIONS: Chest and abdomi swelling, indigestion, excessive sputu difficulty in bowel movements.

ENERGY: slightly cold.

ACTIONS: To expel sputum, stop cough, lubricate lungs, disperse accumulations.

INDICATIONS: Cough with hot sputum, dry lungs, dry cough, lipoma, fibroma, tuberculosis of lymph nodes, carbuncles.

213. **CHINESE:** Zhi-ju-zi 枳椇子 (Japanese raisin tree).

BOTANICAL: Hovenia dulcis Thunberg.

PHARMACEUTICAL: Semen Hoveniae.

PART USED: ripe seed.

DOSAGES: 10 to 15 g.

FLAVOR: sweet and sour.

ENERGY: neutral.

INDICATIONS: Intoxication, mental depression and heat, chronic thirst, vomiting, urination difficulty, constipation.

214. **CHINESE:** Zhi-ma 芝麻 (Hu-ma-ren 胡麻仁; sesame seed).

BOTANICAL: Linum usitatissimum L.

PHARMACEUTICAL: Semen Lini.

PART USED: ripe seed.

DOSAGES: 3 to 10 g.

FLAVOR: sweet.

ENERGY: neutral.

ACTIONS: To tone liver and kidneys, nourish blood, expel wind, lubricate dryness.

INDICATIONS: Weakness after illness, constipation due to dryness, rheumatism, paralysis.

215. **CHINESE:** Zhi-mu 知母 (wind weed).

BOTANICAL: Anemarrhena asphodeloides Bge.

PHARMACEUTICAL: Rhizoma Anemarrhenae.

PART USED: rhizome.

DOSAGES: 6 to 12 g.

FLAVOR: bitter.

ENERGY: cold.

ACTIONS: To clear heat, sedate fire, transform dryness, and moisten intestines.

INDICATIONS: Periodic fever in pulmonary tuberculosis, chronic thirst, constipation.

216. **CHINESE:** Zhi-qiao 枳殼 (unripe citron).

BOTANICAL: Citrus aurantium L./Poncirus trifoliata (L.) Raf./Citrus Wilsonii Tanaka.

PHARMACEUTICAL: Fructus Aurantii F Citri Immaturus Exsiccatus.

PART USED: fruit.

DOSAGES: 3 to 10 g.

FLAVOR: bitter.

ENERGY: slightly cold.

ACTIONS: To promote energy flow, relieve pain, with similar actions as China orange (Zhi-shi) but weaker.

INDICATIONS: Difficult bowel movement, indigestion, copious sputum, chest congestion.

217. **CHINESE:** Zhi-shi 枳實 (China orange).

BOTANICAL: Citrus aurantium L. Poncirus trifoliata Rafinesque Raf. Citrus wilsonii Tanaka.

PHARMACEUTICAL: Fructus Aurantii Immaturus.

PART USED: ripe fruit.

DOSAGES: 3 to 10 g.

FLAVOR: pungent and bitter.

ENERGY: neutral.

ACTIONS: To promote flow of energy and relieve pain, disperse accumulations.

INDICATIONS: Chest and abdominal swelling, indigestion, excessive sputum, difficulty in bowel movements.

218. **CHINESE:** Zhi-zi 梔子 (gardenia).

BOTANICAL: Gardenia jasminoides Ellis. var. radicans (Thunb.) Makino.

PHARMACEUTICAL: Fructus Gardeniae.

PART USED: fruit.

DOSAGES: 3 to 12 g.

FLAVOR: bitter.

ENERGY: cold.

ACTIONS: To clear heat in triple cavity (triple burning space), relieve depression, promote urination, arrest bleeding (fry till charred black).

INDICATIONS: Mental depression, jaundice, sore throat, pink eyes, nosebleed, mouth canker, scanty urine.

219. **CHINESE:** Zhu-li 竹瀝 (bamboo juice).

BOTANICAL: Phyllostachys nigra (Lodd.) Munro var. henonis (Mitf.) Stapf ex Rendle.

PHARMACEUTICAL: Saccus Bambusae.

PART USED: bamboo juice from the middle section of a baked/burned bamboo stick.

DOSAGES: 30 to 60 g.

FLAVOR: sweet and bitter.

ENERGY: cold.

ACTIONS: To clear heat, remove sputum, relieve convulsion, benefit cavities.

INDICATIONS: Stroke, cough due to hot lungs, epilepsy, convulsion, high fever, thirst, tetanus, *zifan* (fetus depression, or irritability with heart palpitations and panic during pregnancy).

220. **CHINESE:** Zhu-ru 竹茹 (bamboo shavings).

BOTANICAL: Phyllostachys nigra (Lodd.) Munro var. henonis (Mitf.) Stapf ex Rendle.

PHARMACEUTICAL: Caulis Bambusae In Taeniam.

PART USED: culm shavings.

DOSAGES: 5 to 10 g.

FLAVOR: sweet.

ENERGY: slightly cold.

ACTIONS: To relieve vomiting and hiccups due to hot stomach, cool the blood, clear heat.

INDICATIONS: Cough, vomiting, bloody urine, insecure fetus, nosebleed, excessive vaginal bleeding.

221. **CHINESE:** Zhu-ye 竹葉 (bamboo leaf).

SCIENTIFIC: Phyllostachys nigra (Lodd.) Munro var. henonis (Mitf.) Stapf ex Rendle.

PHARMACEUTICAL: Folium Bambusae In Taeniam.

PART USED: bamboo leaf.

DOSAGES: 6 to 12 g.

FLAVOR: sweet and light.

ENERGY: cold.

ACTIONS: To clear heat, relieve mental depression, produce fluids, promote urination.

INDICATIONS: Hot diseases, convulsions in children, cough, vomiting of blood, nosebleed, red face, discharge of short and bloody urine, mouth cankers.

222. **CHINESE:** Zi-cao 紫草 (Asian puccoon).

BOTANICAL: Arnebia euchrorma (Royle). Johnst./Lithospermum erythrorhizon. Sieb. et Zucc.

PHARMACEUTICAL: Radix Arnebiae seu Lithospermi.

PART USED: root.

DOSAGES: 10 to 15 g.

FLAVOR: sweet and salty.

ENERGY: cold.

ACTIONS: To clear heat, cool the blood, counteract toxic effects.

INDICATIONS: Prevention of measles, high fever, delirium, vomiting of blood, nosebleed, scabies, carbuncles.

PART III

TREATMENT OF DISORDERS

In this section, you will frequently find a selection of foods listed for both excess and deficiency syndromes, even though the disorder itself may manifest only as one of the two. This is because sometimes you may want to balance a recipe for an excess syndrome with deficiency ingredients, or vice versa (see Chapter 1 for a fuller explanation).

CHAPTER 6

Common Symptoms and Ailments

6.1 Hiccups

1. Cold Syndrome

SYMPTOMS AND SIGNS:

- Constipation.
- Coughing and vomiting of saliva.
- Aversion to cold and talking.
- Dry throat.
- Cold extremities.
- Hiccups with cold extremities, easily started by cold air.
- Loud, forceful hiccups.
- Craving for hot drinks.
- Pale complexion.
- Excessive saliva.
- Severe pain in the joints.
- Thirst but with no desire to drink.
- Pale urine.

2. Hot Syndrome

SYMPTOMS AND SIGNS:

- Constipation or diarrhea.
- Diminished urination.
- Excessive yellow, sticky sputum.
- Dry lips.
- Flatulence with noise.
- Loud hiccups, with dryness and thirst.
- Frequent, short hiccups.
- Light fever.
- Warm limbs.
- Little saliva.
- Love of cold or cold drinks.

- Stool with an offensive smell.
- Overpowering thirst.
- Swollen, red throat with foul liquid product.
- Urine with an offensive smell.
- Vomiting of sour-smelling foods and love of cold drinks.

3. Stomach Indigestion Syndrome

SYMPTOMS AND SIGNS:

- Abdominal pain.
- Abdominal pain eased by massage.
- Abdominal pain aggravated by massage.
- Foul taste in the mouth.
- Offensive-smelling belching after a meal.
- Diarrhea and constipation.
- Loud, forceful hiccups.
- Hot sensations in the center of palms.
- Indigestion.
- Lack of appetite.
- Stomachache.
- Stool with an offensive smell.
- Vomiting.

4. Yin Deficiency Syndrome

SYMPTOMS AND SIGNS:

- Bleeding from gums.
- Constipation.
- Dizziness.
- Dry, small stools.
- Dry sensations in the mouth.
- Dry throat.
- Fatigue.
- Headache in the afternoon.
- Hiccups that occur frequently on an empty stomach.
- Hiccups lacking in force.
- Light fever in the afternoon.
- Night sweats.
- Nosebleed.
- Short streams of reddish urine.
- Underweight.
- Insomnia.
- Swallowing difficulty.
- Toothache.

5. Yang Deficiency Syndrome

SYMPTOMS AND SIGNS:

- Clear, long streams of urine.
- Cold extremities.
- Constipation or diarrhea.
- Diminished urination.
- Discharge of watery-thin stool.
- Fatigue.
- Aversion to cold.
- Headache in the morning.
- Hiccups that occur more easily on an empty stomach.
- Hiccups that are weak and in a low voice.
- Palpitation.
- Normal perspiration due to hot weather or warm clothing.
- Profuse cold perspiration.
- Little energy, and quiet.
- Excessive sleeping.

INGREDIENTS FOR CREATING RECIPES

FOODS FOR EXCESS: litchi nut, pea, fresh ginger.

FOODS FOR DEFICIENCY: sword bean, litchi nut, pea.

HERBS: Ji-nei-jin (membrane of chicken gizzard), Lu-gen (reed rhizome), Ban-xia (half-summer pinellia), Chen-pi (dried tangerine peel), Hua-jiao (Chinese prickly ash), Zhu-ru (bamboo shavings), Shi-di (Japanese persimmon), Ding-xiang (cloves), Dang-shen (root of pilose asiabell), Bei-sha-shen (straight ladybell north), Sha-ren (grains of paradise).

Syndromes of disease and herbs to use:

1. **COLD:** Lu-gen (reed rhizome), Ban-xia (half-summer pinellia), Chen-pi (dried tangerine peel), Hua-jiao (Chinese prickly ash), Shi-di (Japanese persimmon), Ding-xiang (cloves); cook with foods for excess.

2. **HOT**: Ban-xia (half-summer pinellia), Chen-pi (dried tangerine peel), Zhu-ru (bamboo shavings), Shi-di (Japanese persimmon), Ding-xiang (cloves); cook with foods for excess.

3. **STOMACH INDIGESTION:** Ji-nei-jin (membrane of chicken gizzard), Ban-xia (half-summer pinellia), Chen-pi (dried tangerine peel), Shi-di (Japanese persimmon), Ding-xiang (cloves), Sha-ren (grains of paradise); cook with foods for excess.

4. **YIN DEFICIENCY:** Ban-xia (half-summer pinellia), Shi-di (Japanese persimmon), Ding-xiang (cloves), Bei-sha-shen (straight ladybell north); cook with foods for deficiency.

5. **YANG DEFICIENCY:** Ban-xia (half-summer pinellia), Shi-di (Japanese persimmon), Ding-xiang (cloves), Dang-shen (root of pilose asiabell); cook with foods for deficiency.

RECIPE 1

MASTER: Shi-di (Japanese persimmon) 5 pieces.

ASSOCIATE: sword bean 20 g (cut to pieces).

ASSISTANT: fresh ginger 3 slices.

SEASONING: brown sugar.

STEPS:

(1) Boil the first three ingredients in water until cooked.

(2) Add brown sugar to drink.

CONSUMPTION: prepare this recipe for consumption whenever hiccups occur.

INDICATIONS: cold syndrome, stomach indigestion syndrome, yin deficiency syndrome, and yang deficiency syndrome of hiccups.

ANALYSIS: Both Shi-di (Japanese persimmon) and sword bean are noted for their effects on hiccups.

6.2 Insomnia

1. Heart-Spleen Deficiency Syndrome

SYMPTOMS AND SIGNS:

- Abdominal swelling.
- Discharge of watery-thin stool.
- Small or poor appetite.
- Fatigue.
- Forgetfulness.
- Impotence.
- Many dreams.
- Anxiety.
- Nervousness.
- Night sweats.
- Palpitation.
- Shortness of breath
- Dry, sallow complexion.

2. Heart-Kidney Yin Deficiency Syndrome

SYMPTOMS AND SIGNS:

- Deafness.
- Dizziness.
- Flushed face due to fatigue or overexertion.

- Depression.
- Forgetfulness.
- Light but periodic fever ("tidal fever").
- Nervousness.
- Night sweats.
- Palpitation.
- Ringing in ears.
- Seminal emission.
- Stress.

3. Heart-Gallbladder Energy Deficiency Syndrome

SYMPTOMS AND SIGNS:

- Bitter taste in the mouth.
- Depression with nausea.
- Depression with aversion to bright lights.
- Nervousness.
- Easily panicked.
- Disturbed sleep.

4. Sputum Fire Syndrome

SYMPTOMS AND SIGNS:

- Difficult bowel movement or urination.
- Hunger with no appetite.
- Mentally unstable.
- Ringing in ears and hearing difficulties.
- Congested chest.

5. Stomach indigestion Syndrome

SYMPTOMS AND SIGNS:

- Abdominal pain.
- Abdominal pain eased by massage.
- Abdominal pain aggravated by massage.
- Abdominal distension.
- Offensive-smelling belching after a meal.
- Chest and diaphragm congestion and discomfort.
- Diarrhea or constipation.
- Hot sensations in the center of palms.
- Indigestion.
- Lack of appetite.
- Desire for hot drinks, but can drink only a little.
- Nausea.
- Stomachache with swelling and feeling of fullness.
- Foul-smelling stools.
- Vomiting of clear liquid.

INGREDIENTS FOR CREATING RECIPES

FOODS FOR EXCESS: bitter gourd (balsam pear), day lily, wheat bran.

FOODS FOR DEFICIENCY: polished rice, glutinous rice, sparrow, longan nut, grape.

HERBS: Yuan-zhi (slender-leaved milkwort), Wu-wei-zi (magnolia vine fruit), He-huan-pi (mimosa), Suan-zao-ren (jujube), Bai-zi-ren (oriental arborvitae kernel), Ren-shen (Chinese ginseng), Dang-gui (Chinese angelica), Dang-shen (root of pilose asiabell), Da-zao (red date), Cong-bai (welsh onion), Lian-zi (East Indian lotus), Ling-zhi (lucid ganoderma), Fu-pen-zi (wild raspberry), Wu-wei-zi (magnolia vine fruit), Jin-ying-zi (cherokee rose), Sang-shen (mulberry).

Syndromes of disease and herbs to use:

1. **HEART-SPLEEN DEFICIENCY**: Yuan-zhi (slender-leaved milkwort), Wu-wei-zi (magnolia vine fruit), He-huan-pi (mimosa), Suan-zao-ren (jujube), Bai-zi-ren (oriental arborvitae kernel), Ren-shen (Chinese ginseng), Dang-gui (Chinese angelica), Dang-shen (root of pilose asiabell), Dazao (red date), Ling-zhi (lucid ganoderma), Sang-shen (mulberry); cook with foods for deficiency.

2. **HEART-KIDNEY YIN DEFICIENCY:** Yuan-zhi (slender-leaved milkwort), Wu-wei-zi (magnolia vine fruit), He-huan-pi (mimosa), Suan-zao-ren (jujube), Bai-zi-ren (oriental arborvitae kernel), Ren-shen (Chinese ginseng), Dang-shen (root of pilose asiabell), Da-zao (red date), Fu-pen-zi (wild raspberry), Wu-wei-zi (magnolia vine fruit), Jin-ying-zi (cherokee rose), Ling-zhi (lucid ganoderma), Sang-shen (mulberry); cook with foods for deficiency.
3. **HEART-GALLBLADDER DEFICIENCY:** Yuan-zhi (slender-leaved milkwort), Wu-wei-zi (magnolia vine fruit), Ling-zhi (lucid ganoderma); cook with foods for deficiency.
4. **SPUTUM FIRE:** Cong-bai (welsh onion), Lian-zi (East Indian lotus), Ling-zhi (lucid ganoderma); cook with foods for excess.
5. **STOMACH INDIGESTION:** Ren-shen (Chinese ginseng), Dang-shen (root of pilose asiabell), Da-zao (red date); Ling-zhi (lucid ganoderma); cook with foods for excess.

RECIPE 2

MASTER: 100 g Sang-shen (mulberry).

ASSOCIATE: 50 g glutinous rice.

ASSISTANT: 10 g wheat bran.

SEASONING: 2 cubes rock sugar.

STEPS:

(1) Make a decoction of Sang-shen (mulberry) by boiling in water for 30 minutes. Strain and set aside.

(2) Boil glutinous rice in water for 20 minutes, then add wheat bran and rock sugar and the Sang-shen soup to boil together for another five minutes.

CONSUMPTION: drink the soup once daily, one hour before bedtime, for one week as a course of treatment.

INDICATIONS: insomnia due to heart-spleen deficiency or heart-kidney yin deficiency.

ANALYSIS: Sang-shen (mulberry) is a common herb to calm the spirit, essential for sleep; glutinous rice (sweet rice) can tone the spleen, and wheat bran can increase yin energy in the body, contributing to good sleep.

6.3 Ringing in the ears and hearing difficulties

1. Wind Heat Syndrome

SYMPTOMS AND SIGNS:

- Cough.
- Coughing out blood.
- Dizziness.
- Headache.
- Headache with dizziness.
- Sensitivity to light with swelling and dislike of wind.
- Muddy, nasal discharge.
- Nasal congestion.
- Nosebleed.
- Pain in the eyes.
- Pain in the throat.
- Bloodshot eyes.
- Thirst.
- Toothache.
- Yellow urine.
- Yellowish discharge from the nose.

2. Hot Liver Syndrome

SYMPTOMS AND SIGNS:

- Bitter taste in the mouth.
- Hearing difficulties.
- Dry throat.
- Head swelling.
- Haematuria (discharge of urine containing blood).

- Morning sickness.
- Pain in the ribs.
- Partial suppression of lochia.
- Pink eyes with swelling.
- Depression.
- Loud ringing in ears.
- Sour taste in the mouth.
- Spasms.
- Twitching.
- Vaginal discharge with a strong, fishy smell.

3. Damp Phlegm Syndrome

SYMPTOMS AND SIGNS:

- Cough.
- Sputum that can be coughed out easily.
- Discharge of white watery sputum.
- Dizziness.
- Excessive whitish vaginal discharge.
- Frequent coughs during pregnancy that cause and prolong fetal motion.
- Headache.
- Hiccups.
- Pain in the chest.
- Panting.
- Prolonged dizziness.
- Ringing in ears with dizziness.
- Ringing in ears that comes and goes with varying degrees of loudness.
- Sleep a lot.
- Sleeplessness.
- Vomiting.
- Whitish sputum that can be cleared from the throat easily.

4. Kidney Deficiency Syndrome

SYMPTOMS AND SIGNS:

- Chronic backache.
- Deafness.
- Diarrhea.
- Frequent miscarriage.
- Loss of hair.
- Large quantities of urine with no thirst or drink.
- Excessive sleepiness.
- Pain (falling) in the lower abdomen with fondness for massage.
- Ringing in ears and deafness.
- Persistent ringing in ears like the sound of a cicada.
- Toothache.
- Urinary disorders.

INGREDIENTS FOR CREATING RECIPES

FOODS FOR EXCESS: spinach root, black soybean.

FOODS FOR DEFICIENCY: polished rice, black sesame seed.

HERBS: Chen-pi (dried tangerine peel), Fu-ling (tuckahoe; Indian bread), Lian-zi (East Indian lotus), Shu-di (processed glutinous rehmannia), Nu-zhen-zi (wax tree).

Syndromes of disease and herbs to use:

1. **WIND HEAT:** Chen-pi (dried tangerine peel), Lian-zi (East Indian lotus); cook with foods for excess.
2. **HOT LIVER:** Lian-zi (East Indian lotus); cook with foods for excess.
3. **DAMP PHLEGM:** Chen-pi (dried tangerine peel), Fu-ling (tuckahoe; Indian bread); cook with foods for excess.
4. **KIDNEY DEFICIENCY:** Shu-di (processed

glutinous rehmannia), Nu-zhen-zi (wax tree); cook with foods for deficiency.

RECIPE 3

MASTER: 10 g Chen-pi (dried tangerine peel).

ASSOCIATE: 5 g Fu-ling (tuckahoe; Indian bread).

ASSISTANT: 5 g Lian-zi (East Indian lotus).

SEASONING: brown sugar.

STEPS:

(1) Decoct Chen-pi and Fu-ling in water; strain to obtain soup.

(2) Put Lian-zi in the soup to boil again until well cooked.

(3) Season with brown sugar before removing from heat.

CONSUMPTION: serve as a side dish at mealtime, once a day for ten days as a course of treatment.

INDICATIONS: all syndromes of ringing in ears.

ANALYSIS: Chen-pi (dried orange peel) is to promote energy circulation; Fu-ling (tuckahoe; Indian bread) is to tone up the body and drain off water; Lian-zi (East Indian lotus) is to relieve anxiety; brown sugar is to improve the taste of the recipe.

6.4 Chronic fatigue

1. Energy Deficiency

SYMPTOMS AND SIGNS:

- Abdominal pain.
- Irregular heartbeats.
- Dizziness.
- Shallow breathing and weak voice.
- Weak limbs accompanied by a desire to recline.
- Headache.
- Lack of appetite.
- Numbness.
- Menstrual pain in women.
- Ringing in ears.
- Underweight with dry skin.

2. Blood Deficiency Syndrome

SYMPTOMS AND SIGNS:

- Dizziness.
- Fever at night.
- Headache in the afternoon with dizziness.
- Insomnia.
- Pale lips.
- Blurred vision.
- Night sweats.
- Pale complexion.
- Palpitation.
- Underweight with dry skin.

3. Yang Deficiency Syndrome

SYMPTOMS AND SIGNS:

- Excessive or scanty perspiration.
- Cold hands and feet.
- Constipation.
- Diarrhea.
- Edema.
- Aversion to cold.
- Headache in the morning.
- Palpitation.
- Profuse cold perspiration.
- Sleep a lot.

4. Yin Deficiency Syndrome

SYMPTOMS AND SIGNS:

- Bleeding from gums.
- Constipation.

- Dizziness.
- Dry stool.
- Scratchy throat.
- Insomnia.
- Night sweats.
- Nosebleed.
- Scanty, reddish urine.
- Underweight.
- Sore throat.
- Toothache.

INGREDIENTS FOR CREATING RECIPES

FOODS FOR EXCESS: ling in fresh form.

FOODS FOR DEFICIENCY: beef, mutton, polished rice, black sesame seed, sheep or goat's liver, chicken, mussel, ling in cooked form.

HERBS: Dang-shen (root of pilose asiabell), Ren-shen (Chinese ginseng), Huang-qi (membranous milk vetch), Shu-di (processed glutinous rehmannia), Dang-gui (Chinese angelica), Huang-jing (sealwort), Ba-ji-tian (morinda root), Yin-yang-huo (longspur epimendium), Bai-he (lily), Nu-zhen-zi (wax tree).

Syndromes of disease and herbs to use:

1. **ENERGY DEFICIENCY:** Dang-shen (root of pilose asiabell), Ren-shen (Chinese ginseng), Huang-qi (membranous milk vetch); cook with foods for deficiency.
2. **BLOOD DEFICIENCY:** Shu-di (processed glutinous rehmannia), Dang-gui (Chinese angelica); cook with foods for deficiency.
3. **YANG DEFICIENCY:** Ba-ji-tian (morinda root), Yin-yang-huo (longspur epimendium); cook with foods for deficiency.
4. **YIN DEFICIENCY:** Huang-jing (sealwort), Bai-he (lily), Nu-zhen-zi (wax tree); cook with foods for deficiency.

RECIPE 4

MASTER: 5 g Ren-shen (Chinese ginseng).

ASSOCIATE: 5 g Huang-qi (membranous milk vetch).

ASSISTANT: 100 g polished rice, 250 g milk.

SEASONING: none.

STEPS:

(1) Decoct Ren-shen (Chinese ginseng) and Huang-qi (membranous milk vetch) in water; strain to obtain soup.

(2) Boil polished rice until almost cooked. Add milk and the herbal soup to boil for another two minutes.

CONSUMPTION: serve as a side dish at mealtimes.

INDICATIONS: all syndromes of chronic fatigue.

ANALYSIS: This is basically a vegetarian dish. All ingredients are tonics; Ren-shen and Huang-qi and rice are energy tonics, and milk is a yin tonic. Energy tonics are used in this recipe because energy deficiency is responsible for most cases of chronic fatigue.

6.5 Dizziness

1. Liver Fire Upsurging Syndrome

SYMPTOMS AND SIGNS:

- Acute dizziness.
- Bleeding from stomach.
- Congested chest.
- Hearing impairment.
- Dim vision.
- Dry sensations in the mouth.
- Easily angered.
- Headache felt as pain on both sides of the head and in the sockets of the eyes.
- Headache that is severe.
- Hiccups.
- Nosebleed.

- Bloodshot eyes.
- Ringing in ears.
- Disturbed sleep patterns.
- Vomiting with blood.
- Yellow-red urine.

2. **Deficient Yin with Excessive Yang Syndrome**

SYMPTOMS AND SIGNS:

- Coughing with blood.
- Dizziness with ringing in the ears.
- Chronic dizziness.
- Excessive sex drive.
- Hot sensations in the body.
- Insomnia.
- Jumpiness.
- Night sweats.
- Seminal emission.
- Underweight.
- Tidal fever.

3. **Deficiency of Yin and Yang Syndrome**

SYMPTOMS AND SIGNS:

- Cold limbs and sensations in the body.
- Ringing in the ears getting worse on fatigue.
- Fatigue or low energy.
- Palpitation.
- Perspiration with hot sensations in the body easily triggered by physical activities.
- Poor spirits.
- Ringing in ears.
- Skinniness.
- Too lazy to talk.

4. **Spleen Sputum Syndrome**

SYMPTOMS AND SIGNS:

- Abundant saliva.
- Dizziness with heavy sensations in the head.
- Severe dizziness.
- Overweight but eat little.
- Poor appetite.
- Slight fullness of the stomach.
- Suppression of menses in women.
- Weak limbs.

5. **Deficiency of Energy and Blood Syndrome**

SYMPTOMS AND SIGNS:

- Bleeding of various kinds with light-colored blood, often seen in consumptive diseases.
- Dizziness that gets worse on movement.
- Fatigue.
- Impaired vision with "jumpy" images.
- Insomnia.
- Low energy.
- Low voice.
- Numbness of limbs.
- Pale complexion and lips.
- Pale nails.
- Palpitation.

INGREDIENTS FOR CREATING RECIPES

FOODS FOR EXCESS: freshwater clam, black soybean, sunflower.

FOODS FOR DEFICIENCY: beef liver, mussel, chicken.

HERBS: Ju-hua (mulberry-leaved chrysanthemum), Cang-er-zi (achene of Siberian cocklebur), Jue-ming-zi (coffee weed), Gou-teng (gambir), tian-ma, Gan-cao (licorice), Da-zao (red date), Ban-xia (half-summer pinellia), Chen-pi (dried tangerine peel), Mai-dong (lilyturf), Huang-qi (membranous milk vetch), Dang-gui (Chinese angelica), Shan-yao (Chinese yam), Ren-shen (Chinese ginseng), Bei-sha-shen (straight ladybell north), Huang-jing (sealwort), Shu-di (processed glutinous rehmannia).

Syndromes of disease and herbs to use:

1. **LIVER FIRE UPSURGING:** Ju-hua (mulberry-leaved chrysanthemum), Jue-ming-zi (coffee weed); cook with foods for excess.
2. **DEFICIENCT YIN WITH EXCESSIVE YANG:** Gou-teng (gambir), tian-ma, Bei-sha-shen (straight ladybell north), Huang-jing (sealwort); cook with foods for deficiency.
3. **DEFICIENCY OF YIN AND YANG:** Gan-cao (licorice), Ren-shen (Chinese ginseng), Da-zao (red date), Mai-dong (lilyturf); cook with foods for deficiency.
4. **SPLEEN SPUTUM:** Cang-er-zi (achene of Siberian cocklebur), Chen-pi (dried tangerine peel), Ban-xia (half-summer pinellia); cook with foods for excess.
5. **DEFICIENCY OF ENERGY AND BLOOD:** (Shu-di (processed glutinous rehmannia), Huang-qi (membranous milk vetch), Dang-gui (Chinese angelica), Shan-yao (Chinese yam), Bai-zhu (white atractylodes).

RECIPE 5

MASTER: 10 g Dang-shen (root of pilose asiabell), 10 g Bei-sha-shen (straight ladybell north), 15 g Huang-jing (sealwort).

ASSOCIATE: 1 whole chicken (with or without skin).

ASSISTANT: 100 g black soybeans, 50 g peas, peanut oil.

SEASONING: wine, soy sauce, white sugar, salt.

STEPS:

(1) Decoct Dang-shen (root of pilose asiabell), Bei-sha-shen (straight ladybell north), and Huang-jing (sealwort) together for 30 minutes; strain to obtain soup.

(2) Cut up the chicken in eight equal pieces.

(3) Heat frying pan with the peanut oil over high heat. Put in chicken pieces.

(4) When the chicken changes color, season to taste with wine, soy sauce, white sugar, salt, and fry for a short while longer.

(5) Add the herbal soup to the chicken and bring to a boil, cooking for fifteen minutes.

(6) Soak black soybean in water for at least two hours before cooking. Discard water and add 1 cup fresh water to the beans, bring to a boil, then reduce to low heat.

(7) Add the soybeans and peas to the herbal chicken soup and cook until all ingredients are soft.

CONSUMPTION: have as a meal.

INDICATIONS: deficiency syndromes of dizziness.

ANALYSIS: Dang-shen and chicken are both energy tonics; Bei-sha-shen, Huang-jing, and peanut oil are all yin tonics. Thus this recipe is primarily a tonic recipe. Black soybeans promote blood circulation, and the seasonings improve the taste.

6.6 Premature gray hair

1. Innate Deficiency Syndrome

SYMPTOMS AND SIGNS:

- Dizziness.
- Pale tongue.
- Premature gray hair among family members.
- Vision impairment.
- Weak lower back and legs.

2. **Hot Blood Syndrome**

SYMPTOMS AND SIGNS:

- Bleeding of various kinds.
- Nosebleed.
- Skin ulcer.
- Urination difficulty.

INGREDIENTS FOR CREATING RECIPES

FOODS FOR EXCESS: black soybean, processed dried persimmon.

FOODS FOR DEFICIENCY: sesame seed, walnut, mutton.

HERBS: Dang-gui (Chinese angelica), Gou-qi-zi (matrimony vine fruits), He-shou-wu (tuber of multiflower knotweed), Da-zao (red date), Shu-di (processed glutinous rehmannia), Shan-yao (Chinese yam), Tu-si-zi (dodder seed), Sheng-di (dried glutinous rehmannia).

Syndromes of disease and herbs to use:

1. **INNATE DEFICIENCY:** Dang-gui (Chinese angelica) Gou-qi-zi (matrimony vine fruits) He-shou-wu (tuber of multiflower knotweed) Da-zao (red date) Shu-di (processed glutinous rehmannia) Shan-yao (Chinese yam), Tu-si-zi (dodder seed); cook with foods for deficiency.
2. **HOT BLOOD:** Sheng-di (dried glutinous rehmannia), xuan-shen; cook with foods for excess.

RECIPE 6

MASTER: Shu-di (processed glutinous rehmannia), Shan-yao (Chinese yam), Tu-si-zi (dodder seed), 3 g each; 5 g He-shou-wu (tuber of multiflower knotweed).

ASSOCIATE: 3 g walnuts, 5 g black soybeans preferably (presoaked).

ASSISTANT: 500 g mutton, boneless.

SEASONING: green onion, fresh ginger, white pepper, salt.

STEPS:

(1) Wrap the four herbs in a gauze bag.

(2) Put the bag in a pot, and add the green onion, fresh ginger, and white pepper to taste.

(3) Cut up mutton into small pieces and add to the pot.

(4) Add water to the pot and cook over high heat. Bring to a boil, then reduce to low heat to cook until mutton is done.

(5) Remove the gauze bag from the pot and discard.

(6) Soak black soybeans in water for at least two hours before cooking. Discard water and add 1 cup fresh water to the beans, bring to a boil, then reduce to low heat.

(7) Combine all the ingredients and season with salt and pepper.

CONSUMPTION: eat mutton and black soybean and walnuts together as a side dish at mealtimes, once a week for ten weeks as a course of treatment.

INDICATIONS: innate deficiency syndrome of premature gray hair.

ANALYSIS: This is a tonic recipe; all herbs are tonics. Black soybean and walnuts are foods to treat premature gray hair.

RECIPE 7

MASTER: 30 g He-shou-wu (tuber of multiflower knotweed).

ASSOCIATE: 100 g polished rice.

ASSISTANT: 3 Da-zao (red date), 2 g rock sugar.

SEASONING: none.

STEPS:

(1) Decoct He-shou-wu (tuber of multiflower knotweed) in water for thirty minutes; strain to obtain herbal soup.

(2) Boil polished rice, red dates, and rock sugar together in an adequate amount of water.

(3) Add the herbal soup to the rice gruel and eat as a meal.

INDICATIONS: innate deficiency syndrome of premature gray hair.

ANALYSIS: He-shou-wu, a well-known herb to treat gray hair, is a blood tonic. Da-zao (red date) and rock sugar are energy tonics. Rock sugar is also used as a seasoning ingredient to improve the taste without putting on weight.

6.7 Common acne

Common acne normally belongs to the hot syndrome.

SYMPTOMS AND SIGNS:

- Bad breath.
- Bleeding from gums or swollen gums.
- Coughing with yellowish, offensive-smelling sputum.
- Chest pain.
- Dry mouth and stools.
- Fever.
- Easily hungry.
- Nosebleed.
- Perspiring in the head.
- Craving for cold drinks.
- Yellowish urine.

INGREDIENTS FOR CREATING RECIPES

FOODS FOR EXCESS: mung bean, seagrass, Chinese wax gourd, seaweed.

HERBS: Yu-xing-cao (cordate houttuynia), Shan-zha (Chinese hawthorn), Tao-ren (peach kernel), Yi-yi-ren (Job's tears), Dan-shen (purple sage), Bai-he (lily).

1. **HOT:** Yu-xing-cao (cordate houttuynia), Shan-zha (Chinese hawthorn), Tao-ren (peach kernel), Yi-yi-ren (Job's tears), Dan-shen (purple sage); cook with foods for excess.

RECIPE 8

MASTER: 10 g Bai-he (lily).

ASSOCIATE: 100 g mung bean.

ASSISTANT: 5 g rock sugar.

SEASONING: none.

STEPS: Boil the three ingredients in enough water and have with meals.

INDICATIONS: common acne.

ANALYSIS: Bai-he can lubricate and reduce heat in the lungs, mung bean can also reduce heat in the blood, and rock sugar is to both lubricate and tone up energy slightly.

RECIPE 9

MASTER: 9 g Tao-ren (peach kernel).

ASSOCIATE: 30 g Yi-yi-ren (Job's tears).

ASSISTANT: 9 g seagrass, 9 g kelp.

SEASONING: salt.

STEPS:

(1) Boil Tao-ren (peach kernel), seagrass, and kelp in enough water to cover the ingredients for thirty minutes; strain to obtain herbal soup.

(2) Boil Yi-yi-ren (Job's tears) in 2 cups water for a few minutes, add the herbal soup and continue cooking until ingredients are soft.

(3) Season with salt and eat as a porridge.

INDICATIONS: common acne.

ANALYSIS: Tao-ren can disperse the blood so that it does not stagnate to cause acne. Yi-yi-ren can remove water, seagrass and kelp can cool the body and clear pimples, and salt improves the taste.

6.8 Eczema

1. Wind Syndrome

SYMPTOMS AND SIGNS:

- Abnormal perspiration.
- Aversion to wind
- Headache.
- Extremely itchy skin.
- Light cough.
- Nasal discharge.

- Pain in the joints.
- Sneezing.
- Tickle in the throat.

2. **Blood Deficiency Syndrome**

SYMPTOMS AND SIGNS:

- Abdominal pain.
- Dizziness.
- Dry mouth and lips.
- Fever at night.
- Headache in the afternoon with dizziness.
- Insomnia.
- Pale lips.
- Blurred vision.
- Night sweats.
- Pale complexion.
- Palpitation.
- Thin with dry skin.

3. **Hot Fire Syndrome**

SYMPTOMS AND SIGNS:

- Bleeding from gums.
- Cold hands and feet.
- Hot sensations in the center of palms.
- Insomnia.
- Mouth cankers.
- Palpitation.
- Yellowish urine.

INGREDIENTS FOR CREATING RECIPES

FOODS FOR EXCESS: guava, freshwater clam.

FOODS FOR DEFICIENCY: Irish potato.

HERBS: He-shou-wu (tuber of multiflower knotweed), Cang-er-zi (achene of Siberian cocklebur), Qing-dai (blue indigo), Qu-mai (rainbow pink), She-chuang-zi (snake bed seeds), Ai-ye (mugwort), Ye-ju-hua (wild chrysanthemum), Bai-xian-pi (white bark), Yi-yi-ren (Job's tears), Tu-fu-ling (tuckahoe; Indian bread), Pu-gong-ying (Asian dandelion).

Syndromes of disease and herbs to use:

1. **WIND:** Cang-er-zi (achene of Siberian cocklebur), Ai-ye (mugwort), Ye-ju-hua (wild chrysanthemum), Bai-xian-pi (white bark), Yi-yi-ren (Job's tears); cook with foods for excess.

2. **BLOOD DEFICIENCY**: He-shou-wu (tuber of multiflower knotweed), She-chuang-zi (snake bed seeds); cook with foods for deficiency.

3. **HOT FIRE**: Qing-dai (blue indigo), Qu-mai (rainbow pink), Ye-ju-hua (wild chrysanthemum), Bai-xian-pi (white bark), Yu-fu-ling (tuckahoe; Indian bread), Pu-gong-ying (Asian dandelion); cook with foods for excess.

RECIPE 10

MASTER: 15 g Tu-fu-ling (tuckahoe; Indian bread), 30 g Yi-yi-ren (Job's tears), 20 g Pu-gong-ying (Asian dandelion), 3 g Gan-cao (licorice).

ASSOCIATE: 100 g freshwater clam.

ASSISTANT: 50 g Irish potatoes.

SEASONING: salt.

STEPS:

(1) Boil the herbs in enough water to cover for thirty minutes; strain to obtain herbal soup.

(2) Boil freshwater clams and Irish potatoes (peeled and chopped small) in enough water until cooked to make a soup.

(3) Add the herbal soup and have as a porridge.

INDICATIONS: wind syndrome and hot fire syndrome of eczema.

ANALYSIS: This recipe is to deal with excess types of eczema. Tu-fu-ling is to clear heat, Yi-yi-ren is to remove water, and Pu-gong-ying is to eliminate toxic heat and fire. Fresh water clam is a cold food to clear heat, Irish potatoes can heal inflammation, and salt is to improve the taste.

6.9 Psoriasis

1. Dry Blood (internal dryness) Syndrome

SYMPTOMS AND SIGNS:

- Dizziness.
- Numbness of hands and feet.
- Pain in the ribs.
- Spots in front of the eyes.
- Twitching.

2. Hot Blood Syndrome

SYMPTOMS AND SIGNS:

- Bleeding of various kinds.
- Nosebleed.
- Skin ulcer.
- Urination difficulty.

3. Blood Coagulation Syndrome

SYMPTOMS AND SIGNS:

- Abdominal pain.
- Bleeding from gums.
- Chest pain.
- Coughing with blood.
- Lumbago.
- Pain in ribs.
- Palpitation.
- Stomachache.
- Vomiting with blood.

INGREDIENTS FOR CREATING RECIPES

FOODS FOR EXCESS: turnip root-leaf, vinegar, grapefruit, torreyanut.

HERBS: Wu-mei (black plum), Che-qian-zi (Asiatic plantain seed), Yi-yi-ren (Job's tears), Ding-xiang (cloves), Bai-xian-pi (white bark), Ku-shen (bitter sophora), Dan-pi (peony), Dang-gui (Chinese angelica), Mai-dong (lilyturf), Tian-dong (lucid asparagus).

Syndromes of disease and herbs to use:

1. **DRY BLOOD:** Wu-mei (black plum), Mai-dong (lilyturf), Tian-dong (lucid asparagus); cook with foods for excess.
2. **HOT BLOOD:** Che-qian-zi (Asiatic plantain seed), Yi-yi-ren (Job's tears), Bai-xian-pi (white bark), Ku-shen (bitter sophora), Dan-pi (peony); cook with foods for excess.
3. **BLOOD COAGULATION:** Ding-xiang (cloves), Dang-gui (Chinese angelica); cook with foods for excess.

RECIPE 11

MASTER: 15 g Che-qian-zi (Asiatic plantain seed).

ASSOCIATE: 30 g Yi-yi-ren (Job's tears).

ASSISTANT: none.

SEASONING: vinegar, white sugar.

STEPS:

(1) Make a decoction from Che-qian-zi (Asiatic plantain seed); strain to obtain herbal soup.

(2) Add Yi-yi-ren (Job's tears) to the herbal soup.

(3) Season with vinegar and white sugar after removing from heat.

INDICATIONS: hot blood syndrome of psoriasis.

ANALYSIS: Che-qian-zi and Yi-yi-ren are commonly used to treat psoriasis, vinegar is used to control psoriasis, and white sugar (or rock sugar) is to improve the taste.

6.10 Premature aging

Premature aging is normally due to a decline in the functioning of various internal organs, which should be identified and corrected.

INGREDIENTS FOR CREATING RECIPES

FOODS FOR DEFICIENCY: walnut, chicken, duck.

HERBS: He-shou-wu (tuber of multiflower knotweed), Ren-shen (Chinese ginseng), Lu-rong (pilose antler of a young stag), E-jiao (donkey-hide gelatin), Huang-jing (sealwort), Huang-qi (membranous milk vetch), Gou-qi-zi (matrimony vine fruit), Fu-ling (tuckahoe; Indian bread), Nu-zhen-zi (wax tree), Bu-gu-zhi (psoralea), Yin-yang-huo (longspur epimendium), Shi-chang-pu (grass-leaved sweetflag), Du-zhong (eucommia bark), Tu-si-zi (dodder seed), Dong-chong-xia-cao (Chinese caterpillar fungus), Dang-shen (root of pilose asiabell), Da-zao (red date).

RECIPE 12

MASTER: 50 g Dong-chong-xia-cao (Chinese caterpillar fungus).

ASSOCIATE: 50 g Dang-shen (root of pilose asiabell).

ASSISTANT: 50 g Da-zao (red date); 1,500 ml (6 cups) rice wine.

SEASONING: none.

STEPS:

(1) Boil Dong-chong-xia-cao (Chinese caterpillar fungus), Dang-shen (root of pilose asiabell), and Da-zao (red date) together in water for three minutes, then filter. Let cool completely.

(2) Place the herbs in wine and seal the mixture in a wine bottle for at least one month.

(3) Drink a glass of this medicated wine after meals.

INDICATIONS: promoting longevity.

ANALYSIS: Dong-chong-xia-cao is dried fungus growing on the larva of a caterpillar. It is used as both a herb and a food, and is a yang tonic. Chinese people are in the habit of eating it as a general tonic to promote longevity. Dang-shen and Da-zao are both energy tonics. Wine is here used to reinforce the above three ingredients.

6.11 Alzheimer's disease

1. Spleen Sputum Syndrome

SYMPTOMS AND SIGNS:

- Excessive saliva.
- Prone to silence.
- Overweight but eat only a small amount of food.
- Loss of memory.
- Poor appetite.
- Slight fullness of the stomach.
- Sudden crying and laughing.
- Weak limbs.

2. Sputum Congestion and Blood Coagulation Syndrome

SYMPTOMS AND SIGNS:

- Silence alternating with illogical talk.
- Alternating impassiveness with jumpiness.
- Chest pain.
- Heavy sensations.
- Insanity.
- Lumpy spots in the body that do not shift.
- Numbness.
- Prickling sensation and chronic pain in a fixed spot.
- Symptoms get worse in cold weather and better in warm weather.
- Mental fogginess.

3. **Hot Phlegm Syndrome**

SYMPTOMS AND SIGNS:

- History of asthma.
- Worsening chronic dementia.
- Spells of fainting or unconsciousness.
- Cough.
- Discharge of hard, yellowish sputum in lumps.
- Sticky, turbid, and thin stool.
- Discharge of sticky, yellowish sputum in lumps.
- Mental instability.
- Insomnia.
- Stool with a foul odor.
- Vomiting.
- Wheezing.

4. **Spleen-Kidney Yang Deficiency Syndrome**

SYMPTOMS AND SIGNS:

- Listlessness.
- Clear signs of aging.
- Cold hands and feet or cold loins.
- Diarrhea before dawn.
- Diarrhea that consists of sticky and muddy stool.
- Edema that occurs all over the body.
- Fatigue.
- Aversion to cold.
- Frequent urination with clear, whitish urine.
- Incontinence.
- Loss of memory.
- Paralysis of limbs.
- Slow movement.
- Sputum rumbling in the throat with panting.

5. **Liver-Kidney Yin Deficiency Syndrome**

SYMPTOMS AND SIGNS:

- Dizziness.
- Dry eyes or throat.
- Explosive laughter and crying.
- Fatigue.
- Headache with pain in the bony ridge forming the eyebrow.
- Loss of speech.
- Lumbago.
- Night blindness.
- Night sweats.
- Pain in the hypochondrium.
- Heat in the palms of hands and soles of feet.
- Poor memory.
- Trembling hands.
- Insomnia with forgetfulness.
- Weak loins and tibia.

6. **Energy Congestion and Blood Coagulation Syndrome**

SYMPTOMS AND SIGNS:

- Abdominal distention.
- Indifference or apathy.
- Congested chest.
- Forgetfulness.
- Hallucination.
- Excessive sighing.
- Lump in the abdomen that stays in the same region.
- Slow response.
- Sudden fear and nervousness.

INGREDIENTS FOR CREATING RECIPES

FOODS FOR EXCESS: eggplant, celery.

FOODS FOR DEFICIENCY: mutton, longan nut, brown sugar, chestnut, apricot.

HERBS: Rou-cong-rong (saline cistanche), Shi-chang-pu (grass-leaved sweetflag), Shan-yao (Chinese yam), Tu-si-zi (dodder seed), Yu-jin (aromatic turmeric root-tuber), Ban-xia (half-summer pinellia), Chen-pi (dried tangerine peel), Nu-zhen-zi (wax tree), Huang-jing (sealwort).

Syndromes of disease and herbs to use:

1. **SPLEEN SPUTUM:** Shan-yao (Chinese yam), Shi-chang-pu (grass-leaved sweetflag); cook with foods for excess.
2. **SPUTUM CONGESTION AND BLOOD COAGULATION:** Yu-jin (aromatic turmeric root-tuber), Chen-pi (dried tangerine peel), Ban-xia (half-summer pinellia), Shi-chang-pu (grass-leaved sweetflag); cook with foods for excess.
3. **HOT PHLEGM:** Ban-xia (half-summer pinellia), Chen-pi (dried tangerine peel); cook with foods for excess.
4. **SPLEEN-KIDNEY YANG DEFICIENCY:** Tu-si-zi (dodder seed), Rou-cong-rong (saline cistanche), Shan-yao (Chinese yam); cook with foods for deficiency.
5. **LIVER-KIDNEY YIN DEFICIENCY:** Nu-zhen-zi (wax tree), Huang-jing (sealwort); cook with foods for deficiency.
6. **ENERGY CONGESTION AND BLOOD COAGULATION:** Yu-jin (aromatic turmeric root-tuber); cook with foods for excess.

RECIPE 13

MASTER: 15 g Rou-cong-rong (saline cistanche), 10 g Tu-si-zi (dodder seed), 9 g Shi-chang-pu (grass-leaved sweetflag), 9 g Yu-jin (aromatic turmeric root-tuber), 500 g Shan-yao (Chinese yam).

ASSOCIATE: 500 g mutton.

ASSISTANT: 100 g chestnut.

SEASONING: salt.

STEPS:

(1) Cut up Shan-yao (Chinese yam) and mutton in small pieces.

(2) Put all the master ingredients (five herbs) in a gauze bag to boil in a saucepan of water with mutton over high heat, covered, until the mutton is tender.

(3) Reduce to low heat, add Shan-yao and chestnuts to cook for a few minutes longer.

(4) Season with salt before eating.

INDICATIONS: deficiency syndromes of Alzheimer's disease.

ANALYSIS: Rou-cong-rong and Tu-si-zi are yang tonics, Shan-yao is an energy tonic, Shi-chang-pu is a herb normally used to treat mental disorders, Yu-jin can promote blood circulation, mutton can warm the body, and chestnut is good for the kidneys.

6.12 Smoking and intoxication

Smoking and drinking are forms of addiction. Recipes may be created to counteract the addiction and its effects.

INGREDIENTS FOR CREATING RECIPES

FOODS FOR EXCESS: apple, fresh lotus rhizome, mung bean sprout, tea, tofu.

FOODS FOR DEFICIENCY: apple, dried lotus rhizome, oyster, shiitake mushroom, tofu.

HERBS: Ge-gen (kudzu vine).

RECIPE 14

MASTER: 30 g Ge-gen (kudzu vine).

ASSOCIATE: 150 g tofu.

ASSISTANT: 20 g mung bean sprouts.

SEASONING: salt and rice vinegar.

STEPS:

(1) Boil Ge-gen (kudzu vine) in water for 30 minutes; strain to obtain a decoction.

(2) Add tofu and mung bean sprouts to the soup, and bring to a boil for 10 minutes.

(3) Season with salt and rice vinegar. Drink the soup, and eat the tofu and sprouts.

INDICATIONS: smoking and alcoholism.

ANALYSIS: Ge-gen (kudzu vine) is a common herb to cure intoxication and alcoholism, and tofu and mung bean are common foods to cure excessive types of intoxication and alcoholism. In case of deficiency, use foods listed for deficiency instead. Salt and rice vinegar are used to improve the taste.

6.13 Cancers of various kinds

The following foods and herbs have been found to be anticancerous in that they are beneficial in treating all types of cancer.

INGREDIENTS FOR CREATING RECIPES

Foods generally considered beneficial in treatment of cancers may be divided into foods for excess and foods for deficiency.

FOODS FOR EXCESS: tea, apple, ling in fresh form, yellow soybean, pea, common button mushroom, mung bean, shepherd's purse, gold carp.

FOODS FOR DEFICIENCY: shiitake mushroom, apple, ling in cooked form, royal jelly, pea, squash.

FOODS CAPABLE OF DECOMPOSING CARCINOGENIC NITROSAMINE: radish, pea, squash, mung bean sprouts.

FOODS TO INCREASE THE IMMUNE SYSTEM AGAINST CANCERS: common button mushroom, shiitake mushroom, water chestnut, barley, yellow soybean, hyacinth bean (lablab bean), royal jelly.

ANTICANCEROUS FOODS: garlic, mango, white pepper, ling, shepherd's purse.

HERBS CONSIDERED BENEFICIAL TO CANCERS: Bai-ying (white nightshade), Yu-xing-cao (cordate houttuynia), Pu-gong-ying (Asian dandelion), Wei-ling-xian (Chinese clematis), Ban-zhi-lian (barbed skullcap), Ji-xing-zi (seed of garden balsam), Tian-xing-ren (sweet apricot seed), Da-zao (red date), Zi-cao (Asian puccoon), Yi-yi-ren (Job's tears).

RECIPE 15

MASTER: 10 pieces of Da-zao (red dates).

ASSOCIATE: 50 g fresh shiitake mushrooms (25 g in case of dried mushrooms).

ASSISTANT: 10 g mung beans.

SEASONING: salt.

STEPS:

(1) Boil Da-zao (red date), shiitake mushrooms and mung bean sprouts in water until cooked.

(2) Season with salt and remove from heat.

CONSUMPTION: eat the contents and drink the soup.

INDICATIONS: good for cancers of various kinds.

ANALYSIS: Da-zao is an energy tonic to boost the immune system; shiitake mushroom has been found effective in inhibiting the growth of cancers in lab rats, including cerival cancer and liver cancer; mung bean sprouts eliminate toxic heat in the body; and salt is to improve the taste of the recipe.

RECIPE 16

MASTER: 25 g Yi-yi-ren (Job's tears).

ASSOCIATE: 50 g ling.

ASSISTANT: 50 shepherd's purse.

SEASONING: sugar.

STEPS:

(1) Wash shepherd's purse and ling and chop into small pieces.

(2). Boil shepherd's purse and ling in water with Yi-yi-ren (Job's tears).

(3) Season with sugar and remove from heat.

CONSUMPTION: eat at mealtimes.

INDICATIONS: good for cancers of various kinds.

ANALYSIS: Yi-yi-ren is both a herb and a food, widely used to inhibit the growth of cancerous cells of all kinds. The same can be said of ling. Shepherd's purse is to improve the condition of the liver, and sugar is to improve the taste.

RECIPE 17

MASTER: 6 g Tian-xing-ren (sweet apricot seed).

ASSOCIATE: 1 whole duck.

ASSISTANT: 30 g white pepper, 100 g fresh ginger.

SEASONING: salt.

STEPS:

(1) Wash and remove all internal organs from the duck.

(2) Slice the fresh ginger.

(3) Fill the stomach of the duck with Tian-xing-ren (sweet apricot seed), white pepper and the ginger.

(4) Steam the duck for 2 hours in an appropriate pot.

CONSUMPTION: drink the broth from the steaming pot, once daily. Season the duck meat and eat if so desired.

INDICATIONS: cancers of various kinds, esophagus cancer in particular.

ANALYSIS: Tian-xing-ren acts on the lungs, which is why it is more effective for esophagus cancer; duck is a yin tonic good for the respiratory system; white pepper and fresh ginger are to warm the recipe slightly; and salt is to improve the taste, which may be replaced by a different seasoning such as rock sugar. The juice of the duck is better than duck meat because a patient of esophagus cancer may have difficulty swallowing.

RECIPE 18

MASTER: over 150 g gold carp.

ASSOCIATE: 50 g Yi-yi-ren (Job's tears).

ASSISTANT: 2 cloves garlic.

SEASONING: none.

STEPS:

(1) Wash the gold carp and remove scales as you would in normal cooking.

(2) Chop the garlic. Fill the stomach of the carp with the garlic and Yi-yi-ren (Job's tears).

(3) Wrap the carp in aluminum foil to bake in an oven at 250 C° until it is equally dry inside and outside (this will take from 10 to 15 minutes), and grind into powder.

CONSUMPTION: take 3 g each time, 2 to 3 times daily. Put the powder on the tongue and wash down with warm water.

INDICATIONS: cancers of various kinds.

ANALYSIS: All three ingredients in this recipe are to drain off water in the body, ideal for cancers with water retention.

CHAPTER 7 Digestive System

7.1 Gastroduodenal ulcers

1. **Stomach Indigestion Syndrome**

SYMPTOMS AND SIGNS:

- Abdominal pain or swelling that gets better after bowel movement.
- Acid indigestion.
- Belching with poor appetite.
- Discharge of watery thin stool.
- Dry stool.
- Hot sensations in the body.
- Insomnia.
- Red complexion.
- Sour, bad breath.
- Stomachache that gets worse with pressure from the hand.
- Stool with an extremely foul smell.
- Vomiting and diarrhea simultaneously.
- Vomiting with a sour, strong smell and a craving for cold drinks.

2. **Liver-Energy-Attacking-the-Stomach Syndrome**

SYMPTOMS AND SIGNS:

- Abdominal rumbling.
- Belching.
- Chest discomfort.
- Hiccups.
- Irregular bowel movement.
- Pain in inner part of stomach.
- Painful sensations running through ribs on both sides.
- Stomachache that gets worse with emotional upheaval.
- Vomiting of acid or blood.

3. **Stomach Yin Deficiency Syndrome**

SYMPTOMS AND SIGNS:

- Constipation.
- Dry cough.
- Dry lips.
- Dry sensations in the mouth with thirst.

- Hiccups.
- Hot sensations in the limbs.
- Indigestion.
- Insomnia.
- Light but periodic fever not unlike the tide.
- Low fever.
- Pain (burning) in stomach.
- Palpitation.
- Stomachache that gets worse on an empty stomach.
- Vomiting.
- Vomiting with blood.
- No appetite.

4. Spleen-Stomach Yang Deficiency Syndrome

SYMPTOMS AND SIGNS:

- Abdominal pain.
- Cold limbs.
- Diarrhea.
- Fatigue.
- Intermittent hiccups in a low-pitched voice.
- Love of warmth and massage.
- Pain gets worse on fatigue and hunger.
- Pain improves on rest and eating.
- Poor appetite.
- Shortness of breath.
- Stomachache with dull pain.
- Upset stomach.
- Vomiting of undigested foods or acid or clear water.
- Water noise in the stomach.
- Withered, yellowish complexion.

5. Stomach Blood Coagulation Syndrome

SYMPTOMS AND SIGNS:

- Hunger pangs and nausea.
- Pain gets worse on massage.
- Pain in inner part of stomach with prickling sensation and swelling.
- Pain in inner part of stomach, acute after meals, and an aversion to massage.
- Pain in a fixed spot.
- Vomiting with blood.

INGREDIENTS FOR CREATING RECIPES

FOODS FOR EXCESS: fresh ginger, prickly ash, black or white pepper, radish, fresh lotus rhizome.

FOODS FOR DEFICIENCY: rooster, honey, maltose, Irish potato, chicken egg, dried lotus rhizome, wild cabbage.

HERBS: Ren-shen (Chinese ginseng), Gao-liang-jiang (lesser galangal), Wu-jia-pi (slender acanthopanax root bark), Yan-hu-suo (Chinese yanhusuo), Hai-piao-xiao (cuttlebone), Bai-ji (amethyst orchid), Gan-jiang (dried ginger), Gan-cao (licorice), Sha-ren (grains of paradise), Ding-xiang (cloves), Rou-gui (Chinese cassia bark), ju-pi, Bi-bo (long pepper), Zhi-qiao (unripe citron), Shen-qu (digestive tea), Shan-zha (Chinese hawthorn), xiang-fu (nutgrass flatsedge rhizome), Wa-leng-zi (arca shell), Qing-pi (green orange peel), Hou-pu (official magnolia), Bai-zhu (white atractylodes), Fu-ling (tuckahoe; Indian bread), Yu-zhu (Solomon's seal), Shi-hu (orchid), Chen-pi (dried tangerine peel), Bai-shao (white peony), Mai-ya (malt), San-qi (pseudo-ginseng).

Syndromes of disease and herbs to use:

1. **STOMACH INDIGESTION:** Ren-shen (Chinese ginseng), Wu-jia-pi (slender acanthopanax root bark), Gan-cao (licorice); cook with foods for excess.

2. **LIVER ENERGY ATTACKING THE STOMACH:** Yan-hu-suo (Chinese yanhusuo), Hai-piao-xiao (cuttlebone), Bai-ji (amethyst orchid); cook with foods for excess.

3. **STOMACH YIN DEFICIENCY:** Gan-cao (licorice), Wu-jia-pi (slender acanthopanax root bark); cook with foods for deficiency.

4. **SPLEEN-STOMACH YANG DEFICIENCY:** Ren-shen (Chinese ginseng), Gao-liang-jiang (lesser galangal), Wu-jia-pi (slender acanthopanax root bark), Gan-jiang (dried ginger); cook with foods for deficiency.

5. **STOMACH BLOOD COAGULATION:** Yan-hu-suo (Chinese yanhusuo); cook with foods for excess.

RECIPE 19

MASTER: 8 g Wu-jia-pi (slender acanthopanax root bark).

ASSOCIATE: two heads wild cabbage.

ASSISTANT: maltose.

SEASONING: none.

STEPS:

(1) Boil Wu-jia-pi (slender acanthopanax root bark) in water for thirty minutes; strain to obtain a decoction.

(2) Wash wild cabbage leaves and stems with cold water and crush to squeeze out the juice.

(3) Heat the cabbage juice and the Wu-jia-pi soup together, then add maltose to taste.

CONSUMPTION: consume daily for 10 days as a course of treatment.

INDICATIONS: early stage of ulcers, chronic gastric and duodenal ulcers.

ANALYSIS: Wu-jia-pi can bring relief to painful ulcers, wild cabbage is commonly used to treat them, and maltose can help to heal them.

7.2 Gastroptosis (falling stomach)

1. Spleen Deficiency Syndrome

SYMPTOMS AND SIGNS:

- Clear, long streams of urine.
- Diarrhea that is sticky and muddy.
- Anal bleeding.
- Watery-thin stools.
- Eating little.
- Fatigue.
- Hands and feet slightly cold.
- Indigestion.
- Desire to lie down.
- Poor appetite.
- Prolonged diarrhea.
- Puffy eyelids.
- Thin.
- Withered complexion.

2. Deficiency Cold Syndrome

SYMPTOMS AND SIGNS:

- Abdominal rumbling.
- Abdominal swelling and discomfort particularly after a meal.
- Watery stools.
- Love of warmth and massage.
- Nausea.
- Palpitation.
- Vomiting of watery sputum.

3. Disharmony of Liver and Stomach (Liver-Energy-Attacking-the-Stomach) Syndrome

SYMPTOMS AND SIGNS:

- Aching pain or discomfort below the hypochondrium.
- Belching.
- Chronic diarrhea.
- Dizziness.
- Excessive perspiration.
- Hiccups.
- Hunger with no appetite.
- Love of sighing.
- Poor appetite.
- Soft stool.
- Dry mouth with no desire to drink.

4. Stomach Yin Deficiency Syndrome

SYMPTOMS AND SIGNS:

- Constipation.
- Dry cough.
- Dry lips.
- Dry sensations in the mouth with thirst.
- Hiccups.
- Hot sensations in the limbs.
- Indigestion.
- Insomnia.
- Light but periodic fever that rises and falls like a tide.
- Low fever.
- Pain (burning) in stomach.
- Palpitation.
- Stomachache that gets worse on an empty stomach.
- Vomiting.
- Vomiting with blood.
- No appetite.

INGREDIENTS FOR CREATING RECIPES

FOODS FOR EXCESS: fresh lotus rhizome (lotus root).

FOODS FOR DEFICIENCY: rabbit, polished rice, glutinous rice, pork stomach (pork tripe), beef stomach (beef tripe), dried lotus rhizome, chicken.

HERBS: Bai-zhu (white atractylodes), Zhi-shi (China orange), Sheng-ma (skunk bugbane), Chai-hu (hare's ear), Huang-qi (membranous milk vetch), Zhi-qiao (unripe citron), Shan-zha (Chinese hawthorn), Dang-gui (Chinese angelica), Huang-jing (sealwort), He-ye (lotus leaf), Da-zao (red date), Ren-shen (Chinese ginseng).

Syndromes of disease and herbs to use:

1. **SPLEEN DEFICIENCY:** Bai-zhu (white atractylodes), Ren-shen (Chinese ginseng), Sheng-ma (skunk bugbane), Huang-qi (membranous milk vetch); cook with foods for deficiency.
2. **DEFICIENCY COLD:** Bai-zhu (white atractylodes), Chai-hu (hare's ear), Huang-qi (membranous milk vetch); cook with foods for deficiency.
3. **DISHARMONY OF LIVER AND STOMACH:** Zhi-shi (China orange), Zhi-qiao (unripe citron); cook with foods for deficiency or foods for excess.
4. **STOMACH YIN DEFICIENCY:** Huang-jing (sealwort), Dang-gui (Chinese angelica); cook with foods for deficiency.

RECIPE 20

MASTER: 5 g Ren-shen (Chinese ginseng).

ASSOCIATE: 5 Da-zao (red dates).

ASSISTANT: 20 g glutinous rice.

SEASONING: none.

STEPS:

(1) Cook glutinous rice the usual way.

(2) Boil the herbs in water until cooked.

CONSUMPTION: eat the rice together with the herbs.

INDICATIONS: spleen deficiency syndrome of gastroptosis.

ANALYSIS: All three ingredients are energy tonics that can tone up the spleen and restore the falling stomach to its original position.

7.3 Gastroenteritis

1. Cold Dampness Syndrome

SYMPTOMS AND SIGNS:

- Abdominal pain with rumbling.
- Absence of perspiration in hot weather.
- Acute attack of vomiting and diarrhea.
- Clear and watery vaginal discharge with an unusual odor.
- Cold sensations in lower abdominal genital region.
- Cough.
- Coughing out sputum with a low-pitched voice.
- Watery stool with no offensive smell.
- Discharge of sputum that can be coughed out easily.
- Edema in the four limbs.
- Headache.
- Movement difficulty.
- Pain in the body.
- Pain in the joints.
- Scanty, clear urine.
- Stomachache.

2. Summer Heat and Dampness Syndrome

SYMPTOMS AND SIGNS:

- Abdominal fullness.
- Burning sensation in the anus.
- Chest discomfort.
- Diarrhea.
- Fever.
- Forceful discharge of stools during bowel movement.
- Poor appetite.
- Normal perspiration due to hot weather or warm clothing.
- Reddish urine.
- Sudden attack of vomiting and diarrhea.
- Thirst.
- Vomiting of substances with acid.
- Yellowish, watery stool.

3. Stomach Indigestion Syndrome

SYMPTOMS AND SIGNS:

- Abdominal pain or swelling that gets better after a bowel movement.
- Acid reflux and belching with a foul smell.
- Frequent belching with poor appetite.
- Watery thin stool.
- Insomnia.
- Sour, bad breath.
- Stomachache.
- Stool with unusually offensive odor.
- Vomiting and diarrhea.
- Vomiting with a sour, strong smell and a desire for cold drinks.

4. **Spleen-Stomach Yang Deficiency Syndrome**

SYMPTOMS AND SIGNS:

- Abdominal pain.
- Clear urine.
- Cold limbs.
- Diarrhea and vomiting that occur frequently.
- Fatigue.
- Weak hiccups.
- Love of warmth and massage.
- Pain gets worse on fatigue and hunger and gets better on rest and eating.
- Pale complexion.
- Perspiration with cold limbs.
- Poor appetite.
- Shortness of breath.
- Stomachache.
- Upset stomach.
- Vomiting of undigested foods.
- Water noise in the stomach.

INGREDIENTS FOR CREATING RECIPES

FOODS FOR EXCESS: fresh ginger, prickly ash, tea, garlic, radish, buckwheat.

FOODS FOR DEFICIENCY: red bayberry, grape, honey, chicken, beef.

HERBS: Ding-xiang (cloves), Shan-yao (Chinese yam), Fu-ling (tuckahoe; Indian bread), Yi-yi-ren (Job's tears), Qian-shi (water lily), Bai-bian-dou (hyacinth bean), Lian-zi (East Indian lotus), Zhu-ru (bamboo inner skin), Bai-dou-kou (cardamom seed), Huang-bai (cork tree), Fang-feng (Chinese wind shelter), Gan-jiang (dried ginger), Huo-xiang (Korean mint), Gao-liang-jiang (lesser galangal), Wu-mei (black plum), San-qi (pseudo-ginseng), Huang-qi (membranous milk vetch), Huang-jing (sealwort), Dang-shen (root of pilose asiabell).

Syndromes of disease and herbs to use:

1. **COLD DAMPNESS:** Ding-xiang (cloves), Yi-yi-ren (Job's tears), Bai-dou-kou (cardamom seed), Gan-jiang (dried ginger), Huo-xiang (Korean mint), Gao-liang-jiang (lesser galangal); cook with foods for excess.
2. **SUMMER HEAT AND DAMPNESS:** Yi-yi-ren (Job's tears), Bai-bian-dou (hyacinth bean), Lian-zi (East Indian lotus), Zhu-ru (bamboo inner skin), Huang-bai (cork tree), Fang-feng (Chinese wind shelter); cook with foods for excess.
3. **STOMACH INDIGESTION:** Shan-yao (Chinese yam), Fu-ling (tuckahoe; Indian bread), Yi-yi-ren (Job's tears), Bai-dou-kou (cardamom seed), San-qi (pseudo-ginseng), Huang-qi (membranous milk vetch); cook with foods for excess or foods for deficiency.
4. **SPLEEN-STOMACH YANG DEFICIENCY:** Ding-xiang (cloves), Qian-shi (water lily), Gan-jiang (dried ginger), Huang-qi (membranous milk vetch), Huang-jing (sealwort), Dang-shen (root of pilose asiabell); cook with foods for deficiency.

RECIPE 21

MASTER: 50 g Huang-qi (membranous milk vetch).

ASSOCIATE: 400 g grapes.

ASSISTANT: 5 teaspoons honey.

SEASONING: none.

STEPS:

(1) Decoct Huang-qi (membranous milk vetch) in water for 30 minutes; strain to obtain soup.

(2) Wash grapes. Crush and strain to obtain juices.

(3) Mix Huang-qi soup with grape juice and honey. Put the mixture in an earthenware pot and simmer until it is dry and sticky; it will become jelly when cool.

CONSUMPTION: take 3 to 5 g (2 teaspoons) grape jelly each time with warm water before meals, 3 times daily, with reduced dosages and white sugar added to taste for children.

INDICATIONS: gastroenteritis.

ANALYSIS: Huang-qi is a mild energy tonic to improve the function of the intestines; grapes can check diarrhea; and honey is good for inflammation of the intestines.

7.4 Dysentery

1. Superficial Damp Heat Syndrome

SYMPTOMS AND SIGNS:

- Abdominal pain.
- Congested chest.
- Diarrhea with forceful discharge of stool.
- Muddy, yellowish-red stool with a strong odor.
- Excessive perspiration.
- Greasy taste in the mouth.
- Low fever.
- Pain in the joints of four limbs, with swelling and heaviness.
- Perspiration in hands and feet or in the head.
- Red-tinged, scanty urine.
- Retention of urine.
- Swollen tongue.
- Thirst with no desire for drink.
- Yellowish skin not unlike mandarin orange.

2. Toxic-Heat-Penetrating-into-the-Deep-Region Syndrome

SYMPTOMS AND SIGNS:

- Acute abdominal pain.
- Acute onset of various symptoms.
- Breathing difficulty.
- Alternate cold and hot sensations.
- Discharge of pus and blood from anus.
- Bleeding from the mouth.
- Headache that is severe.
- High fever.
- Blurred vision.
- Nosebleed.
- Mental fogginess.
- Severe pain in the whole body.
- Twitching.
- Difficult bowel movement.
- Vomiting of blood.

3. Spleen Yang Deficiency Syndrome

SYMPTOMS AND SIGNS:

- Abdominal pain.
- Chronic bowel movement difficulty.
- Cold sensation in the forehead.
- Dysentery with discharge of pus and blood.
- Edema.
- Hot sensations with nausea.
- Intermittent diarrhea.
- Stomachache.

INGREDIENTS FOR CREATING RECIPES

FOODS FOR EXCESS: tea, tofu.

FOODS FOR DEFICIENCY: beef liver, polished rice, tofu, grape.

HERBS: Yadanzi (brucea fruit), Shan-zha (Chinese hawthorn), Bai-tou-weng (Chinese pulsatilla), Huang-qi (membranous milk vetch), Huang-bai (cork tree), Jin-yin-hua (Japanese honeysuckle), Da-qing-ye (mayflower glorybower leaf), Bing-lang (areca nut), Hou-pu (official magnolia), Bai-shao (white peony), Gan-jiang (dried ginger), Rou-gui (Chinese cassia bark).

Syndromes of disease and herbs to use:

1. **SUPERFICIAL DAMP HEAT:** Bai-tou-weng (Chinese pulsatilla), Huang-qin (skullcap), Huang-bai (cork tree), Jin-yin-hua (Japanese honeysuckle), Da-qing-ye (mayflower glorybower leaf), Hou-pu (official magnolia), Bai-shao (white peony), Bing-lang (areca nut); cook with foods for excess.
2. **TOXIC-HEAT-PENETRATING-INTO-THE-DEEP-REGION:** Bai-tou-weng (Chinese pulsatilla), Huang-qin (skullcap), Huang-bai (cork tree), Jin-yin-hua (Japanese honeysuckle), Da-qing-ye (mayflower glorybower leaf), Hou-pu (official magnolia); cook with foods for excess.
3. **SPLEEN YANG DEFICIENCY:** Gan-jiang (dried ginger), Rou-gui (Chinese cassia bark); cook with foods for deficiency.

RECIPE 22

MASTER: 10 g Bai-tou-weng (Chinese pulsatilla).

ASSOCIATE: 200 g tofu.

ASSISTANT: 50 g beef liver.

SEASONING: rice vinegar.

STEPS:

(1) Boil Bai-tou-weng (Chinese pulsatilla) in water for 30 minutes; strain to obtain soup.

(2) Put tofu and sliced beef liver in the soup, bring to a boil, then lower to a simmer until cooked.

(3) Season to taste with rice vinegar when the soup is cool.

CONSUMPTION: have the soup on an empty stomach once daily.

INDICATIONS: superficial damp heat syndrome of dysentery.

ANALYSIS: Bai-tou-weng is a leading herb to treat dysentery and diarrhea; tofu, which is beneficial to the digestive system, can cool the intestines; beef liver can tone the liver and is good for the stomach and spleen; and rice vinegar can constrict the intestines and check diarrhea.

7.5 Hemorrhoids

1. Damp Heat Syndrome

SYMPTOMS AND SIGNS:

- Abdominal pain.
- Abnormal perspiration.
- Burning sensations and itch in the genital area.
- Diarrhea.
- Painful, watery eyes sensitive to light.
- Pain in the joints.
- Unusual perspiration in hands, feet, or head.
- Retention of urine.
- Discharge of reddish urine.
- Unusual thirst.

2. Hot Blood Syndrome

SYMPTOMS AND SIGNS:

- Abdominal pain.
- Bleeding of various kinds.
- Nosebleed.
- Skin ulcer.
- Urination difficulty.

3. Spleen Energy Deficiency Syndrome

SYMPTOMS AND SIGNS:

- Diarrhea.
- Edema.
- Fatigue.
- Rolled up lips.
- Malnutrition in children.
- Stiffness in the tongue.
- Stomachache.
- Abnormal vaginal discharge in women.
- Vomiting of blood.

INGREDIENTS FOR CREATING RECIPES

FOODS FOR EXCESS: eggplant, cantaloupe, freshwater clam, coriander (Chinese parsley), fig, persimmon, banana, black fungus, water chestnut, Chinese wax gourd, cucumber, fresh lotus rhizome, peanut, tomato, radish, torreyanut, pork gallbladder.

FOODS FOR DEFICIENCY: cantaloupe, tomato, pork, dried lotus rhizome, white fungus, sea cucumber.

HERBS: Huai-hua (Japanese pagoda tree flower), Huai-mi (Japanese pagoda tree flower bud), Huai-jiao (Japanese pagoda tree pod), Ge-hua (kudzu vine flower), Xian-he-cao (agrimony), Jing-jie (Japanese ground-ivy), Di-yu (burnet), Cang-zhu (gray atractylodes), Gan-cao (licorice).

Syndromes of disease and herbs to use:

1. **DAMP HEAT:** Huai-hua (Japanese pagoda tree flower), Huai-mi (Japanese pagoda tree flower bud), Ge-hua (kudzu vine flower), Xian-he-cao (agrimony), Jing-jie (Japanese ground-ivy); cook with foods for excess.
2. **HOT BLOOD**: Huai-hua (Japanese pagoda tree flower), Huai-mi (Japanese pagoda tree flower bud), Ge-hua (kudzu vine flower), Xian-he-cao (agrimony); cook with foods for excess.
3. **SPLEEN ENERGY DEFICIENCY:** Huai-jiao (Japanese pagoda tree pod), Xian-he-cao (agrimony); cook with foods for deficiency.

RECIPE 23

MASTER: 5 g Huai-hua (Japanese pagoda tree flower), 5 g Di-yu (burnet), 10 g Gan-cao (licorice).

ASSOCIATE: 100 g pork.

ASSISTANT: 30 white fungus.

SEASONING: vinegar 1 teaspoonful, salt 1/6 teaspoonful.

STEPS:

(1) Dry roast the three master ingredients and grind into powder.

(2) Cook white fungus in water until soft.

(3) Slice pork. With the white fungus and herbal powder, fry in a pan until pork is cooked.

(4) Season with vinegar and salt to taste.

CONSUMPTION: eat daily for one week as a course of treatment.

INDICATIONS: all syndromes of hemorrhoids.

ANALYSIS: Both Huai-hua and Di-yu are common herbs to treat hemorrhoids; Gan-cao is an energy tonic used to strengthen the intestines; white fungus is a common food to treat hemorrhoids; vinegar can constrict the intestines; and salt can moisten the intestines, thus good for constipation.

7.6 Irritable bowels

1. Liver-Energy-Attacking-the-Spleen Syndrome

SYMPTOMS AND SIGNS:

- Abdominal pain and swelling that gets better after diarrhea.
- Watery diarrhea.
- Mental tension and anxiety.

2. **Spleen-Stomach Energy Deficiency Syndrome**

SYMPTOMS AND SIGNS:

- Diarrhea often triggered by eating cold and greasy foods.
- Watery stools or diarrhea.
- Fatigue.
- Indigestion with poor appetite.
- Withered, yellowish complexion.

3. **Cold Dampness Syndrome**

SYMPTOMS AND SIGNS:

- Cold limbs.
- Watery diarrhea and abdominal pain.
- Aversion to cold.
- Heavy sensations in the body and head.
- Poor appetite.

4. **Energy Stagnation Syndrome**

SYMPTOMS AND SIGNS:

- Severe abdominal pain.
- Constipation.
- Difficult bowel movement.
- Frequent belching.
- Pain in the hypochondrium.

INGREDIENTS FOR CREATING RECIPES

FOODS FOR EXCESS: green tea, tofu, spinach.

FOODS FOR DEFICIENCY: tofu, eggplant, sword bean.

HERBS: Dang-shen (root of pilose asiabell), Bai-zhu (white atractylodes), Fu-ling (tuckahoe; Indian bread), Gan-cao (licorice), Huo-xiang (Korean mint), Lai-fu-zi (radish seed).

Syndromes of disease and herbs to use:

1. **LIVER-ENERGY-ATTACKING-THE-SPLEEN:** Gan-cao (licorice), Huo-xiang (Korean mint), Lai-fu-zi (radish seed); cook with foods for excess.

2. **SPLEEN-STOMACH ENERGY DEFICIENCY:** Dang-shen (root of pilose asiabell), Bai-zhu (white atractylodes), Fu-ling (tuckahoe; Indian bread), Gan-cao (licorice); cook with foods for deficiency.

3. **COLD DAMPNESS:** Huo-xiang (Korean mint), Bai-zhu (white atractylodes); cook with foods for excess.

4. **ENERGY STAGNATION:** Huo-xiang (Korean mint), Lai-fu-zi (radish seed); cook with foods for excess.

RECIPE 24

MASTER: 10 g Dang-shen (root of pilose asiabell), 15 g Bai-zhu (white atractylodes), 15 g Fu-ling (tuckahoe; Indian bread), 5 g Gan-cao (licorice), 15 g Huo-xiang (Korean mint).

ASSOCIATE: 100 g polished rice.

ASSISTANT: 50 g tofu.

SEASONING: brown sugar.

STEPS:

(1) Make a decoction of the five master ingredients; strain to obtain herbal soup.

(2) Cook the polished rice; midway through the cooking, add the tofu to the rice.

(3) When rice is cooked, add the soup.

(4) Season with brown sugar to taste.

CONSUMPTION: eat once a day. (Eat as a meal if you have a poor appetite. If you have a good appetite, eat with something else.)

INDICATIONS: all syndromes of irritable bowels.

ANALYSIS: Dang-shen, Bai-zhu, and Gan-cao are energy tonics to strengthen the bowels; Fu-ling is to strengthen the spleen; Huo-xiang is to harmonize the stomach; polished rice and tofu are also energy tonics; and brown sugar is good for the spleen and also improves the taste.

7.7 Hepatitis

1. **Superficial Damp Heat Syndrome**

SYMPTOMS AND SIGNS:

- Constipation or diarrhea.
- Excessive perspiration.
- Nausea.
- Low fever.
- Pain in the joints of four limbs, with swelling and heaviness.
- Poor appetite.
- Red and scanty urine.
- Retention of urine.
- Swollen tongue.
- Abnormal thirst.
- Vomiting.
- Bright yellowish eyes and skin.

2. **Spleen Dampness Syndrome**

SYMPTOMS AND SIGNS:

- Abdominal swelling.
- Chest discomfort with poor appetite.
- Cold sensations in the body with cold limbs.
- Diarrhea.
- Edema.
- Fatigue.
- Heavy sensations in head.
- Heavy sensations in the body with discomfort.
- Preference for hot drinks.
- Nausea and vomiting.
- Poor appetite.
- Stomach fullness and discomfort.
- Watery stools.
- Dark yellowish eyes and skin.

3. **Liver Energy Congestion Syndrome**

SYMPTOMS AND SIGNS:

- Abdominal obstruction.
- Abdominal pain.
- Anger.
- Convulsion.
- Fatigue.
- Numbness.
- Pain in the hypochondrium.
- Poor appetite.
- Soft stool.
- Stomachache.
- Subjective sensation of object in the throat.
- Vomiting of blood.

4. **Energy Congestion and Blood Coagulation Syndrome**

SYMPTOMS AND SIGNS:

- Abdominal swelling.
- Chronic hepatitis.
- Cirrhosis.
- Congested chest.
- Difficult bowel movement.
- Enlargement of the liver and spleen.
- Love of sighing.
- Lump in the abdomen that stays in a fixed region.
- Poor appetite.
- Wandering pain in the hypochondrium and ribs.

5. Disharmony of Liver and Spleen (Liver-energy-attacking-the-spleen) Syndrome

SYMPTOMS AND SIGNS:

- Abdominal enlargement.
- Abdominal rumbling.
- Aching pain below the hypochondrium.
- Chronic diarrhea.
- Dizziness.
- Excessive perspiration.
- Hungry but able to eat little.
- Poor appetite.
- Soft stool.
- Dry mouth with no desire for drink.

6. Liver-Kidney Yin Deficiency Syndrome

SYMPTOMS AND SIGNS:

- Difficulty in both bowel movement and urination.
- Dizziness.
- Dry eyes or throat.
- Fatigue.
- Headache with pain in the bony ridge forming the eyebrow.
- Lumbago.
- Many dreams.
- Night-blindness.
- Night sweats.
- Pain in the hypochondrium with fondness for massage.
- Hot palms of hands and soles of feet.
- Ringing in the ears.
- Sleeplessness with forgetfulness.
- Weak loins and tibia.

INGREDIENTS FOR CREATING RECIPES

FOODS FOR EXCESS: tomato, carrot, celery, day lily, turnip root leaf, common button mushroom, common carp.

FOODS FOR DEFICIENCY: polished rice, eel, tomato, carrot, chicken egg yolk.

HERBS: Bai-hua-she-she-cao (herb of spreading hedyotis), Yu-mi-xu (corn silk), Chai-hu (hare's ear), Ling-zhi (lucid ganoderma), Yin-chen (capillary artemisia), Qing-dai (blue indigo), Ban-lan-gen (woad), Jue-ming-zi (coffee weed), Da-zao (red date), Chen-pi (dried tangerine peel), Bai-jiang-cao (scabiosa-leaved valerian).

Syndromes of disease and herbs to use:

1. **SUPERFICIAL DAMP HEAT:** bai-hua-she-she-cao (herb of spreading hedyotis), Yu-mi-xu (corn silk), Ban-lan-gen (woad), Qing-dai (blue indigo), Bai-jiang-cao (scabiosa-leaved valerian); cook with foods for excess.
2. **SPLEEN DAMPNESS**: Chen-pi (dried tangerine peel), Yu-mi-xu (corn silk), Ling-zhi (lucid ganoderma); cook with foods for excess.
3. **LIVER ENERGY CONGESTION:** Chai-hu (hare's ear), Ling-zhi (lucid ganoderma), Yin-chen (capillary artemisia), Jue-ming-zi (coffee weed); cook with foods for excess.
4. **ENERGY CONGESTION AND BLOOD COAGULATION:** Ling-zhi (lucid ganoderma); cook with foods for excess.
5. **DISHARMONY OF LIVER AND SPLEEN:** Chen-pi (dried tangerine peel), Ling-zhi (lucid ganoderma); cook with foods for excess or foods for deficiency.
6. **LIVER-KIDNEY YIN DEFICIENCY:** Da-zao (red date), Ling-zhi (lucid ganoderma); cook with foods for deficiency.

RECIPE 25

MASTER: 10 g fresh Yu-mi-xu (corn silk).

ASSOCIATE: one large common carp.

ASSISTANT: 20 g carrots.

SEASONING: fresh ginger root.

STEPS:

(1) Prepare the carp; cut open the stomach and remove internal organs. Rinse.

(2) Cut carrots into small pieces.

(3) Fill the stomach of the carp with Yu-mi-xu and carrots.

(4) Steam or poach the carp until cooked.

(5) Grate ginger, then wrap in gauze and squeeze to get juice. About 1 minute before removing from heat, season the carp with the juice.

CONSUMPTION: eat once every 2 days.

INDICATIONS: hepatitis.

ANALYSIS: all the ingredients in this recipe can promote water flow to remove dampness from the body. Fresh ginger is used to facilitate this action, while also helping to eliminate the odor of the fish.

7.8 Cirrhosis

1. Dampness Syndrome

SYMPTOMS AND SIGNS:

- Abdominal pain and rumbling.
- Diarrhea.
- Diminished urination.
- Dizziness.
- Headache as if the head were wrapped in a wet towel.
- Heavy sensations in the body.
- Preference for hot drinks.
- Quick bowel movement.
- Excessively itchy toes.

2. Damp Heat Syndrome

SYMPTOMS AND SIGNS:

- Abdominal pain.
- Abnormal perspiration.
- Burning sensations and itch in the genital area.
- Diarrhea.
- Pain in the eyes with watering and sensitivity to light.
- Pain in the joints.
- Unusual perspiration in hands, feet, or head.
- Retention of urine.
- Discharge of reddish urine.
- Abnormal thirst.

3. Spleen Dampness Syndrome

SYMPTOMS AND SIGNS:

- Chest discomfort with little appetite.
- Periodic diarrhea.
- Watery stools.
- Edema.
- Heavy sensations in the head.
- Heavy sensations in the body with discomfort.
- Preference for hot drinks.
- Nausea and vomiting.
- Stomach fullness and discomfort.
- Sweet-sticky taste in mouth.
- Little energy to talk or move.

4. Spleen-Kidney Yang Deficiency Syndrome

SYMPTOMS AND SIGNS:

- Chronic diarrhea with stools containing undigested foods.

- Diarrhea at dawn.
- Fatigue.
- Scanty urine with puffiness of limbs.
- Shivering with cold sensations of limbs.
- Sore loins and lower back pain.
- Pale, colorless complexion.

5. Liver-Kidney Yin Deficiency Syndrome

- Difficulty in flexing and extending.
- Dizziness.
- Hot sensations in palms of hands and soles of feet.
- Muscle twitching.
- Numbness of limbs.
- Ringing in ears.

INGREDIENTS FOR CREATING RECIPES

FOODS FOR EXCESS: black soybean, gold and common carp, Chinese wax gourd peel, pear, mung bean.

FOODS FOR DEFICIENCY: pork, pear.

HERBS: Chi-xiao-dou (small red bean), Mu-xiang (costus root), Tao-ren (peach kernel), Shan-zha (Chinese hawthorn), Chen-pi (dried tangerine peel), Zhi-qiao (unripe citron), Yu-mi-xu (corn silk), Gan-sui (Kansui root), lingzhi, Dang-shen (root of pilose asiabell), Fu-ling (tuckahoe; Indian bread), Bai-zhu (white atractylodes), Huang-qi (membranous milk vetch), Sha-ren (grains of paradise), Huang-jing (sealwort), Bai-jiang-cao (scabiosa-leaved valerian).

1. **DAMPNESS:** herbs Chi-xiao-dou (small red bean), Tao-ren (peach kernel), Gan-sui (Kansui root); cook with foods for excess.
2. **DAMP HEAT:** Gan-sui (Kansui root), Sha-ren (grains of paradise), Bai-jiang-cao (scabiosa-leaved valerian); cook with foods for excess.
3. **SPLEEN DAMPNESS:** Mu-xiang (costus root), Shan-zha (Chinese hawthorn), Chen-pi (dried tangerine peel) Zhi-qiao (unripe citron), Yu-mi-xu (corn silk); cook with foods for excess.
4. **SPLEEN-KIDNEY YANG DEFICIENCY:** Dang-shen (root of pilose asiabell), Fu-ling (tuckahoe; Indian bread), Bai-zhu (white atractylodes), Huang-qi (membranous milk vetch); cook with foods for deficiency.
5. **LIVER-KIDNEY YIN DEFICIENCY:** Huang-qi (membranous milk vetch), Dang-shen (root of pilose asiabell), Huang-jing (sealwort); cook with foods for deficiency.

RECIPE 26

MASTER: 20 g Huang-qi (membranous milk vetch), 15 g Huang-jing (sealwort), 15 g Bai-jiang-cao (scabiosa-leaved valerian), 12 g Tao-ren (peach kernel).

ASSOCIATE: 150 g lean pork.

ASSISTANT: 100 g polished rice.

SEASONING: salt, rice wine, green onion, fresh ginger.

STEPS:

(1) Decoct the four master ingredients in water for thirty minutes; strain to obtain herbal soup.

(2) Slice the pork and cook in water with the rice, until both are tender.

(3) Add the herbal soup to pork and rice. Season with salt, rice wine, green onion and fresh ginger to taste before removing from heat.

CONSUMPTION: eat as a main dish.

INDICATIONS: damp heat syndrome and deficiency syndrome of cirrhosis.

ANALYSIS: Huang-qi is an energy tonic; Huang-jing is a yin tonic; both herbs are designed to improve the general condition of the liver. Bai-jiang-cao can protect the liver and improve its condition; it is often used to treat liver cancer as well. Tao-ren promotes blood circulation. Lean pork and polished rice are energy tonics to also help improve the condition of the liver. The seasoning ingredients improve energy circulation in the body with the exception of salt, which is to improve the taste.

7.9 Gallstones

1. Hot Syndrome

SYMPTOMS AND SIGNS:

- Bitter taste in the mouth.
- Deafness.
- Love of sighing.
- Pain in the ribs.

2. Cold Syndrome

SYMPTOMS AND SIGNS:

- Cold limbs.
- Falling of scrotum with hardness, swelling, and pain.
- Aversion to cold.
- Pain in the lower abdomen affecting the testes.

INGREDIENTS FOR CREATING RECIPES

FOODS FOR EXCESS: chicory, celery.

FOODS FOR DEFICIENCY: walnut, sesame oil, rock sugar, polished rice, cuttlefish.

HERBS: Ji-nei-jin (membrane of chicken gizzard), Jin-qian-cao (coin grass), Yu-mi-xu (corn silk), Yi-yi-ren (Job's tears), Yin-chen (capillary artemisia).

Syndromes of disease and herbs to use:

1. **HOT:** Ji-nei-jin (membrane of chicken gizzard), Jin-qian-cao (coin grass), Yu-mi-xu (corn silk), Yin-chen (capillary artemisia); cook with foods for excess.
2. **COLD:** Yi-yi-ren (Job's tears); cook with foods for excess or foods for deficiency.

RECIPE 27

MASTER: 500 g walnuts.

ASSOCIATE: 500 g sesame oil.

ASSISTANT: 500 g rock sugar.

SEASONING: none.

STEPS: Steam the above three ingredients in an earthenware pot for 3 to 4 hours.

CONSUMPTION: eat warm, three times daily before meals, for one week to ten days. In case of a tendency toward diarrhea, reduce sesame oil by half.

INDICATIONS: both syndromes of gallstones.

ANALYSIS: walnut is a food to treat gallstones and stones in the urinary tract; and sesame oil and rock sugar are to lubricate the internal region and facilitate expulsion of the stones.

RECIPE 28

MASTER: 5 g Ji-nei-jin (membrane of chicken gizzard).

ASSOCIATE: none.

ASSISTANT: 100 g polished rice.

SEASONING: white sugar.

STEPS:

(1) Fry Ji-nei-jin over low heat until brownish, then grind into powder.

(2) Boil polished rice and sugar in water. Add the powdered Ji-nei-jin just before the rice is cooked, bring to a boil again, then remove from heat.

CONSUMPTION: eat at mealtimes.

INDICATIONS: hot syndrome of gallstone.

ANALYSIS: Ji-nei-jin can eliminate congestion; it is commonly used to expel stones, including gallstones. Polished rice can promote urination, frequently facilitating expulsion of stones through urination. White sugar is added to improve the taste.

7.10 Constipation

1. Large Intestine Heat Syndrome

SYMPTOMS AND SIGNS:

- Abdominal pain.
- Constipation with bad breath.
- Anal bleeding.
- Dry, hard stool.
- Sticky, muddy stool with a strong odor.
- Dry sensations in the mouth.
- Swollen gums.
- Cracked lips.
- Pain in anal area with swelling and burning sensations.
- Short streams of reddish urine.
- Yellow-colored stool that is watery and has a strong odor.

2. Energy Stagnation Syndrome

SYMPTOMS AND SIGNS:

- Abdominal pain.
- Chest and rib discomfort.
- Chest pain.
- Constipation with a desire to empty the bowels.
- Pain in inner part of stomach with prickling sensation and swelling.
- Pain in the hypochondrium.
- Retention of urine.
- Ringing in ears and hearing difficulty.
- Stomachache.
- Subjective sensation of lump in the throat.
- Swallowing difficulty.
- Bloating and congestion after eating.

3. Cold Large Intestine Syndrome

SYMPTOMS AND SIGNS:

- Abdominal pain.
- Abdominal rumbling.
- Clear, long streams of urine.
- Cold hands and feet.
- Difficult bowel movement.
- Sticky, muddy stool.

4. Energy Deficiency Syndrome

SYMPTOMS AND SIGNS:

- Abdominal pain.
- Constipation with discharge of soft stool.
- Sticky, turbid stool or diarrhea.
- Dizziness.
- Fatigue followed by bowel movement.
- Headache (severe) that occurs with fatigue after labor.
- Periodic headaches, headache in the morning, or prolonged headache.
- Dizziness upon sitting up from a reclining position.
- Blurred vision.
- Numbness.
- Palpitation with anxiety.
- Perspiration in hands and feet.
- Ringing in ears that causes hearing difficulty.
- Trembling of both hands.
- Shortness of breath.
- Thin with dry skin.
- Swallowing difficulty.
- Feeble voice.
- Extremities slightly cold.

5. **Blood Deficiency Syndrome**

SYMPTOMS AND SIGNS:

- Abdominal pain.
- Constipation with discharge of hard stool.
- Difficult bowel movement.
- Dizziness.
- Cracked lips and dry mouth.
- Fatigue.
- Fever.
- Feeling psychologically low.
- Headache in the afternoon.
- Headache with dizziness.
- Pale lips.
- Dizziness upon sitting up from a reclining position.
- Blurred vision.
- Muscle spasms.
- Night sweats.
- Palpitation with anxiety.
- Thin with dry skin.
- Insomnia.
- Spasms.
- Pale complexion.

INGREDIENTS FOR CREATING RECIPES

FOODS FOR EXCESS: peach, carrot, soybean, banana, black fungus, jellyfish, apple, laver, soy milk, celery, radish, seaweed, common carp, shiitake mushroom.

FOODS FOR DEFICIENCY: walnut, sesame seed, peach, carrot, sweet potato, white fungus, sea cucumber, sesame oil, honey, apple, soy milk, polished rice, rock sugar, chicken.

HERBS: Tao-ren (peach kernel), Dang-gui (Chinese angelica), Da-huang (rhubarb), Yu-li-ren (dwarf flowering cherry), Sheng-di (dried glutinous rehmannia), Huo-ma-ren (hemp), Lu-hui (aloe), Gua-lou-ren (snake gourd kernel), Sang-shen (mulberry), Bei-sha-shen (straight ladybell north), Yu-zhu (Solomon's seal), Wu-mei (black plum), Fan-xie-ye (senna leaf).

Syndromes of disease and herbs to use:

1. **LARGE INTESTINE HEAT:** Da-huang (rhubarb), Lu-hui (aloe), Sheng-di (dried glutinous rehmannia), Fan-xie-ye (senna leaf); cook with foods for excess.
2. **ENERGY STAGNATION:** Tao-ren (peach kernel), Da-huang (rhubarb), Yu-li-ren (dwarf flowering cherry), Huo-ma-ren (hemp), Gua-lou-ren (snake gourd kernel), Wu-mei (black plum), Fan-xie-ye (senna leaf); cook with foods for excess.
3. **COLD LARGE INTESTINE:** Huo-ma-ren (hemp), Dang-gui (Chinese angelica); cook with foods for excess.
4. **ENERGY DEFICIENCY:** Sheng-di (dried glutinous rehmannia), Dang-gui (Chinese angelica), Sang-shen (mulberry); cook with foods for deficiency.
5. **BLOOD DEFICIENCY:** Dang-gui (Chinese angelica), Sheng-di (dried glutinous rehmannia), Bei-sha-shen (straight ladybell north), Sang-shen (mulberry), Yu-zhu (Solomon's seal), Wu-mei (black plum); cook with foods for deficiency.

RECIPE 29

MASTER: 5 g Dang-gui (Chinese angelica).

ASSOCIATE: 30 black fungus.

ASSISTANT: 30 g sea cucumber.

SEASONING: salt.

STEPS:

(1) Bake or dry roast Dang-gui (Chinese angelica) until charred brown, then grind into powder.

(2) Steam Dang-gui (Chinese angelica) powder, black fungus, and sea cucumber together until cooked. Season with salt to taste and eat with meals.

INDICATIONS: deficiency syndromes of constipation.

ANALYSIS: Dang-gui, black fungus, and sea cucumber all lubricate the intestines to promote bowel movement. Dang-gui and sea cucumber are both blood tonics, with the latter also being a yin tonic. Salt is to improve the taste. This recipe is to tone up and lubricate the intestines simultaneously.

RECIPE 30

MASTER: 100 g Tao-ren (peach kernel).

ASSOCIATE: 1 chicken.

ASSISTANT: 100 g shiitake mushrooms.

SEASONING: rice wine, white sugar.

STEPS:

(1) Steam Tao-ren (peach kernel) until cooked.

(2) Boil the chicken in water to obtain chicken soup.

(3) Heat the chicken soup (without chicken) with a cup of rice wine and some white sugar.

(4) Add the mushrooms and cooked Tao-ren (peach kernel) to the soup and bring to a boil.

CONSUMPTION: eat with your meal.

INDICATIONS: energy stagnation syndrome of constipation.

ANALYSIS: Tao-ren can break up congestion to promote bowel movement; chicken soup is an energy tonic and easily digested; shiitake mushroom is an energy tonic and good for the stomach; rice wine promotes energy circulation; and white sugar improves the taste.

7.11 Blood in stool

1. Spleen-Unable-to-Govern-the-Blood Syndrome

SYMPTOMS AND SIGNS:

- Blood in urine.
- Bowel movements first, followed by bleeding.
- Anal bleeding of a dark color.
- Sticky, muddy stool or diarrhea.
- Dizziness.
- Mental fatigue.
- Nosebleed.
- Palpitation.
- Poor appetite.
- Pale complexion.
- Shortness of breath.
- Stomach and abdominal distention and fullness.
- Dry, yellowish skin.

2. Large Intestine Damp Heat Syndrome

SYMPTOMS AND SIGNS:

- Abdominal pain.
- Bleeding first, following by bowel movement.
- Bright red blood when bleeding.
- Damp, glossy, and reddened anal area in children.
- Diarrhea with stool containing a mixture of pus and blood.
- Anal bleeding.
- Dysentery.
- Hemorrhoids.
- Pain in anus with swelling and burning sensations.
- Short, reddish streams of urine.

INGREDIENTS FOR CREATING RECIPES

FOODS FOR EXCESS: spinach, black fungus, eggplant, tea.

FOODS FOR DEFICIENCY: polished rice, chestnut, white fungus.

HERBS: Da-zao (red date), He-ye (lotus leaf), Huai-mi (Japanese pagoda tree flower bud), Bai-zi-ren (oriental arborvitae kernel).

Syndromes of disease and herbs to use:

1. **SPLEEN-UNABLE-TO-GOVERN-THE-BLOOD:** Da-zao (red date); cook with foods for deficiency.
2. **LARGE INTESTINE DAMP HEAT:** He-ye (lotus leaf), Huai-mi (Japanese pagoda tree flower bud), Bai-zi-ren (oriental arborvitae kernel); cook with foods for excess.

RECIPE 31

MASTER: 5 g He-ye (lotus leaf), 10 g Da-zao (red date).

ASSOCIATE: 30 g black fungus.

ASSISTANT: 100 g polished rice.

SEASONING: rock sugar.

STEPS:

(1) Wash He-ye (lotus leaf) and boil in water over medium heat with all other ingredients, about 15 minutes.

(2) Discard the He-ye (lotus leaf) and eat with meals.

INDICATIONS: both syndromes of blood in stool.

ANALYSIS: He-ye and black fungus can stop bleeding; polished rice is an energy tonic; and rock sugar can lubricate the internal region and also improve the taste.

7.12 Vomiting

1. Cold Dampness Syndrome

SYMPTOMS AND SIGNS:

- Absence of perspiration in hot weather.
- Cold sensations in lower abdominal-genital region.
- Cough.
- Feeble cough with sputum.
- Diarrhea.
- Discharge of sputum that can be coughed out easily.
- Edema in the four limbs.
- Headache.
- Movement difficulty.
- Nausea.
- Pain in the body.
- Pain in the joints.
- Scanty, clear urine.
- Stomachache.

2. Stomach Indigestion Syndrome

SYMPTOMS AND SIGNS:

- Abdominal pain.
- Abdominal pain that is relieved by massage.
- Abdominal pain with an aversion to massage.
- Belching with offensive odor after a meal.
- Discomfort from chest and diaphragm congestion.
- Diarrhea alternating with constipation.
- Diarrhea in children.
- Hot sensations in the center of palms.
- Lack of appetite.
- Preference for hot drinks, but unable to drink much.
- Malaria.
- Nausea.
- Pain in inner part of stomach with swelling and feeling of fullness.
- Stomachache.
- Stool with an unusual odor.

- Vomiting of clear water or spoiled acid.

3. **Damp Phlegm Syndrome**

SYMPTOMS AND SIGNS:

- Cough.
- Discharge of sputum that can be coughed out easily.
- Discharge of white-watery sputum.
- Dizziness.
- Headache.
- Hiccups.
- Pain in the chest.
- Shortness of breath.
- Prolonged dizziness.
- Excessive sleeping.
- Insomnia.
- Vomiting of watery sputum.
- White, slippery sputum that can be cleared from throat easily.

4. **Stomach Energy Upsurging Syndrome**

SYMPTOMS AND SIGNS:

- Dysphagia (difficulty swallowing).
- Vomiting of all kinds (after eating, some hours later, dry, watery, acid, etc.)
- Hiccups.
- Nausea.
- Upset stomach.

5. **Yang Deficiency Syndrome**

SYMPTOMS AND SIGNS:

- Clear, long streams of urine.
- Cold hands and feet.
- Constipation.
- Diarrhea.
- Diminished urination.
- Watery-thin stool.
- Edema.
- Fatigue.
- Aversion to cold.
- Fingertips often cold.
- Cold limbs and extremities.
- Frequent illness and need for sleep.
- Body curled up when reclining.
- Headache in the morning.
- Palpitation.
- Perspiration like cold water.
- Lack of energy and motivation.
- Excessive need for sleep.
- Vomiting of clear water.
- Vomiting right after a full meal.

6. **Yin Deficiency Syndrome**

SYMPTOMS AND SIGNS:

- Bleeding from gums.
- Constipation.
- Dizziness.
- Dry sensations in the mouth.
- Dry throat.
- Dry vomiting.
- Fatigue.
- Headache in the afternoon.
- Light fever in the afternoon.
- Night sweats.
- Nosebleed.
- Pain in the throat.
- Short, reddish urine.
- Thin.
- Insomnia.

- Swallowing difficulty.
- Toothache.

INGREDIENTS FOR CREATING RECIPES

FOODS FOR EXCESS: chili pepper (cayenne pepper), olive, tea, tomato, fresh ginger, black pepper, prickly ash.

FOODS FOR DEFICIENCY: beef, tomato, walnut.

HERBS: Huo-xiang (Korean mint), Lai-fu-zi (radish seed), Xiao-hui-xiang (fennel seed), Yi-tang (maltose), Bai-bian-dou (hyacinth bean), Ban-xia (half-summer pinellia), Xuan-fu-hua (elecampane), Bei-sha-shen (straight ladybell north), Mai-dong (lilyturf), Da-zao (red date).

Syndromes of disease and herbs to use:

1. **COLD DAMPNESS:** Xiao-hui-xiang (fennel seed), Huo-xiang (Korean mint); cook with foods for excess.
2. **STOMACH INDIGESTION:** Lai-fu-zi (radish seed), Xiao-hui-xiang (fennel seed), Yi-tang (maltose); cook with foods for excess or foods for deficiency.
3. **DAMP SPUTUM:** Bai-bian-dou (hyacinth bean), Ban-xia (half-summer pinellia); cook with foods for excess.
4. **STOMACH ENERGY UPSURGING:** Ban-xia (half-summer pinellia), Xuan-fu-hua (elecampane), Bei-sha-shen (straight ladybell north); cook with foods for excess.
5. **YANG DEFICIENCY:** Yi-tang (maltose), Xiao-hui-xiang (fennel seed); cook with foods for deficiency.
6. **YIN DEFICIENCY:** Da-zao (red date), Yi-tang (maltose), Bei-sha-shen (straight ladybell north), Mai-dong (lilyturf); cook with foods for deficiency.

RECIPE 32

MASTER: 2 Da-zao (red date).

ASSOCIATE: 2 walnuts.

ASSISTANT: 1 tomato.

SEASONING: none.

STEPS:

(1) Crush the walnuts and remove seeds from red dates.

(2) Boil the three ingredients in water until cooked soft.

CONSUMPTION: drink the soup twice daily.

INDICATIONS: yin deficiency syndrome of vomiting.

ANALYSIS: Da-zao is an energy tonic; walnut can lubricate the stomach to prevent dry vomiting; and tomato produces fluids and strengthens the stomach. (No seasoning is listed because the recipe is already sweetened by Da-zao and walnuts).

7.13 Stomachache

1. Liver Energy Congestion Syndrome

SYMPTOMS AND SIGNS:

- Abdominal pain.
- Belching.
- Convulsion.
- Nausea.
- Numbness.
- Stomachache that affects the hypochondrium and gets slightly better on massage.
- Stomachache that gets worse when emotional.
- Subjective sensations of objects in the throat.
- Vomiting of blood.

2. Blood Coagulation Syndrome

SYMPTOMS AND SIGNS:

- Abdominal pain.

- Bleeding from gums.
- Chest pain.
- Coughing with blood.
- Headache.
- Lumbago.
- Pain (acute) around umbilicus unrelieved by massage, with hard spots felt by hands.
- Pain in region between navel and pubic hair with feeling of hardness.
- Pain in the hypochondrium as if being pricked by a needle.
- Pain in the hypochondrium that gets worse after eating.
- Pain in the loins as if being pierced with an awl.
- Pain in the ribs.
- Palpitation with anxiety.
- Spasm.
- Stomachache.
- Swelling and congestion after eating.
- Vomiting of blood.

3. **Stomach Indigestion Syndrome**

SYMPTOMS AND SIGNS:

- Abdominal pain.
- Offensive-smelling belching after a meal.
- Chest and diaphragm congestion and discomfort.
- Diarrhea alternating with constipation.
- Diarrhea in children.
- Hot sensations in the center of palms.
- Indigestion.
- Lack of appetite.
- Preference for hot drinks, but unable to drink much.
- Nausea.
- Pain in inner part of stomach with swelling and feeling of fullness.
- Stomachache that gets worse on massage.
- Stomachache that occurs all of a sudden.
- Stool with an unusually bad smell.
- Vomiting, including of clear water.

4. **Deficiency Cold Syndrome**

SYMPTOMS AND SIGNS:

- Abdominal pain on the right and left sides of navel (umbilicus).
- Cold hands and feet.
- Cold sensations in lower abdominal-genital region.
- Diarrhea with undigested food.
- Fatigue.
- Aversion to cold.
- Tips of fingers appear light red.
- Preference for hot drinks.
- Love of sighing.
- Night sweats.
- Palpitation.
- Emotionally run-down.
- Shortness of breath.
- Feeble vomiting.
- Pale complexion.

5. **Yin Deficiency Syndrome**

SYMPTOMS AND SIGNS:

- Bleeding from gums.
- Burning pain in the stomach.
- Constipation.
- Dry, scanty stool.
- Dry sensations in the mouth.

- Dry throat.
- Fatigue.
- Headache in the afternoon.
- Light fever in the afternoon.
- Night sweats.
- Nosebleed.
- Pain in the throat.
- Pain in the throat that is red and swollen.
- Hot palms of hands and soles of feet.
- Short, reddish urine.
- Thin.
- Insomnia.
- Stomachache that gets worse when the stomach is empty.
- Toothache.

INGREDIENTS FOR CREATING RECIPES

FOODS FOR EXCESS: pork gallbladder, gold or common carp, yellow soybean, fresh ginger, papaya, black pepper, coriander (Chinese parsley), prickly ash, mung bean, sunflower, fig.

FOODS FOR DEFICIENCY: oyster, white sugar, chicken egg, sesame oil, sword bean.

HERBS: Xiao-hui-xiang (fennel seed), Sha-ren (grains of paradise), Shan-zha (Chinese hawthorn), Hai-piao-xiao (cuttlebone), Pi-pa-ye (loquat leaf), Ju-pi (tangerine peel), Da-zao (red date), Rou-gui (Chinese cassia bark).

Syndromes of disease and herbs to use:

1. **LIVER ENERGY CONGESTION:** Sha-ren (grains of paradise), Hai-piao-xiao (cuttlebone), Pi-pa-ye (loquat leaf); cook with foods for excess.
2. **BLOOD COAGULATION:** Sha-ren (grains of paradise), Ju-pi (tangerine peel); cook with foods for excess.
3. **STOMACH INDIGESTION:** Shan-zha (Chinese hawthorn), Ju-pi (tangerine peel); cook with foods for excess.
4. **DEFICIENCY COLD:** Rou-gui (Chinese cassia bark), Xiao-hui-xiang (fennel seed), Wu-jia-pi (slender acanthopanax root bark); cook with foods for excess or foods for deficiency.
5. **YIN DEFICIENCY:** Wu-jia-pi (slender acanthopanax root bark), Shan-zha (Chinese hawthorn), Da-zao (red date); cook with foods for deficiency.

RECIPE 33

MASTER: 6 g Rou-gui (Chinese cassia bark), 9 g Shan-zha (Chinese hawthorn).

ASSOCIATE: 30 g brown sugar.

ASSISTANT: none

SEASONING: none

STEPS:

(1) Boil Shan-zha in water for twenty minutes, then add Rou-gui.

(2) Remove from heat when Shan-zha is cooked; strain to obtain herbal soup.

(3) Add brown sugar to the soup and stir.

CONSUMPTION: drink at mealtimes.

INDICATIONS: deficiency and cold syndromes of stomachache.

ANALYSIS: Rou-gui can warm the stomach and Shan-zha can promote digestion. Brown sugar is an associate ingredient, instead of a seasoning, because it plays the important role of promoting blood circulation to relieve stomachache.

RECIPE 34

MASTER: 10 g Ju-pi or Chen-pi (dried tangerine peel).

ASSOCIATE: 1 gold or common carp.

ASSISTANT: 30 g fresh ginger.

SEASONING: black pepper, salt.

STEPS:

(1) Clean the carp, cut open the belly, and remove the viscera. Rinse the belly cavity clean.

(2) Put Ju-pi, fresh ginger, and black pepper in a gauze bag and place inside the fish. (Use toothpicks to seal the fish belly.)

(3) Poach the fish in water until cooked.

(4) Remove the gauze bag and discard.

CONSUMPTION: eat the fish and drink the soup.

INDICATIONS: all syndromes of stomachache.

ANALYSIS: both Ju-pi and Chen-pi are tangerine peel. Ju-pi is dried tangerine peel, a few months to a year old, while Chen-pi is old tangerine peel, which may be as old as ten years or more. The older the peel, the more effective it is. Tangerine peel can promote energy circulation to relieve stomachache; carp can strengthen the spleen; fresh ginger can warm the stomach and promote energy circulation; and black pepper and salt can improve the taste.

NOTE: If gold carp is not available, another kind of carp may be used.

7.14 Abdominal pain

1. Cold Spleen Syndrome

SYMPTOMS AND SIGNS:

- Acute onset of chronic abdominal pain.
- Abdominal pain.
- Abdominal pain intensifies with coldness, improves with warmth.
- Cold hands and feet.
- Yellowish, dark skin.
- Diarrhea with cool sensations in the body.
- Watery-thin stool.
- Edema.
- Indigestion.
- Pale lips.
- Sweet taste in the mouth.
- Poor appetite.
- Prolonged diarrhea.
- Runny, thin saliva.
- Vomiting.

2. Deficiency Cold Syndrome

SYMPTOMS AND SIGNS:

- Chronic abdominal pain.
- Abdominal pain that intensifies with coldness, improves with warmth.
- Abdominal pain that intensifies with hunger.
- Cold hands and feet.
- Cold sensations in lower abdominal-genital region.
- Diarrhea with undigested food.
- Fatigue.
- Aversion to cold.
- Preference for hot drinks.
- Frequent sighing.
- Night sweats.
- Palpitation.
- Emotionally run-down.
- Shortness of breath.
- Feeble, slow vomiting.
- Pale complexion.

3. Excess Heat Syndrome

SYMPTOMS AND SIGNS:

- Chronic abdominal pain.
- Abdominal pain that intensifies with massage.
- Abdominal pain with burning sensations.
- Thirst with inability to drink much.
- Forceful hiccups.
- Red and swollen sore throat.
- Forceful vomiting sore throat.

4. **Stomach Indigestion Syndrome**

SYMPTOMS AND SIGNS:

- Abdominal pain that gets worse with massage and improves after bowel movement.
- Belching with a bad odor after a meal.
- Diarrhea alternating with constipation.
- Hot sensations in the center of palms.
- Indigestion.
- Lack of appetite.
- Preference for hot drinks, but able to drink little.
- Nausea.
- Pain in inner part of stomach with swelling and feeling of fullness.
- Stomachache.
- Stool with an unusually bad smell.
- Vomiting, especially of clear water.

5. **Energy Stagnation Syndrome**

SYMPTOMS AND SIGNS:

- Abdominal pain that improves with release of intestinal gas.
- Belching or hiccups.
- Chest and rib discomfort.
- Chest pain.
- Constipation with a desire to empty the bowel.
- Pain in inner part of stomach with prickling sensation and swelling.
- Pain in the hypochondrium.
- Retention of urine.
- Ringing in ears and deafness.
- Stomachache.
- Subjective sensation of lump in the throat.
- Swallowing difficulty.
- Bloating and congestion after eating.

6. **Blood Coagulation Syndrome**

SYMPTOMS AND SIGNS:

- Abdominal pain as if being pricked by a needle.
- Abdominal pain in a fixed region.
- Bleeding from gums.
- Chest pain.
- Coughing with blood.
- Headache.
- Lumbago.
- Pain (acute) around umbilicus resisting massage, with hard spots felt by hands.
- Pain in region between navel and pubic hair with feeling of hardness.
- Pain in the hypochondrium.
- Pain in the loins as if being pierced with an awl.
- Pain in the ribs.
- Palpitation with insecure feeling.
- Spasm.
- Stomachache.
- Stroke.
- Swelling and congestion after eating.
- Vomiting of blood.

INGREDIENTS FOR CREATING RECIPES

FOODS FOR EXCESS: litchi nut, fresh ginger, chili pepper (cayenne pepper), coriander (Chinese parsley), wine, garlic, tea, tofu.

FOODS FOR DEFICIENCY: litchi nut, mutton, brown sugar, honey, rock sugar, beef, chicken, tofu.

HERBS: Gan-cao (licorice), Gan-jiang (dried ginger), Ren-shen (Chinese ginseng), Bai-zhu (white atractylodes), Zhi-shi (China orange), Rou-gui (Chinese cassia bark), Shen-qu (digestive tea), Lai-fu-zi (radish seed), Dang-gui (Chinese angelica).

Syndromes of disease and herbs to use:

1. **COLD SPLEEN:** Gan-jiang (dried ginger), Rou-gui (Chinese cassia bark); cook with foods for deficiency or foods for excess.
2. **DEFICIENCY COLD:** Gan-cao (licorice), Gan-jiang (dried ginger), Ren-shen (Chinese ginseng), Bai-zhu (white atractylodes), Rou-gui (Chinese cassia bark); cook with foods for deficiency.
3. **EXCESS HEAT:** Gan-cao (licorice); cook with foods for excess.
4. **STOMACH INDIGESTION:** Gan-cao (licorice), Ren-shen (Chinese ginseng), Bai-zhu (white atractylodes), Shen-qu (digestive tea), Lai-fu-zi (radish seed); cook with foods for excess or foods for deficiency.
5. **ENERGY STAGNATION:** Zhi-shi (China orange); cook with foods for excess.
6. **BLOOD COAGULATION:** Gan-jiang (dried ginger), Zhi-shi (China orange); cook with foods for excess.

RECIPE 35

MASTER: 5 g Gan-jiang (dried ginger), 5 g Rou-gui (Chinese cassia bark).

ASSOCIATE: 50 g mutton.

ASSISTANT: 5 g garlic.

SEASONING: salt.

STEPS:

(1) Make a decoction of Gan-jiang (dried ginger) and Rou-gui (Chinese cassia bark) together; strain to obtain herbal soup.

(2) Crush garlic, slice the mutton, and cook them together.

(3) Add herbal soup and boil for another two minutes.

(4) Season with salt to taste.

CONSUMPTION: drink the soup and eat the mutton at mealtimes.

INDICATIONS: cold spleen syndrome of abdominal pain.

ANALYSIS: All the ingredients are very warm or hot; they are good for cold spleen syndrome of abdominal pain, with the exception of salt, which is to improve the taste and also cool down the formula slightly.

7.15 Diarrhea

1. Cold Dampness Syndrome

SYMPTOMS AND SIGNS:

- Absence of perspiration in hot weather.
- Cold sensations in lower abdominal-genital region.
- Cough.
- Feeble coughing with sputum.
- Diarrhea with an unusual odor.
- Discharge of sputum that can be coughed out easily.
- Edema in the four limbs.
- Headache.
- Movement difficulty.
- Pain anywhere in the body.
- Pain in the joints.
- Scanty, clear urine.
- Stomachache.

2. Superficial Damp Heat Syndrome

SYMPTOMS AND SIGNS:

- Burning sensation and itch in the genital area or burning sensation in the anus.
- Diarrhea with forceful discharge of stool.
- Discharge of yellowish red stool that is turbid and has a strong odor.
- Excessive perspiration.

- Feeling low.
- Frequent itch and pain in the vaginal area.
- Low fever.
- Pain in the joints of the four limbs, with swelling and heaviness.
- Paralysis.
- Perspiration in hands and feet or in the head.
- Reddish, scanty urine.
- Retention of urine.
- Short, reddish urine.
- Swollen tongue.
- Thirst.
- Yellowish skin color.

3. Stomach Indigestion Syndrome

SYMPTOMS AND SIGNS:

- Abdominal pain that gets better following bowel movement.
- Offensive-smelling belching after a meal.
- Discomfort from chest and diaphragm congestion.
- Diarrhea alternating with constipation.
- Diarrhea with an unusually offensive odor.
- Hot sensations in the center of palms.
- Indigestion.
- Lack of appetite.
- Preference for hot drinks, but able to drink little.
- Nausea.
- Pain in inner part of stomach with swelling and feeling of fullness.
- Stomachache.
- Stool with an offensive smell.
- Vomiting, especially of clear water.

4. Liver-Energy-Attacking-the-Spleen Syndrome

SYMPTOMS AND SIGNS:

- Abdominal distention.
- Abdominal pain.
- Abdominal rumbling.
- Chronic diarrhea.
- Diarrhea immediately after abdominal pain starts.
- Tired spirits.
- Hunger with inability to eat.
- Thirst with inability to drink.

5. Spleen Dampness Syndrome

SYMPTOMS AND SIGNS:

- Chest discomfort and poor appetite.
- Diarrhea that comes and goes.
- Watery stools.
- Edema.
- Heavy sensations in head as if the head were covered with something.
- Heavy sensations in the body with discomfort.
- Preference for hot drinks.
- Nausea and vomiting.
- Stomach fullness and discomfort.
- Sweet-sticky taste in mouth.
- Lack of energy to talk or move.

6. Spleen-Kidney Yang Deficiency Syndrome

SYMPTOMS AND SIGNS:

- Physically weak with no energy to talk.
- Cold hands and feet.
- Cold loins.

- Diarrhea before dawn.
- Diarrhea immediately after pain occurs.
- Diarrhea with sticky, muddy stool.
- Dysentery.
- Little appetite.
- Edema, especially one that occurs all over the body.
- Fatigue.
- Aversion to cold.
- Normal feeling of comfortableness after bowel movement.
- Weakness in the four limbs.
- Frequent urination with clear, white urine.
- Mental fatigue.
- Sputum rumbling and shortness of breath.

INGREDIENTS FOR CREATING RECIPES

FOODS FOR EXCESS: apple, green and dried guava, sorghum, pear, prune, garlic, fresh lotus rhizome, tea, fresh ginger, buckwheat.

FOODS FOR DEFICIENCY: chestnut, apple, pear, dried lotus rhizome, wheat, chicken egg, longan nut, polished rice, glutinous rice, beef, walnut.

HERBS: Wu-mei (black plum), Lian-zi (East Indian lotus), Qian-shi (water lily), Bai-tou-weng (Chinese pulsatilla), Jin-ying-zi (Cherokee rose), Bai-zhu (white atractylodes), Gan-jiang (dried ginger), Shan-yao (Chinese yam).

Syndromes of disease and herbs to use:

1. **COLD DAMPNESS:** Qian-shi (water lily), Wu-mei (black plum), Jin-ying-zi (Cherokee rose); cook with foods for excess.
2. **SUPERFICIAL DAMP HEAT:** Qian-shi (water lily), Wu-mei (black plum), Lian-zi (East Indian lotus), Bai-tou-weng (Chinese pulsatilla), Jin-ying-zi (Cherokee rose); cook with foods for excess.
3. **STOMACH INDIGESTION:** Qian-shi (water lily), Wu-mei (black plum), Jin-ying-zi (Cherokee rose); cook with foods for excess or foods for deficiency.
4. **LIVER-ENERGY-ATTACKING-THE-SPLEEN:** Qian-shi (water lily), Wu-mei (black plum), Bai-tou-weng (Chinese pulsatilla), Jin-ying-zi (Cherokee rose); cook with foods for excess or foods for deficiency.
5. **SPLEEN DAMPNESS:** Qian-shi (water lily), Wu-mei (black plum), Bai-zhu (white atractylodes), Jin-ying-zi (Cherokee rose); cook with foods for excess or foods for deficiency.
6. **SPLEEN-KIDNEY YANG DEFICIENCY:** Qian-shi (water lily), Wu-mei (black plum), Bai-zhu (white atractylodes), Jin-ying-zi (Cherokee rose), Shan-yao (Chinese yam); cook with foods for deficiency.

RECIPE 36

MASTER: 60 g Shan-yao (Chinese yam).

ASSOCIATE: 1 cup glutinous rice.

ASSISTANT: 1\2 cup buckwheat groats.

SEASONING: white sugar.

STEPS:

(1) Grind 60 g yam into a fine powder.

(2) Cook glutinous rice and buckwheat in water as you would in ordinary cooking, about 20 minutes.

(3) Mix the three ingredients well.

(4) Boil 4 teaspoonfuls of this mixture in ample water—up to 4 cups—with some white sugar to make a cream to eat at breakfast each morning. (The more water you use, the longer this will take.)

INDICATIONS: spleen-kidney yang deficiency syndrome of diarrhea.

ANALYSIS: Shan-yao is an energy tonic, commonly used to stop diarrhea; glutinous rice is also an energy tonic, sticky to help constrict the intestine and slow down intestinal movement; buckwheat can improve digestion; and white sugar improves the taste.

RECIPE 37

MASTER: 10 g Qian-shi (water lily).

ASSOCIATE: 1 cup polished rice.

ASSISTANT: 1/2 cup wheat flour.

SEASONING: salt.

STEPS:

(1) Cut Qian-shi (water lily) in small pieces.

(2) Make a congee with the Qian-shi, polished rice, and wheat.

(3) Season with salt before eating.

INDICATIONS: all syndromes of diarrhea.

ANALYSIS: Qian-shi can constrict the intestine to slow intestinal movement and check diarrhea; polished rice is an energy tonic and promotes digestion; and wheat also checks diarrhea.

CHAPTER 8

Respiratory System

8.1 Bronchitis

1. Spleen-Dampness-Attacking-the-Lungs Syndrome

SYMPTOMS AND SIGNS:

- Cough.
- Sputum that can be coughed out easily.
- Watery white sputum.
- Weak arms and legs.
- Heavy and foggy sensations in the head.
- Heavy sensations in the limbs and trunk.
- Inability to lie on back due to coughing and shortness of breath.
- Poor appetite.
- Shortness of breath.
- Swelling of hands and feet.
- Vomiting.

2. Liver-Fire-Attacking-the-Lungs Syndrome

SYMPTOMS AND SIGNS:

- Cough that causes pain in the hypochondrium.
- Cough with sticky sputum.
- Cough with blood.
- Dry throat.
- Painful sensations running through chest and ribs.
- Shortness of breath.
- Red face.
- Sputum with blood.
- Excessive thirst.
- Vomiting of blood.

INGREDIENTS FOR CREATING RECIPES

FOODS FOR EXCESS: water chestnut, radish, pear, fresh lotus rhizome.

FOODS FOR DEFICIENCY: (would be used in cases of chronic bronchitis): duck egg, chicken egg, honey, pear, dried lotus rhizome, walnut.

HERBS: Xing-ren (apricot kernel), Jie-geng (kikio root), Ting-li-zi (seed of pepperweed), Ma-huang (Chinese ephedra), Di-gu-pi (root bark of Chinese wolfberry), Tian-nan-xing (serrated arum), Kuan-dong-hua (coltsfoot), Bai-he (lily), Yu-xing-cao (cordate houttuynia), Chuan-bei (tendril-leaved fritillary bulb), Zi-su-ye (purple perilla leaf), Gan-jiang (dried ginger), Chen-pi (dried tangerine peel), Ju-hua (mulberry-leaved chrysanthemum), Sang-ye (mulberry leaf), Wu-bei-zi (Chinese nutgall), Ju-hong (tangerine peel, red outer layer), Ban-xia (half-summer pinellia), Fu-ling (tuckahoe; Indian bread), Dong-gua-ren (wax gourd seed), Gan-cao (licorice), Jin-yin-hua (Japanese honeysuckle).

Syndromes of disease and herbs to use:

1. **SPLEEN-DAMPNESS-ATTACKING-THE-LUNGS:** Xing-ren (apricot kernel), Ting-li-zi (seed of pepperweed), Ma-huang (Chinese ephedra), Tian-nan-xing (serrated arum), Kuan-dong-hua (coltsfoot), Chuan-bei (tendril-leaved fritillary bulb), Zi-su-ye (purple perilla leaf), Gan-jiang (dried ginger), Chen-pi (dried tangerine peel), Wu-bei-zi (Chinese nutgall), Ju-hong (tangerine peel, red outer layer), Ban-xia (half-summer pinellia), Fu-ling (tuckahoe; Indian bread), Gan-cao (licorice); cook with foods for excess.
2. **LIVER-FIRE-ATTACKING-THE-LUNGS:** Xing-ren (apricot kernel), Jie-geng (kikio root), Di-gu-pi (root bark of Chinese wolfberry), Yu-xing-cao (cordate houttuynia), Chuan-bei (tendril-leaved fritillary bulb), Ju-hua (mulberry-leaved chrysanthemum), Sang-ye (mulberry leaf), Wu-bei-zi (Chinese nutgall), Dong-gua-ren (wax gourd seed), Gan-cao (licorice), Jin-yin-hua (Japanese honeysuckle); cook with foods for excess.

RECIPE 38

MASTER: 10 g Xing-ren (apricot kernel).

ASSOCIATE: 5 g Gan-cao (licorice).

ASSISTANT: 1 clove garlic.

SEASONING: none.

STEPS:

(1) Crush Xing-ren (apricot kernel) and garlic.

(2) Boil the three ingredients in water until cooked, then drain.

CONSUMPTION: drink the soup in two servings for one day.

INDICATIONS: both syndromes of bronchitis.

ANALYSIS: Xing-ren and Gan-cao are good for cough and bronchitis, while garlic can also relieve cough, including whooping cough.

8.2 Bronchial asthma

1. Cold-Phlegm-Obstructing-the-Lungs Syndrome

SYMPTOMS AND SIGNS:

- Cold limbs.
- Congested chest with a choking sensation.
- Cough with thin, watery sputum.
- Preference for hot or warm drinks.
- No perspiration.
- Pain in the chest.
- Shortness of breath.
- Swollen lungs.
- Wheezing.

2. Sputum Heat Accumulation in the Lungs Syndrome

SYMPTOMS AND SIGNS:

- Acute respiration or gasping for air.
- Cough with yellowish, sticky sputum.
- Shortness of breath.
- Swollen lungs.
- Excessive thirst and preference for cold drinks.
- Wheezing.

3. Lung Dampness Syndrome

SYMPTOMS AND SIGNS:

- Congested chest.
- Copious, sticky phlegm.
- Cough with breathing difficulties.

- Insomnia.
- Nausea.
- Palpitation.
- Poor appetite.
- Vomiting.
- Thinness.

4. Lungs-Unable-to-Direct-Energy-Downward Syndrome

SYMPTOMS AND SIGNS:

- Cough.
- Discharge of copious whitish, sticky sputum.
- Dislike of cold.
- Dry throat without thirst.
- Inability to lie on the back due to coughing and shortness of breath.
- More exhaling than inhaling.
- Pain in the throat.
- Palpitation.
- Scanty, bloody urine.
- Distention in the lower abdomen.
- Wheezing that persists or occurs all of a sudden.
- Wheezing triggered or intensified by moving around.

5. Lung Energy Deficiency Syndrome

SYMPTOMS AND SIGNS:

- Breathing difficulty.
- Cold limbs.
- Common cold.
- Cough.
- Excessive perspiration.
- Fatigue.
- Fear of cold.
- Aversion to wind.
- Light wheezing.
- Low, feeble voice.
- Shortness of breath.
- Normal urination without interruption.
- Sputum that is copious, clear, and watery.
- Swollen lungs.
- Too lazy to talk.

6. Loss-of-Kidneys'-Capacity-for-Absorbing-Inspiration Syndrome

SYMPTOMS AND SIGNS:

- Breathing difficulty.
- Cold limbs.
- Aversion to cold.
- Cold extremities.
- Frequent urination.
- More inhaling than exhaling.
- Shortness of breath.
- Shortness of breath that is triggered or intensified by moving around.
- Normal perspiration due to hot weather or warm clothing.
- Swollen lungs.
- Wheezing.
- Whitish sputum.

INGREDIENTS FOR CREATING RECIPES

FOODS FOR EXCESS: pear, Chinese wax gourd, radish, lotus root.

FOODS FOR DEFICIENCY: pear, white fungus, walnut, duck egg, chestnut.

HERBS: Ban-xia (half-summer pinellia), Chen-pi (dried tangerine peel), Ma-huang (Chinese ephedra), Gan-jiang (dried ginger), Gan-cao (licorice), Ling-zhi (lucid ganoderma), Zhe-bei (Zhe fritillary bulb), Bai-guo (ginkgo), Dong-chong-xia-cao (Chinese caterpillar fungus), Chuan-bei (tendril-leaved fritillary bulb), Xing-ren (apricot kernel), Qian-hu (purple-flowered peucedanum), Shi-gao (gypsum), Ju-hong (red outer layer of tangerine peel), Ren-shen (Chinese ginseng), Huang-qi (membranous milk vetch).

Syndromes of disease and herbs to use:

1. **COLD-PHLEGM-OBSTRUCTING-THE-LUNGS:** Ling-zhi (lucid ganoderma), Zhe-bei (Zhe fritillary bulb), Chuan-bei (tendril-leaved fritillary bulb); cook with foods for excess.
2. **SPUTUM HEAT ACCUMULATED IN THE LUNGS:** Qian-hu (purple-flowered peucedanum), Ling-zhi, Shi-gao (gypsum); cook with foods for excess.
3. **LUNG DAMPNESS:** Ban-xia (half-summer pinellia), Chen-pi (dried tangerine peel), Ling-zhi (lucid ganoderma); cook with foods for excess.
4. **LUNGS-UNABLE-TO-DIRECT-ENERGY-DOWNWARD:** Chuan-bei (tendril-leaved fritillary bulb), Zhe-bei (Zhe fritillary bulb), Ju-hong (red outer layer of tangerine peel), Chen-pi (dried tangerine peel), Dong-chong-xia-cao (Chinese caterpillar fungus); cook with foods for deficiency.
5. **LUNG ENERGY DEFICIENCY:** Gan-cao (licorice), Ling-zhi (lucid ganoderma), Ren-shen (Chinese ginseng), Huang-qi (membranous milk vetch), Dong-chong-xia-cao (Chinese caterpillar fungus); cook with foods for deficiency.
6. **LOSS-OF-KIDNEYS'-CAPACITY-FOR-ABSORBING-INSPIRATION:** Ren-shen (Chinese ginseng), Huang-qi (membranous milk vetch), Ling-zhi (lucid ganoderma), Dong-chong-xia-cao (Chinese caterpillar fungus); cook with foods for deficiency.

RECIPE 39

MASTER: 10 g Chuan-bei (tendril-leaved fritillary bulb), roasted.

ASSOCIATE: 1 large pear.

ASSISTANT: 30 g brown sugar.

SEASONING: rice wine.

STEPS:

(1) Grind Chuan-bei (tendril-leaved fritillary bulb) into powder.

(2) Put brown sugar and the whole pear (unpeeled) in a large pot of boiling water; when the sugar has melted, add the ground powder.

(3) Season with rice wine.

CONSUMPTION: have two servings daily.

IINDICATIONS: all syndromes of bronchial asthma.

ANALYSIS: Chuan-bei is to relieve cough and shortness of breath; pear can lubricate the lungs and relieve cough and asthma; and the rice wine can speed up the effects of the recipe.

8.3 Bronchiectasis (dilation of bronchi)

1. Wind-Heat-Attacking-the-Lungs Syndrome

SYMPTOMS AND SIGNS:

- Cough.
- Chest pain.
- Pain in the throat.
- Blood in sputum.
- Thirst with a preference for cold drinks.
- Red tongue.

2. Liver-Fire-Attacking-the-Lungs Syndrome

SYMPTOMS AND SIGNS:

- Cough.
- Coughing with blood.

- Blood in sputum.
- Vomiting of blood.

3. Hot-Sputum-Obstructing-the-lungs Syndrome

SYMPTOMS AND SIGNS:

- Fever.
- Blood in sputum.
- Yellowish sputum.
- Wheezing.
- Shortness of breath.
- Cough.

4. Yin-Deficiency-with-Abundant-Fire Syndrome

SYMPTOMS AND SIGNS:

- Dry throat.
- Toothache.
- Night sweats.
- Coughing with blood.
- Fever.

INGREDIENTS FOR CREATING RECIPES

FOODS FOR EXCESS: spinach, asparagus, tomato, lemon, radish, pear, carrot, banana.

FOODS FOR DEFICIENCY: glutinous rice, red dates, honey, tofu, rock sugar, bird's nest, kidney bean, white fungus.

HERBS: Sang-ye (mulberry leaf), Ju-hua (mulberry-leaved chrysanthemum), Xing-ren (apricot kernel), Zhe-bei (Zhe fritillary bulb), Gan-cao (licorice), Huang-qin (skullcap), Sang-bai-pi (root bark of white mulberry), Di-gu-pi (root bark of Chinese wolfberry), Da-huang (rhubarb), Bai-ji (amethyst orchid), Lu-gen (reed rhizome), Ban-xia (half-summer pinellia), Yi-yi-ren (Job's tears), Bai-he (lily), Sheng-di (dried glutinous rehmannia), Mai-dong (lilyturf), Bai-shao (white peony), Huang-jing (sealwort).

Syndromes of disease and herbs to use:

1. **WIND-HEAT-ATTACKING-THE-LUNGS:** Sang-ye (mulberry leaf), Ju-hua (mulberry-leaved chrysanthemum), Xing-ren (apricot kernel), Zhe-bei (Zhe fritillary bulb), Gan-cao (licorice).
2. **LIVER-FIRE-ATTACKING-THE-LUNGS:** Huang-qin (skullcap), Sang-bai-pi (root bark of white mulberry), Di-gu-pi (root bark of Chinese wolfberry), Da-huang (rhubarb), Bai-ji (amethyst orchid).
3. **HOT-SPUTUM-OBSTRUCTING-THE-LUNGS:** Zhe-bei (Zhe fritillary bulb), Lu-gen (reed rhizome), Ban-xia (half-summer pinellia), Yi-yi-ren (Job's tears).
4. **YIN-DEFICIENCY-WITH-ABUNDANT-FIRE:** Bai-he (lily), Sheng-di (dried glutinous rehmannia), Mai-dong (lilyturf), Gan-cao (licorice), Bai-shao (white peony), Bai-ji (amethyst orchid), Huang-jing (sealwort).

RECIPE 40

MASTER: 15 g Bai-ji (amethyst orchid).

ASSOCIATE: 100 g glutinous rice.

ASSISTANT: 5 red dates.

SEASONING: 25 g honey.

STEPS:

(1) Bake Bai-ji until the herb is toasted brown, then grind into power.

(2) Cook glutinous rice, red dates, and honey in 3 cups of water until the rice is 80% cooked. Add the herbal powder, then lower heat and continue to cook for 5 minutes.

CONSUMPTION: Eat warm as a main dish for lunch, once a day for ten days as a course of treatment.

INDICATIONS: bronchiectasis, coughing out or vomiting of blood, tuberculosis.

ANALYSIS: Bai-ji can constrict the lungs and stop bleeding; glutinous rice is a yin tonic good for dry cough; red date is an energy tonic that can strengthen the lungs; and honey can lubricate the lungs.

8.4 Emphysema

1. Lung-Kidney Yang Deficiency Syndrome

SYMPTOMS AND SIGNS:

- Clear, thin sputum.
- Cough in feeble voice.
- Lumbago.
- Shortness of breath getting worse on movement.
- Perspiration with cold limbs.
- Ringing in ears.
- Shortness of breath.

2. Lung-Kidney Yin Deficiency Syndrome

SYMPTOMS AND SIGNS:

- Cough.
- Hot sensations in palms of hands and soles of feet.
- Night sweats.
- Shortness of breath.
- Thirst with craving for drink.
- Tidal fever.

INGREDIENTS FOR CREATING RECIPES

FOODS FOR EXCESS: kiwi fruit (Chinese gooseberry), fresh ginger.

FOODS FOR DEFICIENCY: polished rice, walnut.

HERBS: Chuan-bei (tendril-leaved fritillary bulb), Lai-fu-zi (radish seed), Ban-xia (half-summer pinellia), Zi-su-zi (purple perilla seed), Rou-gui (Chinese cassia bark), Chen-pi (dried tangerine peel).

Syndromes of disease and herbs to use:

1. **LUNG-KIDNEY YANG DEFICIENCY:** Chuan-bei (tendril-leaved fritillary bulb), Lai-fu-zi (radish seed), Ban-xia (half-summer pinellia), Zi-su-zi (purple perilla seed), Rou-gui (Chinese cassia bark), Chen-pi (dried tangerine peel); cook with foods for deficiency.

2. **LUNG-KIDNEY YIN DEFICIENCY:** Chuan-bei (tendril-leaved fritillary bulb), Lai-fu-zi (radish seed), Ban-xia (half-summer pinellia), Zi-su-zi (purple perilla seed), Chen-pi (dried tangerine peel); cook with foods for deficiency.

RECIPE 41

MASTER: 10 g Chuan-bei (tendril-leaved fritillary bulb).

ASSOCIATE: 60 g polished rice.

ASSISTANT: white sugar.

SEASONING: none

STEPS:

(1) Grind Chuan-bei (tendril-leaved fritillary bulb) into powder.

(2) Boil polished rice and white sugar until cooked to make congee.

(3) Add the herbal powder to the congee and bring to a boil again for a few minutes.

CONSUMPTION: eat warm at mealtimes.

INDICATIONS: both syndromes of emphysema.

ANALYSIS: Chuan-bei is a common herb to treat lung disorders, including emphysema; polished rice is an energy tonic; and white sugar can lubricate the lungs.

8.5 Pneumonia

1. Wind Warm Superficial Syndrome

SYMPTOMS AND SIGNS:

- Acute onset of various symptoms.
- Cough.
- Dry mouth or thirst.
- Aversion to cold.

- High fever.
- Light thirst.
- Nasal discharge.
- Slight aversion to cold.
- Nasal congestion.
- Wheezing from the throat.

2. Sputum Energy Heat Syndrome

SYMPTOMS AND SIGNS:

- Cough and shortness of breath.
- Coughing with bloody, clear sputum.
- Discharge of copious yellowish and sticky sputum.
- Dry mouth with no desire to drink.
- Prolonged high fever.
- Light cough.
- Difficult, rapid breathing.
- Scanty urine.
- Shivering.
- Rusty-colored sputum.
- Thirst.
- Wheezing with sputum noise.

3. Pericardium Heat Syndrome

SYMPTOMS AND SIGNS:

- Slow and dull in response.
- Chest pain.
- Slightly cold limbs.
- Difficulty in speech.
- High fever.
- Hearing difficulties.
- Vision difficulties.
- Incontinence of both bowels and bladder.
- Apathy.
- Mental fogginess.
- Sputum noise in the throat.
- Twitching.

4. Extreme-Heat-Generating-Wind-in-the-Liver Syndrome

SYMPTOMS AND SIGNS:

- Convulsions.
- Faint.
- Feeling troubled, quick-tempered, and anxious.
- High fever.
- Muscular tightening.
- Red complexion.
- Stiff neck and/or limbs.
- Twitching or spasms in the limbs.
- Dry tongue.

INGREDIENTS FOR CREATING RECIPES

FOODS FOR EXCESS: garlic, pear, water chestnut, fresh lotus rhizome.

FOODS FOR DEFICIENCY: rock sugar, pear, dried lotus rhizome.

HERBS: Yu-xing-cao (cordate houttuynia), Jie-geng (kikio root), Ma-huang (Chinese ephedra), Xing-ren (apricot kernel), Sang-bai-pi (root bark of white mulberry), Chuan-bei (tendril-leaved fritillary bulb), Gan-cao (licorice), Lu-gen (reed rhizome), Shi-gao (gypsum), Jin-yin-hua (Japanese honeysuckle), Ju-hua (mulberry-leaved chrysanthemum), Sang-ye (mulberry leaf), Zhu-li (bamboo liquid).

Syndromes of disease and herbs to use:

1. **WIND WARM SUPERFICIAL:** Sang-bai-pi (root bark of white mulberry), Gan-cao (licorice), Ju-hua (mulberry-leaved chrysanthemum), Sang-ye (mulberry leaf); cook with foods for excess.

2. **SPUTUM ENERGY HEAT:** Sang-bai-pi (root bark of white mulberry), Xing-ren (apricot kernel), Chuan-bei (tendril-leaved fritillary bulb), Shi-gao (gypsum), Jin-yin-hua (Japanese honeysuckle), Jie-geng (kikio root), Zhu-li (bamboo liquid); cook with food for excess.

3. **PERICARDIUM HEAT:** Gan-cao (licorice), Yu-xing-cao (cordate houttuynia), Lu-gen (reed rhizome), Shi-gao (gypsum), Jin-yin-hua (Japanese honeysuckle), Ju-hua (mulberry-leaved chrysanthemum), Sang-ye (mulberry leaf); cook with foods for excess.

4. **EXTREME-HEAT-GENERATING-WIND-IN-THE-LIVER:** Yu-xing-cao (cordate houttuynia), Lu-gen (reed rhizome), Shi-gao (gypsum), Jin-yin-hua (Japanese honeysuckle), Ju-hua (mulberry-leaved chrysanthemum), Sang-ye (mulberry leaf); cook with foods for excess.

RECIPE 42

MASTER: 60 g Lu-gen (reed rhizome), 30 g Zhu-li (bamboo liquid).

ASSOCIATE: 50 g polished rice.

ASSISTANT: 2 cubes rock sugar.

SEASONING: none.

STEPS:

(1) Decoct Lu-gen (reed rhizome); strain to obtain herbal soup.

(2) Add polished rice and water and bring to a boil, then add Zhu-li (bamboo liquid) and rock sugar to boil for five more minutes.

CONSUMPTION: eat at mealtimes.

INDICATIONS: heat and sputum syndromes of pneumonia.

ANALYSIS: Lu-gen can clear heat and sedate fire, good for removal of lung heat; Zhu-li is cold and can remove hot sputum; and rock sugar can lubricate the lungs.

8.6 Pulmonary tuberculosis

1. **Lung Yin Deficiency Syndrome**

SYMPTOMS AND SIGNS:

- Asthma.
- Cough.
- Cough with or without little sputum.
- Coughing with blood.
- Discharge of scanty, sticky sputum.
- Dry sensations in the mouth.
- Hoarseness.
- Light but periodic fever not unlike the tide.
- Night sweats.
- Hot hands and feet.
- Insomnia.
- Sputum with blood.
- Cheek region appears red in the afternoon.

2. **Deficiency Fire Syndrome**

SYMPTOMS AND SIGNS:

- Coughing with bloody sputumn.
- Dry cough with little phlegm.
- Dry sensations in the mouth.
- Dry throat.
- Depression.
- Forgetfulness.
- Hot sensations from within.
- Hot sensations in body, center of hands and feet, and warm skin and muscles.
- Illness attacks slowly but with a longer duration (chronic illness).

- Light but periodic fever not unlike the tide.
- Night sweats.
- Pain in the throat.
- Ringing in ears.
- Insomnia.
- Sore loins.
- Sputum with blood.
- Toothache.

3. Deficiency of Energy and Yin Syndrome

SYMPTOMS AND SIGNS:

- Cold sensations with aversion to wind.
- Dry cough with scanty sputum.
- Dry mouth.
- Discharge of dry stools.
- Edema in the face and limbs.
- Excessive perspiration.
- Fatigue.
- Frequent vomiting.
- Hot sensations in the palms of hands and soles of feet.
- Mild stomachache with distension.
- Night sweats.
- Palpitation.
- Poor appetite.
- Scanty urine.
- Sore throat.
- Thirst.

INGREDIENTS FOR CREATING RECIPES

FOODS FOR EXCESS: peach, garlic, seaweed, carrot.

FOODS FOR DEFICIENCY: peach, oyster, sea cucumber, honey, white fungus, bird's nest, chicken, beef, royal jelly.

HERBS: Wu-wei-zi (magnolia vine fruit), He-shou-wu (tuber of multiflower knotweed), Dang-shen (root of pilose asiabell), Yi-yi-ren (Job's tears), Gan-cao (licorice), Zhi-mu (wind weed), Tian-dong (lucid asparagus), Bai-ji (amethyst orchid), Bai-bu (wild asparagus), Bai-he (lily), Kuan-dong-hua (coltsfoot), Shan-yao (Chinese yam), Bai-guo (ginkgo).

Syndromes of disease and herbs to use:

1. **LUNG YIN DEFICIENCY:** Wu-wei-zi (magnolia vine fruit), He-shou-wu (tuber of multiflower knotweed), Dang-shen (root of pilose asiabell), Gan-cao (licorice), Tian-dong (lucid asparagus); cook with foods for deficiency.
2. **DEFICIENCY FIRE**: Zhi-mu (wind weed), Bai-ji (amethyst orchid), Bai-bu (wild asparagus), Kuan-dong-hua (coltsfoot), Bai-guo (ginkgo); cook with foods for excess or foods for deficiency.
3. **DEFICIENCY OF YIN AND ENERGY:** He-shou-wu (tuber of multiflower knotweed), Dang-shen (root of pilose asiabell), Yi-yi-ren (Job's tears), Gan-cao (licorice), Bai-he (lily), Shan-yao (Chinese yam), Tian-dong (lucid asparagus); cook with foods for deficiency.

RECIPE 43

MASTER: 30 g Wu-wei-zi (magnolia vine fruit).

ASSOCIATE: 100 g white fungus.

ASSISTANT: 100 g rock sugar.

SEASONING: none.

STEPS:

(1) Put Wu-wei-zi (magnolia vine fruit) and white fungus in a large earthenware pot to boil in water over low heat for 2 hours; strain to obtain soup.

(2) Boil the soup over low heat until thick, then add rock sugar to dissolve.

(3) Store in the refrigerator.

CONSUMPTION: take 10 to 20 ml in warm water before meals, twice daily.

INDICATIONS: pulmonary tuberculosis.

ANALYSIS: Wu-wei-zi acts on the lungs; it is often used to treat tuberculosis, cough, and asthma, all of which are associated with the lungs. White fungus is a yin tonic; it can lubricate the lungs also and is used to treat dry cough and tuberculosis. Rock sugar can eliminate sputum and lubricate the lungs.

8.7 Respiratory allergies

1. Lung Energy Deficiency and Cold Syndrome

SYMPTOMS AND SIGNS:

- Breathing difficulty.
- Common cold.
- Cough.
- Excessive perspiration.
- Fatigue.
- Aversion to cold.
- Frequent sneezing.
- Impaired sense of smell.
- Light wheezing.
- Feeble voice.
- Nasal congestion.
- Severe itch in the nose.
- Shortness of breath.
- Normal urination.
- Sputum that is copious, clear, and watery.
- Too lazy to talk.

2. Spleen-Lung Energy Deficiency Syndrome

SYMPTOMS AND SIGNS:

- Abdominal distention.
- Clear nasal discharge.
- Cough.
- Coughing with sputum and saliva.
- Decreased appetite.
- Decreased sense of smell.
- Diarrhea that is sticky, muddy.
- Discharge of copious, clear and watery sputum.
- Little appetite and indigestion.
- Tired limbs.
- Fatigue.
- Prolonged cough.
- Rapid panting.
- Shortness of breath.
- Thin and feeble.

3. Kidney Yang Deficiency Syndrome

SYMPTOMS AND SIGNS:

- Allergies all year round.
- Cold feet or cold loins and legs.
- Cold sensations in the genital area or in the muscles.
- Diarrhea before dawn.
- Diarrhea with sticky, muddy stool.
- Discharge of watery thin stool.
- Edema.
- Fatigue.
- Frequent urination at night.
- Frequent sneezing with clear nasal discharge.
- Impotence in men.
- Infertility in women.
- Lack of appetite.
- Palpitation.
- Shortness of breath

- Perspiration in the forehead.
- Retention of urine.
- Ringing in ears.
- Shortness of breath.
- Wheezing.

4. Kidney Yin Deficiency Syndrome

SYMPTOMS AND SIGNS:

- Allergies all year round.
- Cold hands and feet.
- Cough with or without sputum containing blood.
- Hearing difficulty.
- Dizziness.
- Dry sensations in the mouth particularly at night.
- Dry throat.
- Fatigue.
- Depression with fever.
- Fever at night with burning sensations in internal organs.
- Hot sensations in the center of hands and feet.
- Night sweats.
- Pain in the heel.
- Pain in the loins (lumbago).
- Retention of urine.
- Ringing in ears.
- Insomnia.
- Spots in front of the eyes.
- Thirst.

INGREDIENTS FOR CREATING RECIPES

FOODS FOR EXCESS: garlic, fresh ginger, carrot.

FOODS FOR DEFICIENCY: royal jelly, chicken, beef, chestnut.

HERBS: Huang-qi (membranous milk vetch), Fang-feng (Chinese wind shelter), Bai-zhu (white atractylodes), Ge-gen (kudzu vine), Cong-bai (Welsh onion), Dan-pi (peony).

Syndromes of disease and herbs to use:

1. **LUNG ENERGY DEFICIENCY AND COLD:** Huang-qi (membranous milk vetch), Bai-zhu (white atractylodes), Fang-feng (Chinese wind shelter), Ge-gen (kudzu vine), Cong-bai (Welsh onion), Dan-pi (peony); cook with foods for deficiency or foods for excess.
2. **SPLEEN-LUNG ENERGY DEFICIENCY:** Huang-qi (membranous milk vetch), Bai-zhu (white atractylodes); cook with foods for deficiency.
3. **KIDNEY YANG DEFICIENCY:** Huang-qi (membranous milk vetch), Bai-zhu (white atractylodes); cook with foods for deficiency.
4. **KIDNEY YIN DEFICIENCY:** Huang-qi (membranous milk vetch), Bai-zhu (white atractylodes); cook with foods for deficiency.

RECIPE 44

MASTER: 5 g Huang-qi (membranous milk vetch), 10 g Fang-feng (Chinese wind shelter), 5 g Bai-zhu (white atractylodes).

ASSOCIATE: 100 g beefsteak.

ASSISTANT: 10 g royal jelly.

SEASONING: none.

STEPS:

(1) Boil the three master ingredients in water, then strain to obtain herbal soup.

(2) Cook beef as you would normally.

(3) Pour the herbal soup and royal jelly over the beefsteak and cook over low heat until warm.

CONSUMPTION: eat the steak at mealtimes.

INDICATIONS: all syndromes of respiratory allergies.

ANALYSIS: Huang-qi and Bai-zhu are energy tonics that can tone the lungs to increase immunity, and fang-feng can assist the body in resistance to the attack of external pathogens. Beef and royal jelly are also energy tonics that can boost the immune system.

8.8 Cough

1. **Wind Cold Syndrome**

SYMPTOMS AND SIGNS:

- Normal breathing through the nose.
- Clear discharge from nose.
- Cough with heavy throat clearing and clear sputum.
- Diarrhea.
- Aversion to cold.
- Dizziness.
- Facial paralysis.
- Headache with dizziness.
- Hoarseness at the beginning of an illness.
- Loss of voice.
- Nosebleed.
- Nasal congestion.
- Vomiting.

2. **Wind Heat Syndrome**

SYMPTOMS AND SIGNS:

- Cough with sticky sputum or blood.
- Dizziness.
- Fever in children.
- German measles in children.
- Headache with dizziness.
- Intolerance of light in both eyes, with swelling and aversion to wind.
- Muddy nasal discharge.
- Nosebleed.
- Pain in the eyes.
- Pain in the throat.
- Red eyes.
- Ringing in ears and hearing impairment.
- Thirst.
- Toothache.
- Yellowish urine.
- Yellowish nasal discharge.

3. **Dry Heat Syndrome**

SYMPTOMS AND SIGNS:

- Constipation.
- Cough with no sputum.
- Cough with a little sputum that is difficult to clear out.
- Dry nose or throat.
- Thirst.

4. **Damp Phlegm Syndrome**

SYMPTOMS AND SIGNS:

- Cough that stops after sputum is cleared.
- Abundant sputum that can be coughed out easily.
- Discharge of watery sputum.
- Dizziness.
- Headache.
- Hiccups.
- Pain in the chest.
- Panting.
- Prolonged dizziness.
- Excessive sleeping or insomnia.
- Vomiting.
- Slippery sputum that can be cleared from the throat easily.

5. **Liver Fire Upsurging Syndrome**

SYMPTOMS AND SIGNS:

- Bleeding from stomach.
- Cough with a sensation of something moving upward in the throat.
- Depressed with feeling of hot sensations.
- Dizziness, acute or otherwise.
- Easily angered.
- Headache on both sides of the head and eye sockets.
- Headache that is severe.
- Nosebleed.
- Red eyes.
- Ringing in ears.
- Insomnia or excessive sleep.
- Yellowish red urine.

6. **Yin Deficiency Syndrome**

SYMPTOMS AND SIGNS:

- Bleeding from gums.
- Constipation.
- Dizziness.
- Scanty stools.
- Dry cough or dry throat with little sputum.
- Dry sensations in the mouth.
- Fatigue.
- Headache in the afternoon.
- Light tidal fever that attacks in the afternoon.
- Night sweats.
- Nosebleed.
- Hot hands and feet.
- Underweight.
- Insomnia.
- Swallowing difficulty.
- Toothache.

INGREDIENTS FOR CREATING RECIPES

FOODS FOR EXCESS: pear, fresh lotus rhizome, prune, banana, tea, jellyfish, radish, radish leaf, lemon, carrot, apple, seaweed.

FOODS FOR DEFICIENCY: pear, dried lotus rhizome, apricot, honey, white fungus, white sugar, lemon, broomcorn, apple.

HERBS: Xing-ren (apricot kernel), Shan-yao (Chinese yam), Bei-sha-shen (straight ladybell north), Bai-he (lily), Ju-hua (mulberry-leaved chrysanthemum), Bai-guo (ginkgo), Yi-tang (maltose), Wu-wei-zi (magnolia vine fruit).

Syndromes of disease and herbs to use:

1. **WIND COLD**: Xing-ren (apricot kernel), Bai-he (lily); cook with foods for excess.
2. **WIND HEAT:** Xing-ren (apricot kernel), Ju-hua (mulberry-leaved chrysanthemum); cook with foods for excess.
3. **DRY HEAT:** Xing-ren (apricot kernel), Ju-hua (mulberry-leaved chrysanthemum), Bei-sha-shen (straight ladybell north), Yi-tang (maltose); cook with foods for excess or foods for deficiency.
4. **DAMP PHLEGM:** Xing-ren (apricot kernel), Bai-guo (ginkgo); cook with foods for excess.
5. **LIVER FIRE UPSURGING:** Ju-hua (mulberry-leaved chrysanthemum), Xing-ren (apricot kernel); cook with foods for excess.
6. **YIN DEFICIENCY:** Wu-wei-zi (magnolia vine fruit). Bei-sha-shen (straight ladybell north), Bai-he (lily), Yi-tang (maltose); cook with foods for deficiency.

RECIPE 45

MASTER: 5 g Wu-wei-zi (magnolia vine fruit).

ASSOCIATE: 1 apple.

ASSISTANT: 3 teaspoons honey.

SEASONING: none.

STEPS: Put the three ingredients in an earthenware pot and steam for one hour.

CONSUMPTION: eat at mealtimes or as a dessert.

INDICATIONS: yin deficiency syndrome of cough.

ANALYSIS: Wu-wei-zi acts on the lungs; it is often used to treat tuberculosis, cough, and asthma, all of which are associated with the lungs. Apple can lubricate the lungs to relieve cough, and honey is a yin tonic that can lubricate dryness.

RECIPE 46

MASTER: 5 g Bai-guo (ginkgo).

ASSOCIATE: 200 g radish.

ASSISTANT: 1 large gold or common carp.

SEASONING: black pepper.

STEPS:

(1) Crush Bai-guo (ginkgo) to boil in water for 30 minutes; strain to obtain soup.

(2) Peel and cut radish into small pieces.

(3) Remove internal organs from carp.

(4) Over water, steam radish and carp together.

(5) Pour the Bai-guo (ginkgo) soup over the radish and carp.

CONSUMPTION: eat at mealtimes (good for one serving).

INDICATIONS: damp sputum syndrome of cough.

ANALYSIS: Bai-guo is commonly used to remove sputum and suppress cough; radish can clear sputum; gold carp can eliminate dampness in the body; and black pepper assists the carp in eliminating dampness while also improving the taste.

RECIPE 47

MASTER: 10 g Yi-tang (maltose).

ASSOCIATE: 1 large pear.

ASSISTANT: 50 g fresh ginger.

SEASONING: black pepper.

STEPS:

(1) Peel the pear and fresh ginger and cut into small pieces.

(2) Put pear, fresh ginger, and Yi-tang (maltose) and two cups of water into a saucepan to boil for 30 minutes.

CONSUMPTION: divide into two servings for one-day consumption.

INDICATIONS: yin deficiency syndrome of cough.

ANALYSIS: Yi-tang is an energy tonic. It can also lubricate dryness to suppress cough. Pear can lubricate dryness, clear heat, and suppress cough, while fresh ginger can promote energy circulation. Black pepper can assist fresh ginger in promoting energy circulation.

8.9 Common cold and flu

1. Wind Cold Syndrome

SYMPTOMS AND SIGNS:

- Absence of perspiration in hot weather.
- Normal breathing through the nose.
- Clear nasal discharge.
- Cough with heavy, unclear sounds and clear sputum.
- Diarrhea.
- Aversion to cold.
- Dizziness.
- Headache with dizziness.
- Hoarseness at the beginning of illness.
- Itch in the throat.
- Light fever.
- Loss of voice.
- Nosebleed.
- Pain in the body shifting around with no fixed region.
- Pain in the joints.

- Nasal congestion.
- Vomiting.

2. **Wind Heat Syndrome**

SYMPTOMS AND SIGNS:

- Cough with yellowish phlegm.
- Strong fever and a mild or less severe chill.
- Headache with dizziness.
- Light sensitivity in both eyes, with swelling and aversion to wind.
- Muddy nasal discharge.
- Nosebleed.
- Pain in the eyes.
- Pain in the throat.
- Perspiration.
- Red eyes.
- Thirst.
- Toothache.
- Yellowish urine.
- Yellowish nasal discharge.

3. **Summer Heat Syndrome**

SYMPTOMS AND SIGNS:

- Chest discomfort.
- Constipation.
- Cough.
- Dizziness.
- Dry lips or dry sensations in the mouth.
- Fatigue.
- Depression and thirst.
- Heavy sensations in the head.
- High fever.
- Nausea and vomiting.
- No perspiration.
- Difficult urination with reddish urine.
- Difficult and rapid breathing.
- Normal perspiration due to hot weather or warm clothing.
- Profuse perspiration.
- Scanty, reddish urine.
- Thirst.

INGREDIENTS FOR CREATING RECIPES

FOODS FOR EXCESS: fresh ginger, tea, tofu, yellow soybean, fermented black soybean, coriander (Chinese parsley), green onion.

FOODS FOR DEFICIENCY: brown sugar, polished rice, glutinous rice, rock sugar, honey, tofu.

HERBS: Da-qing-ye (mayflower glorybower leaf), Ju-hua (mulberry-leaved chrysanthemum), Bo-he (peppermint), Sang-ye (mulberry leaf), Niu-bang-zi (burdock), Jin-yin-hua (Japanese honeysuckle), Ge-gen (kudzu vine), Huang-qin (skullcap), Ban-lan-gen (woad), Cong-bai (Welsh onion), Zi-su-ye (purple perilla leaf), Lu-gen (reed rhizome), Jing-jie (Japanese ground-ivy), Bai-bian-dou (hyacinth bean).

Syndromes of disease and herbs to use:

1. **WIND COLD:** Jing-jie (Japanese ground-ivy), Cong-bai (Welsh onion), Zi-su-ye (purple perilla leaf); cook with foods for excess.
2. **WIND HEAT:** Ju-hua (mulberry-leaved chrysanthemum), Da-qing-ye (mayflower glorybower leaf), Bo-he (peppermint), Sang-ye (mulberry leaf), Niu-bang-zi (burdock), Ge-gen (kudzu vine), Huang-qin (skullcap), Ban-lan-gen (woad), Lu-gen (reed rhizome); cook with foods for excess.
3. **SUMMER HEAT:** Jin-yin-hua (Japanese honeysuckle), Ju-hua (mulberry-leaved chrysanthemum), Da-qing-ye (mayflower glorybower leaf), Ban-lan-gen (woad), Lu-gen (reed rhizome), Bai-bian-dou (hyacinth bean); cook with foods for excess.

RECIPE 48

MASTER: 30 g Yi-yi-ren (Job's tears), 30 g Bai-bian-dou (hyacinth bean).

ASSOCIATE: 100 g polished rice.

ASSISTANT: none.

SEASONING: none.

STEPS: Boil the three ingredients to make a congee.

CONSUMPTION: eat at mealtimes.

INDICATIONS: summer heat syndrome of common cold and flu.

ANALYSIS: Yi-yi-ren and Bai-bian-dou can both eliminate dampness, while the latter also clears heat; both are good for common cold and flu due to the presence of heat and dampness in summer. Polished rice is an energy tonic to boost body energy. (Seasoning is not suggested here because the recipe stands on its own without it. Green onion may be used to improve the taste if so desired.

RECIPE 49

MASTER: 10 g Jing-jie (Japanese ground-ivy), 9 g Zi-su-ye (purple perilla leaf).

ASSOCIATE: 9 g fresh ginger.

ASSISTANT: 20 g brown sugar.

SEASONING: none.

STEPS:

(1) Decoct Jing-jie (Japanese ground-ivy), Zi-su-ye (purple perilla leaf), and fresh ginger in water; strain to obtain herbal soup.

(2) Dissolve brown sugar in boiling water and mix with the soup.

CONSUMPTION: drink anytime.

INDICATIONS: wind cold syndrome of common cold and flu.

ANALYSIS: Jing-jie and Zi-su-ye can counteract wind and cold; fresh ginger can induce perspiration, which is good for the common cold and flu; and brown sugar is to improve the taste.

RECIPE 50

MASTER: 10 g Niu-bang-zi (burdock), 10 g Sang-ye (mulberry leaf).

ASSOCIATE: 100 g polished rice.

ASSISTANT: 100 g honey.

SEASONING: none.

STEPS:

(1) Decoct the two master ingredients; strain to obtain herbal soup.

(2) Boil polished rice in water to make a congee.

(3) Pour herbal soup and honey into congee and mix well.

CONSUMPTION: eat at mealtimes.

INDICATIONS: wind heat syndrome of common cold and flu.

ANALYSIS: Niu-bang-zi and Sang-ye can clear heat and remove wind in the lungs; polished rice is an energy tonic; and honey lubricates dryness in the lungs.

CHAPTER 9

Cardiovascular System

9.1 High cholesterol

1. Superficial Damp Heat Syndrome

SYMPTOMS AND SIGNS:

- Abdominal swelling or pain.
- Burning sensation and itch in the genitals or burning sensation in the anal area.
- Congested chest.
- Diarrhea that consists of forceful discharge of stool.
- Discharge of yellowish-red stool, turbid and with a foul odor.
- Edema.
- Excessive perspiration.
- Feeling miserable.
- Frequent itch and pain in the vulva.
- Pain in the joints, with swelling and heaviness.
- Perspiration in hands and feet or in the head area.
- Scanty, bloody urine or retention of urine.
- Swollen tongue.
- Thirst.
- Yellowish skin not unlike mandarin orange.

2. Spleen Sputum Syndrome

SYMPTOMS AND SIGNS:

- Abdominal swelling.
- Abundant saliva.
- Coughing with watery sputum.
- Overweight with little food intake.
- Fatigue.
- Poor appetite.
- Slight distension of the stomach.
- Suppression of menses.
- Weak limbs.

3. Hot Stomach Syndrome

SYMPTOMS AND SIGNS:

- Bad breath.
- Bleeding gums.
- Easily hungry.

- Swollen gums.
- Hiccups.
- Morning sickness.
- Nosebleed.
- Pain in the gums with swelling.
- Pain in the throat.
- Perspiring in the head.
- Stomachache.
- Thirst and craving for cold drinks.
- Vomiting.
- Vomiting with blood.
- Vomiting immediately after eating.

4. **Liver Fire Upsurging Syndrome**

SYMPTOMS AND SIGNS:

- Dizziness, especially acute.
- Bleeding from stomach.
- Congested chest.
- Hearing difficulties.
- Foggy vision.
- Dry sensations in the mouth.
- Feeling hasty and quick-tempered or anxious at bedtime.
- Easily angry.
- Headache on both sides of the head and in the sockets of the eyes.
- Severe headache.
- Hiccups.
- Nosebleed.
- Pain in the chest and the hypochondrium.
- Bloodshot eyes.
- Ringing in ears.
- Insomnia or excessive sleeping.
- Vomiting of blood.
- Yellowish-red urine.

5. **Spleen-Kidney Yang Deficiency Syndrome**

SYMPTOMS AND SIGNS:

- Abdominal swelling.
- Cold hands and feet or cold loins.
- Diarrhea before dawn.
- Diarrhea with sticky, muddy stool.
- Eating little.
- Edema, especially one that occurs all over the body.
- Fatigue.
- Aversion to cold.
- Visual impairment, with "flying objects" in front of eyes.
- Weak limbs.
- Frequent clear urination.
- Lumbago.
- Mental fatigue.
- Over 65 years old.
- Sputum caught in the throat with shortness of breath.

6. **Deficiency of Energy and Blood Syndrome**

SYMPTOMS AND SIGNS:

- Bleeding of various kinds with light-colored blood, often seen in consumptive diseases.
- Chest pain or congestion.
- Dizziness.
- Fatigue.
- Visual impairment as in "flying objects" in front of the eyes.
- Insomnia.

- Low energy.
- Feeble voice.
- Numbness in the limbs.
- Pale complexion and lips.
- Pale nails.
- Palpitation.
- Ringing in the ears.

INGREDIENTS FOR CREATING RECIPES

FOODS FOR EXCESS: kelp, seaweed, corn, celery, black fungus, carrot.

FOODS FOR DEFICIENCY: mussel, onion, shiitake mushroom.

HERBS: Ze-xie (water plantain), Da-zao (red date), Shan-zha (Chinese hawthorn), Ling-zhi (lucid ganoderma), Jin-yin-hua (Japanese honeysuckle), He-shou-wu (tuber of multiflower knotweed).

Syndromes of disease and herbs to use:

1. **SUPERFICIAL DAMP HEAT:** Ze-xie (water plantain), Ling-zhi (lucid ganoderma); cook with foods for excess.
2. **SPLEEN SPUTUM:** Ling-zhi (lucid ganoderma), Ze-xie (water plantain), Jin-yin-hua (Japanese honeysuckle); cook with foods for excess.
3. **HOT STOMACH:** Ling-zhi (lucid ganoderma), Jin-yin-hua (Japanese honeysuckle); cook with foods for excess.
4. **LIVER FIRE UPSURGING:** Ze-xie (water plantain), Ling-zhi (lucid ganoderma), Jin-yin-hua (Japanese honeysuckle); cook with foods for excess.
5. **SPLEEN-KIDNEY YANG** deficiency: He-shou-wu (tuber of multiflower knotweed), Ling-zhi (lucid ganoderma); cook with foods for deficiency.
6. **DEFICIENCY OF ENERGY AND BLOOD:** Da-zao (red date), He-shou-wu (tuber of multiflower knotweed), Ling-zhi (lucid ganoderma); cook with foods for deficiency.

RECIPE 51

MASTER: He-shou-wu (tuber of multiflower knotweed).

ASSOCIATE: 50 g polished rice.

ASSISTANT: 10 g Da-zao (red date).

SEASONING: white sugar.

STEPS:

(1) Bake He-shou-wu (tuber of multiflower knotweed) until dry; grind into powder.

(2) Boil polished rice, Da-zao (red date), and white sugar together in water to make a congee.

(3) Add the ground herb powder to the congee, bring to a boil again for a few minutes, then remove from heat.

CONSUMPTION: eat at mealtimes.

INDICATIONS: deficiency syndromes of high cholesterol.

ANALYSIS: He-shou-wu can reduce cholesterol levels; Da-zao is an energy tonic that helps the master ingredient to perform its function of reducing cholesterol levels; and white sugar is to improve the taste.

RECIPE 52

MASTER: 8 g Ze-xie (water plantain).

ASSOCIATE: 10 g black fungus, 250 g tofu.

ASSISTANT: 30 g carrot, 150 g shiitake mushrooms.

SEASONING: fresh ginger, salt, sesame oil.

STEPS:

(1) Decoct Ze-xie (water plantain) in water; strain to obtain herbal soup.

(2) Wash black fungus in warm water, cut up the tofu, carrot, and shiitake mushrooms.

(3) Put black fungus, carrot, and mushrooms in water and bring to a boil, then add the herbal soup.

(3) Season with fresh ginger, salt, and sesame oil before removing from heat.

CONSUMPTION: eat at mealtimes.

INDICATIONS: the first four syndromes of high cholesterol.

ANALYSIS: Ze-xie can remove dampness and reduce cholesterol level; black fungus and tofu cool the blood; carrot reduces dampness, and shiitake mushroom reduces cholesterol level. The three seasonings are present to improve the taste.

9.2 Hypertension

1. Liver Fire Syndrome

SYMPTOMS AND SIGNS:

- Bitter taste in the mouth.
- Blood pressure rises easily during anger or stress.
- Discharge of yellowish, scanty urine.
- Dry mouth.
- Hot temper.
- Bloodshot eyes.
- Flushed face.
- Severe headache.
- Vertigo.

2. Liver-Kidney Yin Deficiency Syndrome with Liver Yang Upsurging

SYMPTOMS AND SIGNS:

- Blood pressure rises easily during fatigue and stress.
- Discharge of bloody, scanty urine.
- Hot temper.
- Insomnia.
- Lumbago.
- Many dreams.
- Numbness in the limbs.
- Pain in the legs.
- Ringing in the ears.
- Seminal emission in men.
- Vertigo.

3. Deficiency of Yin and Yang Syndrome with Yang Moving Upward

SYMPTOMS AND SIGNS:

- Blurred vision.
- Cold limbs.
- Dry mouth.
- Frequent urination at night.
- Heavy breathing on walking.
- Insomnia.
- Light headache.
- Lumbago.
- Many dreams.
- Perspiration.
- Ringing in the ears.
- Slightly flushed face.
- Muscle twitching.
- Vertigo.
- Weak legs.

INGREDIENTS FOR CREATING RECIPES

FOODS FOR EXCESS: celery, onion, jellyfish, jellyfish skin, garlic, carrot, kelp, black fungus, banana, tomato, pea, vinegar, wild rice gall (water oats gall), apple, pear, persimmon, water chestnut, kelp, mung bean, broad bean, preserved duck egg, spinach, Chinese wax gourd, grass carp, hair vegetable.

FOODS FOR DEFICIENCY: white fungus, tomato, rock sugar, apple, pear, mussel, common carp, pork kidney, sea cucumber.

HERBS: Sang-bai-pi (root bark of white mulberry), Shan-zha (Chinese hawthorn), Ju-hua (mulberry-leaved chrysanthemum), Yu-mi-xu (corn silk), Ye-ju-hua (wild chrysanthemum), Xia-ku-cao (self heal), He-shou-wu (tuber of multiflower knotweed), Sang-ji-sheng (mistletoe), Jue-ming-zi (coffee weed), Da-zao (red date), Ge-gen (kudzu vine), Huang-qin (skullcap), Gou-teng (gambir), Mu-li (oyster shell).

Syndromes of disease and herbs to use:

1. **LIVER FIRE:** Sang-bai-pi (root bark of white mulberry), Ju-hua (mulberry-leaved chrysanthemum), Ye-ju-hua (wild chrysanthemum), Xia-ku-cao (self heal), Jue-ming-zi (coffee weed), Yu-mi-xu (corn silk), Ge-gen (kudzu vine), Huang-qin (skullcap), Gou-teng (gambir), Mu-li (oyster shell); cook with foods for excess.
2. **LIVER-KIDNEY YIN DEFICIENCY WITH LIVER YANG UPSURGING:** He-shou-wu (tuber of multiflower knotweed), Sang-ji-sheng (mistletoe), Da-zao (red date), Ju-hua (mulberry-leaved chrysanthemum), Ye-ju-hua (wild chrysanthemum), Xia-ku-cao (self heal); cook with foods for deficiency or foods for excess.
3. **DEFICIENCY OF YIN AND YANG:** He-shou-wu (tuber of multiflower knotweed), Sang-ji-sheng (mistletoe), Da-zao (red date); cook with foods for deficiency.

RECIPE 53

MASTER: 10 g Xia-ku-cao (self heal).
ASSOCIATE: 120 g jellyfish skin.
ASSISTANT: 300 g water chestnuts.
SEASONING: salt.
STEPS:

(1) Decoct Xia-ku-cao (self heal) in water for 30 minutes; strain to obtain about 1,000 ml soup.

(2) Wash jellyfish skin to remove salt and also water chestnuts (with peel on) and crush them.

(3) Boil jellyfish skin and water chestnuts in the herbal soup until it is reduced to 250 ml, then strain.

CONSUMPTION: drink 125 ml on an empty stomach, twice daily.

INDICATIONS: liver fire syndrome of hypertension.

ANALYSIS: Xia-ku-cao can reduce blood pressure due to liver fire; jellyfish skin acts on the liver and relieves headache; water chestnut clears heat; and salt clears heat and improves taste. In Western medicine, salt is regarded as capable of causing high blood pressure, but it is used in this recipe only as a seasoning. The amount used should be minimal, about 1/5 teaspoonful.

RECIPE 54

MASTER: 10 g Gou-teng (gambir).

ASSOCIATE: 15 g hair vegetable.

ASSISTANT: 1 preserved duck egg.

SEASONING: salt.

STEPS:

(1) Decoct Gou-teng (gambir) in water for one hour; strain to obtain 2 to 3 cups of soup.

(2) Wash the hair vegetable and add to the soup. Cook for 5 minutes, then add the duck egg (with shell removed) to cook for a few more minutes.

(3) Season with salt.

CONSUMPTION: eat once daily for as long as necessary.

INDICATIONS: liver fire syndrome of hypertension.

ANALYSIS: Gou-teng can reduce blood pressure due to liver fire; hair vegetable can clear heat; and preserved duck egg is cold and can clear fire. See recipe 53 for comment on salt.

RECIPE 55

MASTER: 10 g Sang-ji-sheng (mistletoe).

ASSOCIATE: 30 g sea cucumber.

ASSISTANT: 10 g rock sugar.

SEASONING: black pepper.

STEPS:

(1) Decoct Sang-ji-sheng (mistletoe) in water for one hour; strain to obtain three cups of soup.

(2) Boil sea cucumber in the herbal soup until soft and tender.

(3) Add rock sugar to the soup to dissolve.

(4) Season with black pepper.

CONSUMPTION: eat the contents and drink the soup at mealtimes.

INDICATIONS: deficiency syndrome of hypertension.

ANALYSIS: Sang-ji-sheng, a yin tonic, can reduce blood pressure. Sea cucumber can nourish the blood and lubricate dryness, rock sugar can lubricate dryness also, and black pepper is added to improve the taste.

9.3 Hypotension

1. Heart Yang Deficiency Syndrome

SYMPTOMS AND SIGNS:

- Cold sensations.
- Fatigue.
- Easily anxious with rapid heartbeat.
- Female.
- Extremely cold hands and feet.
- Over 60 years old.
- Pain in the chest.
- Pain in the heart.
- Palpitation with anxiety.
- Profuse perspiration.
- Systolic pressure below a reading of 90 mm.

2. Spleen-Stomach Yang Deficiency Syndrome

SYMPTOMS AND SIGNS:

- Abdominal pain.
- Abdominal swelling after meals.
- Cold limbs.
- Diarrhea.
- Fatigue.
- Feeble intermittent hiccups.
- Preference for warmth and massage.
- Pain gets worse with fatigue and hunger.
- Pain improves with rest and eating.
- Palpitation.
- Poor appetite.
- Shortness of breath.
- Stomachache.
- Indigestion.
- Vomiting of undigested foods.
- Water noise in the stomach.
- Sallow and dry complexion.

3. Spleen-Kidney Deficiency Syndrome

SYMPTOMS AND SIGNS:

- Hearing loss.
- Diarrhea.
- Difficult urination.
- Dizziness.
- Fatigue of the four limbs.
- Forgetfulness.
- Insomnia.
- Blurred vision.
- Palpitation.
- Ringing in the ears.
- Shortness of breath.
- Sallow complexion.

4. Deficiency of Energy and Yin Syndrome

SYMPTOMS AND SIGNS:

- Constipation.
- Dizziness.
- Dry cough with scanty sputum.

- Dry mouth.
- Discharge of dry stools.
- Excessive perspiration.
- Fatigue.
- Fever.
- Frequent vomiting.
- Hot sensations in the palms of hands and soles of feet.
- Mild stomachache with distension.
- Palpitation.
- Poor appetite.
- Scanty urine.
- Sore throat.
- Thirst.
- Too lazy to talk.

5. Heart-Kidney Yang Deficiency Syndrome

SYMPTOMS AND SIGNS:

- Cold limbs.
- Cold sweats.
- Discharge of watery thin stool.
- Edema.
- Frequent urination particularly at night.
- Top-heavy sensation.
- Pain in the chest.
- Palpitation.
- Nervousness.
- Shock.

INGREDIENTS FOR CREATING RECIPES

FOODS FOR DEFICIENCY: chicken, chicken egg, beef, longan nut, mutton, walnut, lime.

HERBS: Ren-shen (Chinese ginseng), Mai-dong (lilyturf), Fu-ling (tuckahoe; Indian bread), Suan-zao-ren (jujube), Lian-zi (East Indian lotus), Rou-gui (Chinese cassia bark), Gan-jiang (dried ginger), Gan-cao (licorice), Huang-jing (sealwort), Ju-pi (tangerine peel), Wu-wei-zi (magnolia vine fruit), Huang-qi (membranous milk vetch), Bei-sha-shen (straight ladybell north), Bai-zhu (white atractylodes), Yu-zhu (Solomon's seal), Shu-di (processed glutinous rehmannia), Dang-shen (root of pilose asiabell), Tu-si-zi (dodder seed), Gou-qi-zi (matrimony vine fruit), Rou-cong-rong (saline cistanche), Shan-yao (Chinese yam), Bai-he (lily).

Syndromes of disease and herbs to use:

1. **HEART YANG DEFICIENCY:** Ren-shen (Chinese ginseng), Rou-gui (Chinese cassia bark), Gan-jiang (dried ginger), Bai-zhu (white atractylodes), Dang-shen (root of pilose asiabell), Tu-si-zi (dodder seed), Rou-cong-rong (saline cistanche), Shan-yao (Chinese yam); cook with foods for deficiency.
2. **SPLEEN-STOMACH YANG DEFICIENCY:** Ren-shen (Chinese ginseng), Rou-gui (Chinese cassia bark), Gan-jiang (dried ginger), Bai-zhu (white atractylodes), Dang-shen (root of pilose asiabell), Tu-si-zi (dodder seed), Rou-cong-rong (saline cistanche); cook with foods for deficiency.
3. **SPLEEN-KIDNEY DEFICIENCY:** Ren-shen (Chinese ginseng), Dang-shen (root of pilose asiabell), Fu-ling (tuckahoe; Indian bread), Suan-zao-ren (jujube), Gan-cao (licorice), Huang-jing (sealwort), Shan-yao (Chinese yam); cook with foods for deficiency.
4. **DEFICIENCY OF ENERGY AND YIN:** Bai-he (lily), Ren-shen (Chinese ginseng), Mai-dong (lilyturf), Suan-zao-ren (jujube), Lian-zi (East Indian lotus), Gan-cao (licorice), Huang-jing (sealwort), Wu-wei-zi (magnolia vine fruit), Huang-qi (membranous milk vetch), Bei-sha-shen (straight ladybell north), Bai-zhu (white atractylodes), Yu-zhu (Solomon's seal), Gou-qi-zi (matrimony vine fruit); cook with foods for deficiency.
5. **HEART-KIDNEY YANG DEFICIENCY:** Ren-shen (Chinese ginseng), Rou-gui (Chinese cassia bark), Gan-jiang (dried ginger), Bai-zhu (white atractylodes), Dang-shen (root

of pilose asiabell), Tu-si-zi (dodder seed), Rou-cong-rong (saline cistanche); cook with foods for deficiency.

RECIPE 56

MASTER: 6 g Ren-shen (Chinese ginseng), 15 g Mai-dong (lilyturf), 15 g Huang-jing (sealwort), 12 g Ju-pi (tangerine peel), 9 g Gan-cao (licorice), 9 g Wu-wei-zi (magnolia vine fruit).

ASSOCIATE: 100 g polished rice.

ASSISTANT: none.

SEASONING: none.

STEPS:

(1) Decoct the six master ingredients; strain to obtain herbal soup.

(2) Add polished rice and more water to the herbal soup; bring to a boil until cooked to make a congee.

CONSUMPTION: divide into two servings to consume in one day.

INDICATIONS: all syndromes of hypotension.

ANALYSIS: Ginseng is an energy tonic, and thus increases blood pressure. Mai-dong and Huang-jing are both yin tonics; Gan-cao is an energy tonic; and Wu-wei-zi can water the kidneys. The six master ingredients work together as a team. Polished rice is an energy tonic to assist the master ingredients in increasing blood pressure. See also comments for recipe 34.

9.4 Arteriosclerosis

1. Deficient Yin with Excessive Yang Syndrome

SYMPTOMS AND SIGNS:

- Bitter taste in the mouth.
- Chest congestion.
- Dizziness.
- Dry throat.
- Easily angry.
- Headache.
- Hypertension.
- Numbness in the four limbs.
- Obstructed vision.
- Pain in the heart region.

2. Kidney Yin Deficiency Syndrome

SYMPTOMS AND SIGNS:

- Cold hands and feet.
- Cough with bloody sputum.
- Hearing difficulty.
- Dizziness.
- Dry sensations in the mouth or dry throat.
- Fatigue.
- Depression and anxiety with fever.
- Fever at night with burning sensations in internal organs.
- Frequent urination at night.
- Hot sensations in any part of the body.
- Night sweats.
- Pain in the heel.
- Pain in the loins (lumbago).
- Pain in the tibia.
- Ringing in ears.
- Seminal emission mostly without erotic dreams.
- Insomnia.
- Sore loins and weak legs.
- Spots in front of the eyes.
- Thirst.
- Toothache or loose teeth.

3. **Cold Syndrome**

SYMPTOMS AND SIGNS:

- Congested chest.
- Dizziness with fatigue.
- Irregular heartbeat.
- Palpitation with shortness of breath.
- Periodic pain in the heart region.
- Sore loins with weak legs.

4. **Sputum Congestion Syndrome**

SYMPTOMS AND SIGNS:

- Cold limbs.
- Congested chest.
- Palpitation with nervousness.
- Perspiration that stops quickly.
- Sudden pricking and choking pain in the heart region, sometimes affecting the back.

5. **Heart Yang Prolapse Syndrome**

SYMPTOMS AND SIGNS:

- Blue complexion.
- Chest congestion.
- Cold sweat.
- Cold limbs.
- Continual severe pain in the heart region.
- Fainting.

INGREDIENTS FOR CREATING RECIPES

FOODS FOR EXCESS: banana, peach, watermelon, water chestnut, sunflower, tomato, eggplant, celery, apple, black sesame seed, persimmon, jellyfish, spinach, black fungus, soy milk, onion, laver, tofu.

FOODS FOR DEFICIENCY: peach, sea cucumber, tomato, apple, pork, buckwheat, duck egg, soy milk, polished rice, rabbit, tofu.

HERBS: Ling-zhi (lucid ganoderma), Shan-zha (Chinese hawthorn), He-shou-wu (tuber of multiflower knotweed), Ru-xiang (frankincense), Mo-yao (myrrh), Gua-lou (snake gourd), Gui-zhi (cinnamon stick), Mu-xiang (costus root), Lian-zi-xin (lotus plumule).

Syndromes of disease and herbs to use:

1. **DEFICIENT YIN WITH EXCESSIVE YANG:** Ling-zhi (lucid ganoderma), He-shou-wu (tuber of multiflower knotweed), Lian-zi-xin (lotus plumule); cook with foods for deficiency or foods for excess.
2. **KIDNEY YIN DEFICIENCY:** Ling-zhi (lucid ganoderma), He-shou-wu (tuber of multiflower knotweed), Lian-zi-xin (lotus plumule); cook with foods for deficiency.
3. **COLD:** Ling-zhi (lucid ganoderma), Gui-zhi (cinnamon stick), Mu-xiang (costus root); cook with foods for excess.
4. **SPUTUM CONGESTION:** Gua-lou (snake gourd), Mo-yao (myrrh), Ru-xiang (frankincense), Mu-xiang (costus root); cook with foods for excess.
5. **HEART YANG PROLAPSE:** Gua-lou (snake gourd), Gui-zhi (cinnamon stick), Mu-xiang (costus root); cook with foods for deficiency.

RECIPE 57

MASTER: 500 g Gui-zhi (cinnamon stick).

ASSOCIATE: 250 g honey.

ASSISTANT: none.

SEASONING: none.

STEPS:

(1) Decoct Gui-zhi (cinnamon stick) in water; strain and obtain herbal soup.

(2) Over low heat, mix honey with herbal soup to boil until thick and sticky.

(3) Store in a glass jar.

CONSUMPTION: take 20 g each time, three times daily.

INDICATIONS: heart yang prolapse syndrome of arteriosclerosis.

ANALYSIS: Gui-zhi, a heart tonic and heart muscle relaxant, is a common herb to treat arteriosclerosis and heart disease in general. Honey can relieve pain and lubricate dryness.

9.5 Coronary heart disease

1. Heart Blood Coagulation Syndrome

SYMPTOMS AND SIGNS:

- Chest congestion.
- Chronic backache.
- Cold hands and feet.
- Excessive perspiration.
- Pain in the chest.
- Needle pricking sensation in the heart and chest.
- Pale complexion.
- Palpitation.
- Excessive perspiration.
- Poor appetite.
- Shortness of breath.

2. Energy Congestion and Blood Coagulation Syndrome

SYMPTOMS AND SIGNS:

- Abdominal swelling.
- Chest pain and backache.
- Chest pain that comes and goes as if being pricked by a needle.
- Congested chest.
- Liver disease.
- Love of sighing.
- Lump in the abdomen that stays in the same region.
- Shortness of breath.
- Ulcer.

3. Liver-Kidney Yin Deficiency Syndrome

SYMPTOMS AND SIGNS:

- Chest pain, particularly at night.
- Difficulty in both bowel movement and urination.
- Dizziness.
- Dry eyes, throat, or mouth.
- Fatigue.
- Headache with pain in the bony ridge forming the eyebrow.
- Lumbago.
- Night-blindness.
- Night sweats.
- Pain in the hypochondrium.
- Hot hands and feet.
- Paralysis.
- Period pain.
- Insomnia with forgetfulness.
- Weak loins and tibia.
- Withered complexion.

4. Deficiency of Yin and Yang Syndrome

SYMPTOMS AND SIGNS:

- Cold limbs and cold sensations in the body.
- Fatigue.
- Frequent urination at night.
- Low energy.
- Pain in the heart.
- Palpitation.
- Perspiration with hot sensations in the body easily triggered by physical activities.

- Poor appetite.
- Poor spirits.
- Ringing in ears.
- Underweight.
- Too lazy to talk.
- Restless sleep due to pain.

INGREDIENTS FOR CREATING RECIPES

FOODS FOR EXCESS: pea, garlic, seaweed, kelp, black fungus.

FOODS FOR DEFICIENCY: wheat, longan nut, honey, oyster.

HERBS: Lian-zi (East Indian lotus), Shan-zha (Chinese hawthorn), Fu-ling (tuckahoe; Indian bread), Suan-zao-ren (jujube), Ju-hua (mulberry-leaved chrysanthemum), Tao-ren (peach kernel), Rou-gui (Chinese cassia bark), Gan-jiang (dried ginger), He-shou-wu (tuber of multiflower knotweed), Chen-pi (dried tangerine peel), Ren-shen (Chinese ginseng), Dan-shen (purple sage), Hong-hua (safflower), Bai-he (lily), Sang-shen (mulberry).

Syndromes of disease and herbs to use:

1. **HEART BLOOD COAGULATION:** Shan-zha (Chinese hawthorn), Lian-zi (East Indian lotus), Tao-ren (peach kernel), Dan-shen (purple sage), Hong-hua (safflower); cook with foods for excess.

2. **ENERGY CONGESTION AND BLOOD COAGULATION:** Chen-pi (dried tangerine peel), Tao-ren (peach kernel), Dan-shen (purple sage), Hong-hua (safflower), Ju-hua (mulberry-leaved chrysanthemum); cook with foods for excess.

3. **LIVER-KIDNEY YIN DEFICIENCY:** Fu-ling (tuckahoe; Indian bread), Suan-zao-ren (jujube), He-shou-wu (tuber of multiflower knotweed), Ren-shen (Chinese ginseng), Sang-shen (mulberry), Bai-he (lily); cook with foods for deficiency.

4. **DEFICIENCY OF YIN AND YANG:** Suan-zao-ren (jujube), He-shou-wu (tuber of multiflower knotweed), Ren-shen (Chinese ginseng), Sang-shen (mulberry), Rou-gui (Chinese cassia bark), Gan-jiang (dried ginger), Bai-he (lily); cook with foods for deficiency.

RECIPE 58

MASTER: 30 g Shan-zha (Chinese hawthorn).

ASSOCIATE: 50 g seaweed.

ASSISTANT: 50 g wheat.

SEASONING: white sugar or rock sugar.

STEPS:

(1) Crush Shan-zha (Chinese hawthorn), bake until dry, then grind into powder.

(2) Boil seaweed and wheat in water to make soup.

(3) Add the herbal powder to the soup.

(4) Season with white sugar.

CONSUMPTION: Have at mealtimes.

INDICATIONS: heart blood coagulation syndrome of coronary heart disease.

ANALYSIS: Shan-zha, widely used to treat coronary heart disease, is an effective heart tonic in that it can activate the blood and bring down blood pressure. Seaweed can soften up hardness; wheat checks excessive perspiration and reduces internal heat; and white sugar or rock sugar improve the taste.

9.6 Arrhythmia (irregular heartbeat)

1. Heart Energy Deficiency Syndrome

SYMPTOMS AND SIGNS:

- Congested chest.
- Pale complexion.
- Palpitation and nervousness.
- Perspiration.
- Shortness of breath.

2. Deficiency of Energy and Yin Syndrome

SYMPTOMS AND SIGNS:

- Fatigue.
- Hot sensations in palms of hands and soles of feet and in the middle of chest.
- Insomnia with many dreams.
- Palpitation and nervousness.
- Tidal fever and night sweats.

3. Energy Deficiency and Blood Coagulation Syndromes

SYMPTOMS AND SIGNS:

- Fatigue.
- Pain in the heart region.
- Palpitation with nervousness.
- Shortness of breath.

4. Yin Deficiency with Abundant Fire Syndrome

SYMPTOMS AND SIGNS:

- Dizziness.
- Dry mouth and tongue.
- Insomnia with forgetfulness.
- Palpitation with mental depression.
- Ringing in ears.

5. Heart-Spleen Deficiency Syndrome

SYMPTOMS AND SIGNS:

- Abdominal swelling.
- Dizziness.
- Edema with scanty urine.
- Nausea.
- Palpitation and forgetfulness.
- Poor appetite.

6. Damp Phlegm Syndrome

SYMPTOMS AND SIGNS:

- Abdominal swelling with congested chest.
- Cough with excessive sputum.
- Dizziness with heavy sensations in the head.
- Nausea.
- Palpitation with nervousness.
- Poor appetite.

7. Spleen-Kidney Yang Deficiency Syndrome

SYMPTOMS AND SIGNS:

- Cold sensations in the body and limbs.
- Edema with scanty urine.
- Fat tongue.
- Fatigue.
- Pale complexion.
- Palpitation with nervousness.

INGREDIENTS FOR CREATING RECIPES

FOODS FOR EXCESS: celery, pea, water chestnut, peach, sunflower.

FOODS FOR DEFICIENCY: rock sugar, honey, glutinous rice, pork, sea cucumber, apple.

HERBS: Yu-zhu (Solomon's seal), Lian-zi-xin (lotus plumule), Ren-shen (Chinese ginseng), Da-zao (red date), Bai-zhu (white atractylodes), Gan-cao (licorice), Gui-zhi (cinnamon stick), Hong-hua (safflower), Tao-ren (peach kernel), Chuan-xiong (hemlock parsley), Yuan-zhi (slender-leaved milkwort), Bai-zi-ren (oriental arborvitae kernel), He-shou-wu (tuber of multiflower knotweed), Mu-li (oyster shell), Tian-nan-xing (serrated arum), Bai-ji (amethyst orchid), Wu-wei-zi (magnolia vine fruit), Wu-zhu-yu (evodia), rou-dou-kou.

Syndromes of disease and herbs to use:

1. **HEART ENERGY DEFICIENCY:** Ren-shen (Chinese ginseng), Bai-zhu (white atractylodes), Gan-cao (licorice), Gui-zhi (cinnamon stick); cook with foods for deficiency.

2. **DEFICIENCY OF ENERGY AND YIN:** Gan-cao (licorice), Gui-zhi (cinnamon stick), Da-zao (red date), Ren-shen (Chinese ginseng); cook with foods for deficiency.

3. **ENERGY DEFICIENCY AND BLOOD COAGULATION:** Ren-shen (Chinese ginseng), Bai-zhu (white atractylodes), Hong-hua (safflower), Tao-ren (peach kernel), Chuan-xiong (hemlock parsley); cook with foods for deficiency or foods for excess.

4. **YIN DEFICIENCY WITH ABUNDANT FIRE:** Yu-zhu (Solomon's seal), Lian-zi-xin (lotus plumule), Yuan-zhi (slender-leaved milk-wort), Da-zao (red date), Bai-zi-ren (oriental arborvitae kernel); cook with foods for deficiency or foods for excess.

5. **HEART-SPLEEN DEFICIENCY:** Gui-zhi (cinnamon stick), He-shou-wu (tuber of multiflower knotweed), Mu-li (oyster shell); cook with foods for deficiency.

6. **DAMP PHLEGM:** Tian-nan-xing (serrated arum), Bai-ji (amethyst orchid); cook with foods for excess.

7. **SPLEEN-KIDNEY YANG DEFICIENCY**: Wu-wei-zi (magnolia vine fruit), Wu-zhu-yu (evodia), rou-dou-kou, Ren-shen (Chinese ginseng); cook with foods for deficiency.

RECIPE 59

MASTER: 9 g Ren-shen (Chinese ginseng), 30 g Lian-zi-xin (lotus plumule).

ASSOCIATE: 30 g longan nut meat, 10 g Da-zao (red date).

ASSISTANT: 100 g polished rice.

SEASONING: white sugar (or rock sugar).

STEPS:

(1) Cut Ren-shen (Chinese ginseng) in small pieces to decoct over low heat for two hours.

(2) Boil longan nut meat, Da-zao, Lian-zi-xin, and polished rice together in water to make a congee.

(3) Combine the decoction of Ren-shen and congee.

(4) Season with white sugar.

INDICATIONS: deficiency syndromes of arrhythmia.

CONSUMPTION: Have at mealtimes.

ANALYSIS: Ren-shen is an energy tonic and heart tonic; Lian-zi-xin is an effective heart tonic and can reduce blood pressure; longan nut meat is a blood tonic; Da-zao and polished rice are energy tonics; and white sugar (or rock sugar) improves the taste.

CHAPTER

10

Urogenital System

10.1 Urinary infections

Urinary infections include pyelonephritis, urethritis, cystitis, and prostatitis.

1. Lower-Burning-Space Damp Heat Syndrome

SYMPTOMS AND SIGNS:

- Frequent desire to urinate.
- Frequent short streams of reddish-colored urine.
- Low fever in the afternoon.
- Nausea or vomiting.
- Pain on urination.
- Poor appetite.
- Seminal emission.
- Dryness in the mouth and throat but no desire to drink.
- Yellowish, turbid urine.

2. Spleen Deficiency Syndrome

SYMPTOMS AND SIGNS:

- Abdominal pain with a fondness for massage.
- Belching.
- Clear, long streams of urine.
- Diarrhea with sticky, muddy stool.
- Rectal bleeding.
- Discharge of copious sputum.
- Discharge of hard stool followed by sticky, muddy stool.
- Discharge of watery-thin stool.
- Little appetite.
- Edema.
- Overweight but little intake of food.
- Fatigue.
- Hands and feet slightly cold.
- Indigestion.
- Desire to lie down.
- No pain or burning sensation on urination.
- Prolonged diarrhea.
- Puffy eyelids.
- Underweight.

3. **Kidney Deficiency Syndrome.**

SYMPTOMS AND SIGNS:

- Chronic backache.
- Clear vaginal discharge.
- Hearing difficulty.
- Diarrhea.
- Falling hair.
- Large quantities of urine without excessive fluid intake.
- Unusual sleepiness.
- No pain or burning sensation on urination.
- Pain (falling) in the lower abdomen with fondness for massage.
- Ringing in ears.
- Ringing in ears and hearing difficulties.
- Seminal emission.
- Toothache.

INGREDIENTS FOR CREATING RECIPES

FOODS FOR EXCESS: corn, mung bean, sunflower stem.

FOODS FOR DEFICIENCY: wheat, walnut, chicken egg, pork kidney.

HERBS: Cong-bai (Welsh onion), Bai-guo (ginkgo), Che-qian-zi (Asiatic plantain seed), Long-dan-cao (gentian), Shi-wei (stony reed), Qu-mai (rainbow pink), Bian-xu (knot grass), Tong-cao (rice-paper plant), Chi-xiao-dou (small red bean [similar to azuki bean]), Jin-qian-cao (coin grass), Pu-gong-ying (Asian dandelion), Bai-zhu (white atractylodes), Shu-di (processed glutinous rehmannia).

Syndromes of disease and herbs to use:

1. **LOWER BURNING SPACE DAMP HEAT:** Che-qian-zi (Asiatic plantain seed), Long-dan-cao (gentian), Tong-cao (rice-paper plant), Chi-xiao-dou (small red bean), Shi-wei (stony reed), Bai-guo (ginkgo), Cong-bai (Welsh onion), Qu-mai (rainbow pink), Bian-xu (knot grass), Tong-cao (rice-paper plant), Jin-qian-cao (coin grass), Pu-gong-ying (Asian dandelion); cook with foods for excess.
2. **SPLEEN DEFICIENCY:** Pu-gong-ying (Asian dandelion), Bian-xu (knot grass), Bai-zhu (white atractylodes); cook with foods for deficiency.
3. **KIDNEY DEFICIENCY:** Pu-gong-ying (Asian dandelion), Bian-xu (knot grass), Shu-di (processed glutinous rehmannia); cook with foods for deficiency.

RECIPE 60

MASTER: 10 g Tong-cao (rice-paper plant).

ASSOCIATE: 50 g mung beans, soaked in water beforehand.

ASSISTANT: 50 g wheat flour.

SEASONING: rock sugar.

STEPS:

(1) Decoct Tong-cao (rice-paper plant); strain to obtain herbal soup.

(2) Boil mung beans, wheat flour, and the rock sugar in water to make a congee.

(3) Combine the congee with the herbal soup.

CONSUMPTION: have at mealtimes.

INDICATIONS: damp heat syndrome of urinary infections.

ANALYSIS: Tong-cao and mung bean can promote urination and clear heat, which is good for urinary infections due to damp heat. Wheat can also clear heat, and rock sugar improves the taste.

10.2 Cystitis (infection of the bladder)

Cystitis is mostly due to bladder damp heat.

1. **Bladder Damp Heat Syndrome**

SYMPTOMS AND SIGNS:

- Burning sensations and itch in the genital area.

- Dribbling urination.
- Incontinence of urine.
- Fatigue.
- Frequent urination.
- Pale complexion.

INGREDIENTS FOR CREATING RECIPES

FOODS FOR EXCESS: watermelon, cucumber, Chinese wax gourd, mung bean, bitter gourd (balsam pear), radish.

HERBS: Yi-yi-ren (Job's tears), Chi-xiao-dou (small red bean), Gan-cao-shao (licorice fine root), Zhu-ye (bamboo leaf), Che-qian-zi (Asiatic plantain seed), Bai-wei (white rose), Qu-mai (rainbow pink), Hua-shi (talc).

Syndrome of disease and herbs to use:

1. **BLADDER DAMP HEAT:** Yi-yi-ren (Job's tears), Chi-xiao-dou (small red bean), Gan-cao-shao (licorice fine root), Zhu-ye (bamboo leaf), Che-qian-zi (Asiatic plantain seed), Bai-wei (white rose), Qu-mai (rainbow pink), Hua-shi (talc); cook with food for excess.

RECIPE 61

MASTER: 30 g Hua-shi (talc), 10 g Qu-mai (rainbow pink).

ASSOCIATE: 100 g polished rice.

ASSISTANT: none.

SEASONING: none.

STEPS:

(1) Put Hua-shi (talc) in a gauze bag to decoct with Qu-mai (rainbow pink); strain to obtain herbal soup.

(2) Boil rice in water to make a congee.

(3) Mix congee with the herbal soup.

CONSUMPTION: have at mealtimes.

INDICATIONS: bladder damp heat syndrome of cystitis.

ANALYSIS: Hua-shi and Qu-mai can promote urination and heal cystitis; polished rice can remove dampness, which is beneficial to cystitis.

10.3 Prostatitis (inflammation of the prostate gland)

1. Damp Heat Syndrome

SYMPTOMS AND SIGNS:

- Abdominal pain.
- Abnormal perspiration.
- Burning sensations and itch in the genital area.
- Diarrhea.
- Dribbling urination.
- Dry stool.
- Pain in the eyes with watering and sensitivity to light.
- Pain in the joints.
- Pain on urination.
- Perspiration in hands, feet, or head.
- Retention of urine or discharge of reddish-colored urine.
- Distention of the lower abdomen.
- Normal or unusual thirst.

2. Yin Deficiency with Abundant Fire Syndrome

SYMPTOMS AND SIGNS:

- Dizziness.
- Dry mouth and tongue.
- Easily angry.
- Hot sensations in palms of hands and soles of feet.
- Insomnia with forgetfulness.
- Palpitation with mental depression.
- Perspiration.
- Ringing in ears.

3. Energy Congestion and Blood Coagulation Syndrome

SYMPTOMS AND SIGNS:

- Abdominal distention.
- Aching pain in the lower abdomen.
- Chronic stones.
- Colic pain on urination.
- Congested chest.
- Dribbling after urination.
- Love of sighing.
- Lump in the abdomen that stays in the same region.
- Pain across the loins or in the tail bone.
- Pain on urination.

4. Deficiency of Yin and Yang Syndrome

SYMPTOMS AND SIGNS:

- Cold limbs and cold sensations in the body.
- Fatigue.
- Frequent urination at night.
- Low energy.
- Pain in the heart.
- Palpitation.
- Perspiration with hot sensations in the body easily triggered by physical activities.
- Poor appetite.
- Poor spirits.
- Ringing in ears.
- Underweight.
- Too lazy to talk.
- Wake up at night due to pain.

INGREDIENTS FOR CREATING RECIPES

FOODS FOR EXCESS: seaweed, sunflower, torreyanut, litchi nut, common carp.

FOODS FOR DEFICIENCY: litchi nut, pork, royal jelly, duck.

HERBS: Ju-he (tangerine seed), Shan-zha (Chinese hawthorn), Dan-shen (purple sage), Hong-hua (safflower), Ze-lan (water-horehound), Tao-ren (peach kernel), Bai-zhi (angelica), Zhi-zi (gardenia), Xiao-hui-xiang (fennel seed), Da-zao (red date), Sheng-di (dried glutinous rehmannia).

Syndromes of disease and herbs to use:

1. **DAMP HEAT:** zao-xiu, Zhi-zi (gardenia), Bai-zhi (angelica); cook with foods for excess.
2. **YIN DEFICIENCY WITH ABUNDANT FIRE:** Zhi-zi (gardenia), Sheng-di (dried glutinous rehmannia); cook with foods for deficiency.
3. **ENERGY CONGESTION AND BLOOD COAGULATION:** Shan-zha (Chinese hawthorn), Dan-shen (purple sage), Hong-hua (safflower), Ze-lan (water-horehound), Tao-ren (peach kernel), Ju-he (tangerine seed); cook with foods for excess.
4. **DEFICIENCY OF YIN AND YANG:** Xiao-hui-xiang (fennel seed), Da-zao (red date); cook with foods for deficiency.

RECIPE 62

MASTER: 5 g Che-qian-zi (Asiatic plantain seed), 5 g Zhi-zi (gardenia).

ASSOCIATE: 30 g seaweed.

ASSISTANT: 25 g royal jelly.

SEASONING: none.

STEPS:

(1) Decoct Che-qian-zi (Asiatic plantain seed) and Zhi-zi (gardenia); strain to obtain herbal soup.

(2) Boil seaweed in water for a few minutes.

(3) Add royal jelly and the seaweed to the herbal soup.

CONSUMPTION: eat at mealtimes.

INDICATIONS: damp heat syndrome of prostatitis.

ANALYSIS: Che-qian-zi can remove dampness and Zhi-zi can clear heat; the two herbs work together, good for prostatitis due to damp heat. Seaweed can also eliminate dampness, and royal jelly is a yin tonic beneficial to the prostate gland. Any seasoning may be used except salt, which should be kept to a minimum.

10.4 Nephritis

1. Spleen-Dampness-Attacking-the-Lungs Syndrome

SYMPTOMS AND SIGNS:

- Abdominal distention with watery stool.
- Cough.
- Discharge of sputum that can be coughed out easily.
- Discharge of watery, white sputum.
- Weak limbs.
- Aversion to cold.
- Heavy sensations in head as if the head were wrapped up.
- Heavy sensations in the limbs and trunk.
- Inability to lie on back.
- Normal or light perspiration.
- Poor appetite.
- Severe edema particularly in the head and face and the upper half of body.
- Shortness of breath.
- Sore throat.
- Swelling of hands and feet.
- Vomiting.

2. Spleen-Kidney Yang Deficiency Syndrome

SYMPTOMS AND SIGNS:

- Extreme abdominal distension.
- Ascites.
- Physically weak and too lazy to talk.
- Cold hands and feet.
- Cold loins.
- Diarrhea before dawn.
- Diarrhea with sticky, muddy stool.
- Edema that occurs all over the body.
- Fatigue.
- Fear of cold.
- Weak limbs.
- Frequent urination with clear urine.
- Mental fatigue.
- Poor appetite.
- Scanty, clear urine.
- Sputum rumbling with shortness of breath.

3. Deficiency of Energy and Blood Syndrome

SYMPTOMS AND SIGNS:

- Abdominal swelling followed by severe edema.
- Bleeding of various kinds with light-colored blood, often seen in consumptive diseases.
- Dizziness.
- Edema manifested as a slight depression in the skin when finger pressure is applied.
- Fatigue.
- "Flying objects" in front of the eyes.
- Insomnia.
- Low energy.

- Feeble voice.
- Numbness of limbs.
- Pale complexion and lips.
- Pale nails.
- Palpitation.
- Scanty urine.

4. Liver-Kidney Yin Deficiency Syndrome

SYMPTOMS AND SIGNS:

- Blurred vision.
- Difficulty in both bowel movement and urination.
- Dizziness.
- Dry eyes.
- Dry throat.
- Fatigue.
- Headache with pain in the bony ridge forming the eyebrow.
- Lumbago.
- Night-blindness.
- Night sweats.
- Pain in the hypochondrium.
- Hot hands and soles of feet.
- Paralysis.
- Ringing in ears.
- Insomnia with forgetfulness.
- Weak loins and tibia.
- Withered complexion.

INGREDIENTS FOR CREATING RECIPES

FOODS FOR EXCESS: common or gold carp, Chinese wax gourd and its peel, black soybean, watermelon and its peel, black pepper, water spinach, day lily, prickly ash, frog, garlic.

FOODS FOR DEFICIENCY: black sesame seed, chicken egg, duck, litchi nuts.

HERBS: Shu-di (processed glutinous rehmannia), Shan-yao (Chinese yam), Yu-mi-xu (corn silk), Bai-mao-gen (cogon satintail), Dang-shen (root of pilose asiabell), Huang-qi (membranous milk vetch), Zhi-mu (wind weed), Sha-ren (grains of paradise), Bi-bo (long pepper), Shang-lu (pokeberry), Yu-xing-cao (cordate houttuynia), Sang-bai-pi (root bark of white mulberry), Yi-mu-cao (Siberian motherwort), Da-ji (Japanese thistle), Xiao-ji (cornfield thistle), Bai-zhu (white atractylodes), Hou-pu (official magnolia), Mu-xiang (costus root), Dang-gui (Chinese angelica), Bai-shao (white peony), Wu-mei (black plum), Chi-xiao-dou (small red bean), Sheng-di (dried glutinous rehmannia).

Syndromes of disease and herbs to use:

1. **SPLEEN-DAMPNESS-ATTACKING-THE-LUNGS:** Dang-shen (root of pilose asiabell), Huang-qi (membranous milk vetch), Sha-ren (grains of paradise), yumixu, Sha-ren (grains of paradise), Shang-lu (pokeberry), Yu-xing-cao (cordate houttuynia), Sang-bai-pi (root bark of white mulberry), Yi-mu-cao (Siberian motherwort), Da-ji (Japanese thistle), Xiao-ji (cornfield thistle), Chi-xiao-dou (small red bean); cook with foods for excess.
2. **SPLEEN-KIDNEY YANG DEFICIENCY:** Bi-bo (long pepper), Bai-zhu (white atractylodes), Hou-pu (official magnolia), Mu-xiang (costus root); cook with foods for deficiency.
3. **DEFICIENCY OF ENERGY AND BLOOD:** Shu-di (processed glutinous rehmannia), Dang-gui (Chinese angelica), Bai-zhu (white atractylodes), Bai-shao (white peony); cook with foods for deficiency.
4. **LIVER-KIDNEY YIN DEFICIENCY:** Shu-di (processed glutinous rehmannia), Sheng-di (dried glutinous rehmannia), Bai-shao (white peony), Wu-mei (black plum); cook with foods for deficiency.

RECIPE 63

MASTER: 15 g Sang-bai-pi (root bark of white mulberry), 60 g Chi-xiao-dou (small red bean), soaked ahead of time.

ASSOCIATE: none.

ASSISTANT: none.

SEASONING: none.

STEPS:

(1) Decoct Sang-bai-pi; strain to obtain herbal soup.

(2) Boil Chi-xiao-dou in water until cooked.

(3) Add the herbal soup to the beans.

CONSUMPTION: eat the beans and drink the soup.

INDICATIONS: spleen dampness syndrome of nephritis.

ANALYSIS: Both Sang-bai-pi and Chi-xiao-dou can promote water flow and heal nephritis. (Note that the two ingredients take some time to cook, because Sang-bai-pi is the bark of a tree, and Chi-ziao-dou is a bean.) As in this case, a recipe may contain only master ingredients; it need not contain all four categories of ingredients.

10.5 Urinary stones

Urinary stones usually manifest as pain across the loins, abdominal pain, pricking pain on urination, and blood in the urine.

1. Lower-Burning-Space Damp Heat Syndrome

SYMPTOMS AND SIGNS:

- Pain affecting the lower abdomen or radiating toward the genitals.
- Colic pain in the abdomen and across the loins.
- Dribbling after urination.
- Frequent desire to urinate.
- Frequent urination with short, reddish-colored streams.
- Low fever in the afternoon.
- Nausea or vomiting.
- Pain on urination.
- Poor appetite.
- Seminal emission.
- Dry throat and mouth with no desire to drink.
- Yellowish, turbid urine.

2. Energy Congestion and Blood Coagulation Syndrome

SYMPTOMS AND SIGNS:

- Abdominal distention.
- Aching pain in the lower abdomen.
- Chronic stones.
- Colic pain on urination.
- Congested chest.
- Dribbling after urination.
- Love of sighing.
- Lump in the abdomen that stays in the same region.
- Pain across the loins.
- Pain on urination.

3. Spleen-Kidney Yang Deficiency Syndrome

SYMPTOMS AND SIGNS:

- Chronic stones.
- Cold hands and feet.
- Cold loins.
- Diarrhea before dawn.
- Diarrhea with sticky, muddy stool.
- Eating little.
- Edema that occurs all over the body.
- Fatigue.

- Aversion to cold.
- Weak limbs.
- Frequent clear urination.
- Mental fatigue.
- Sputum rumbling with shortness of breath.

INGREDIENTS FOR CREATING RECIPES

FOODS FOR EXCESS: corn, corn root and leaf, day lily root, sunflower stem, radish.

FOODS FOR DEFICIENCY: walnut, sesame oil, rock sugar, honey.

HERBS: Shi-wei (stony reed), Han-lian-cao (ink plant), Jin-qian-cao (coin grass), Yu-mi-xu (corn silk), Di-fu-zi (summer cypress), Che-qian-zi (Asiatic plantain seed), Hua-shi (talc), Bai-mao-gen (cogon satintail), Da-zao (red date).

Syndromes of disease and herbs to use:

1. **LOWER-BURNING-SPACE DAMP HEAT:** Shi-wei (stony reed), yumixu, Di-fu-zi (summer cypress), Che-qian-zi (Asiatic plantain seed), Hua-shi (talc), Bai-mao-gen (cogon satintail); cook with foods for excess.

2. **ENERGY CONGESTION AND BLOOD COAGULATION:** Di-fu-zi (summer cypress); cook with foods for excess.

3. **SPLEEN-KIDNEY YANG DEFICIENCY:** Han-lian-cao (ink plant), Da-zao (red date); cook with foods for deficiency.

RECIPE 64

MASTER: 30 g Yu-mi-xu (corn silk), 30 Bai-mao-gen (cogon satintail).

ASSOCIATE: 100 g polished rice.

ASSISTANT: 5 g Da-zao (red date).

SEASONING: none.

STEPS:

(1) Decoct Yu-mi-xu (corn silk) and Bai-mao-gen (cogon satintail), strain to obtain herbal soup.

(2) Remove seeds from Da-zao (red date).

(3) Boil polished rice and Da-zao (red date) in water to make a congee.

(4) Mix congee with the herbal soup.

CONSUMPTION: eat at mealtime.

INDICATIONS: damp heat syndrome of urinary stone.

ANALYSIS: Yu-mi-xu is effective for the treatment of gallstones and urinary stones; Bai-mao-gen can promote urination and expel urinary stones; polished rice can remove dampness; and Da-zao is an energy tonic.

10.6 Impotence

1. Deficiency Fire Syndrome

SYMPTOMS AND SIGNS:

- Cough with blood.
- Dry cough without sputum.
- Cough with sticky phlegm.
- Dry sensations in the mouth or throat.
- Feeling depressed.
- Forgetfulness.
- Hot sensations in body, center of hands and feet, warm skin and muscles.
- Illness attacks slowly but with a longer duration (chronic illness).
- Light but periodic fever not unlike the tide.
- Night sweats.
- Sore throat
- Ringing in ears.
- Seminal emission with dreams.
- Insomnia.
- Sore loins.
- Sputum with blood.
- Strong sexual desire with premature ejaculation.
- Toothache.

2. Spleen Deficiency Syndrome

SYMPTOMS AND SIGNS:

- Chronic diarrhea.
- Chronic dysentery.
- Lack of firm erection.
- Poor appetite.
- Prolapse of any internal organ.
- Prolapse of rectum.
- Shortness of breath.

3. Kidney Yang Deficiency Syndrome

SYMPTOMS AND SIGNS:

- Cold feet, cold loins and legs, or cold sensations in the genital area.
- Diarrhea before dawn.
- Diarrhea that consists of sticky, muddy stool.
- Dizziness.
- Edema.
- Excessive perspiration.
- Fatigue.
- Frequent urination at night.
- Panting.
- Perspiration in the forehead.
- Retention of urine.
- Ringing in ears.
- Scanty urine.
- Seminal emission.
- Shortness of breath.

INGREDIENTS FOR CREATING RECIPES

FOODS FOR DEFICIENCY: sparrow, lobster, Chinese chive, walnut, sparrow egg, mutton, sea cucumber, mussel, shrimp, oyster, loach, pork, mutton, sea cucumber.

HERBS: Ge-jie (gecko), Zhi-mu (wind weed), Huang-bai (cork tree), Sheng-di (dried glutinous rehmannia), Bai-zhu (white atractylodes), Shan-yao (Chinese yam), Tu-si-zi (dodder seed), She-chuang-zi (snake bed seeds), Du-zhong (eucommia bark), Yin-yang-huo (longspur epimendium).

Syndromes of disease and herbs to use:

1. **DEFICIENCY FIRE:** Zhi-mu (wind weed), Huang-bai (cork tree), Sheng-di (dried glutinous rehmannia); cook with foods for excess or foods for deficiency.
2. **SPLEEN DEFICIENCY:** Bai-zhu (white atractylodes), Shan-yao (Chinese yam); cook with foods for deficiency.
3. **KIDNEY YANG DEFICIENCY:** Tu-si-zi (dodder seed), She-chuang-zi (snake bed seeds), Du-zhong (eucommia bark), Yin-yang-huo (longspur epimendium); cook with foods for deficiency.

RECIPE 65

MASTER: 15 g Du-zhong (eucommia bark).

ASSOCIATE: 100 g walnuts.

ASSISTANT: rice wine.

SEASONING: brown sugar.

STEPS:

(1) Grind Du-zhong (eucommia bark) into a powder.

(2) Crush walnuts into small pieces to mix with the herbal powder.

(3) Add two spoonfuls of water to the mixture and steam until cooked. Add rice wine and steam for another two minutes.

(4) Season with brown sugar.

CONSUMPTION: divide into three servings. Have one serving per day to be taken hot before bedtime.

INDICATION: kidney yang deficiency syndrome of impotence.

ANALYSIS: Du-zhong is a highly effective kidney yang tonic to strengthen erection; walnut is also a kidney yang tonic to reinforce the effect of Du-zhong; rice wine is to speed up the effect of the other ingredients; and brown sugar improves the taste.

10.7 Seminal emission and premature ejaculation

1. Deficiency Fire Syndrome

SYMPTOMS AND SIGNS:

- Coughing with blood.
- Dry cough without sputum.
- Coughing with sticky phlegm.
- Dry sensations in the mouth.
- Dry throat.
- Feeling miserable.
- Forgetfulness.
- Hot sensations in body, center of hands and feet, warm skin and muscles.
- Illness attacks slowly but with a longer duration (chronic illness).
- Light but periodic fever not unlike the tide.
- Night sweats.
- Pain in the throat.
- Ringing in ears.
- Seminal emission with erotic dreams.
- Insomnia.
- Lumbago.
- Sputum with blood.
- Toothache.

2. Superficial Damp Heat Syndrome

SYMPTOMS AND SIGNS:

- Abdominal pain.
- Burning sensation and itch in the genital area or burning sensation in the anus.
- Congested chest.
- Diarrhea that consists of forceful discharge of stool.
- Discharge of yellowish red stool, turbid and with a foul odor.
- Edema.
- Semen and urine mixed during ejaculation.
- Excessive perspiration, especially in the hands, feet, or face.
- Frequent itch and pain in the genital region.
- Low fever.
- Pain in the joints, with swelling and heaviness.
- Pain inside the penis.
- Reddish scanty urine.
- Retention of urine.
- Seminal emission that occurs frequently.
- Thirst.

3. Kidney Yin Deficiency Syndrome

SYMPTOMS AND SIGNS:

- Cold extremeties.
- Cough with sputum containing blood or coughing out fresh blood.
- Loss of hearing.
- Dizziness.
- Dry mouth or throat.
- Fatigue.
- Depression and anxiety, with fever.
- Fever at night with burning sensations in internal organs.
- Hot sensations in any part of the body.

- Night sweats.
- Pain in the heel.
- Lumbago.
- Pain in the tibia.
- Ringing in ears.
- Seminal emission mostly without dreams.
- Insomnia.
- Sore loins and weak legs.
- Spots in front of the eyes.
- Thirst.
- Toothache or loose teeth.

4. Kidney Energy Deficiency Syndrome

SYMPTOMS AND SIGNS:

- Cold sensations in the genital area.
- Hearing loss.
- Dizziness.
- Fatigue.
- Headache.
- Impotence.
- Lumbago.
- Prolonged dizziness.
- Ringing in ears.
- Seminal emission that occurs spontaneously as if semen were seeping out.

INGREDIENTS FOR CREATING RECIPES

FOODS FOR EXCESS: radish, day lily, yellow soybean, cucumber, seaweed, carrot.

FOODS FOR DEFICIENCY: rock sugar, oyster, shrimp, duck, sea cucumber, walnut, mussel, pork kidney, glutinous rice, chicken, longan nut.

HERBS: Rou-cong-rong (saline cistanche), Fu-pen-zi (wild raspberry), Wu-wei-zi (magnolia vine fruit), Zhi-mu (wind weed), Qian-shi (water lily), Shan-yao (Chinese yam), Lian-zi (East Indian lotus), Huang-bai (cork tree), Sheng-di (dried glutinous rehmannia), Shan-zhu-yu (fruit of medicinal cornel).

Syndromes of disease and herbs to use:

1. **DEFICIENCY FIRE:** Zhi-mu (wind weed), Huang-bai (cork tree), Sheng-di (dried glutinous rehmannia); cook with foods for excess or foods for deficiency.
2. **SUPERFICIAL DAMP HEAT:** Huang-bai (cork tree), Lian-zi (East Indian lotus); cook with foods for excess.
3. **KIDNEY YIN DEFICIENCY:** Fu-pen-zi (wild raspberry), Wu-wei-zi (magnolia vine fruit), Qian-shi (water lily), Shan-yao (Chinese yam); cook with foods for deficiency.
4. **KIDNEY ENERGY DEFICIENCY:** Rou-cong-rong (saline cistanche), Fu-pen-zi (wild raspberry), Wu-wei-zi (magnolia vine fruit), Qian-shi (water lily), Shan-yao (Chinese yam); cook with foods for deficiency.

RECIPE 66

MASTER: 15 g Lian-zi (East Indian lotus).

ASSOCIATE: 30 g glutinous rice.

ASSISTANT: 5 g brown sugar.

SEASONING: none.

STEPS:

(1) Grind Lian-zi (East Indian lotus) into powder.

(2) Boil together the Lian-zi powder, glutinous rice, and brown sugar in 3 cups of water to make a congee.

CONSUMPTION: eat on an empty stomach.

INDICATIONS: deficiency syndromes of seminal emission.

ANALYSIS: Lian-zi can control seminal emission and urination through its constrictive effects. Glutinous rice is sticky in nature, also able to constrict semen to check seminal emission. Brown sugar is a spleen tonic. No seasoning is required because the recipe tastes quite good as is.

RECIPE 67

MASTER: 5 g Huang-bai (cork tree).

ASSOCIATE: 50 g radish.

ASSISTANT: 50 g yellow soybeans, soaked beforehand.

SEASONING: salt.

STEPS:

(1) Boil Huang-bai (cork tree), radish, and yellow soybeans together in enough water until cooked.

(2) Remove Huang-bai (cork tree) from the soup. Add salt to taste.

CONSUMPTION: eat the radish and yellow soybeans, and drink the soup at mealtimes.

INDICATIONS: damp heat syndrome of seminal emission.

ANALYSIS: Huang-bai can remove damp heat; radish has a cool energy, which can assist Huang-bai in clearing heat; and yellow soybean can eliminate dampness. Salt is to clear heat and improve taste.

10.8 Blood in urine

1. **Heart Fire Syndrome**

SYMPTOMS AND SIGNS:

- Bleeding from gums.
- Burning sensations on urination.
- Cold hands and feet.
- Bleeding from the mouth.
- Dribbling after urination.
- Feeling depressed.
- Hot sensations in the center of the palms.
- Morning sickness.
- Mouth canker.
- Drowsy.
- Palpitation.
- Ulcer on the tongue and canker in the mouth.
- Seminal emission.
- Short streams of urine.
- Insomnia.
- Bloody urine that is bright-red.
- Yellowish red urine.

2. **Damp Heat Syndrome**

SYMPTOMS AND SIGNS:

- Abdominal pain.
- Burning sensation and itch in the genital area.
- Congested chest.
- Diarrhea.
- Low fever.
- Fresh, red-colored bloody urine.
- Perspiration in hands and feet.
- Reddish, scanty urine.
- Inability to urinate normally.
- Short streams of reddish urine.
- Swollen tongue.
- Unusual thirst.

3. **Deficiency of Energy and Blood Syndrome**

SYMPTOMS AND SIGNS:

- Bleeding of various kinds with light-colored blood, often seen in consumptive diseases.
- Dizziness.
- Fatigue.
- "Flying objects" in front of the eyes.
- Insomnia.
- Low energy.
- Feeble voice.

- No burning sensation on urination.
- Numbness in the limbs.
- Pale complexion and lips.
- Pale nails.
- Palpitation.

4. Kidney Deficiency Syndrome

SYMPTOMS AND SIGNS:

- Asthma.
- Chronic backache.
- Clear, watery vaginal discharge.
- Hearing loss.
- Diarrhea.
- Unusual hair loss.
- Large quantities of urine with no thirst or drink.
- Unusual sleepiness.
- No burning sensation on urination.
- Pain (falling) in the lower abdomen with fondness for massage.
- Ringing in ears.
- Ringing in ears and hearing loss.
- Seminal emission.
- Toothache.

INGREDIENTS FOR CREATING RECIPES

FOODS FOR EXCESS: gold carp, persimmon, spinach, peanut, lotus root, radish, cucumber.

FOODS FOR DEFICIENCY: chestnut, sea cucumber, sugar cane, beef, chicken, duck.

HERBS: Lian-zi (East Indian lotus), Bai-mao-gen (cogon satintail), Mu-tong (akebi), Dan-pi (peony), Zhi-zi (gardenia), da-ji, Xiao-ji (cornfield thistle), Huang-bai (cork tree), Shi-wei (stony reed), Huang-qi (membranous milk vetch), Shu-di (processed glutinous rehmannia), Shan-zhu-yu (fruit of medicinal cornel).

Syndromes of disease and herbs to use:

1. **HEART FIRE:** Lian-zi (East Indian lotus), Bai-mao-gen (cogon satintail), Mu-tong (akebi), Dan-pi (peony), Zhi-zi (gardenia), Shi-wei (stony reed); cook with foods for excess.
2. **DAMP HEAT FLOWING DOWNWARD:** Lian-zi (East Indian lotus), Bai-mao-gen (cogon satintail), Mu-tong (akebi), Dan-pi (peony), Zhi-zi (gardenia), da-ji, Xiao-ji (cornfield thistle), Huang-bai (cork tree), Shi-wei (stony reed); cook with foods for excess.
3. **DEFICIENCY OF ENERGY AND BLOOD:** Huang-qi (membranous milk vetch), Dang-gui (Chinese angelica), Bai-zhu (white atractylodes); cook with foods for deficiency.
4. **KIDNEY DEFICIENCY:** Shu-di (processed glutinous rehmannia), Shan-zhu-yu (fruit of medicinal cornel); cook with foods for deficiency.

RECIPE 68

MASTER: 30 g Lian-zi (East Indian lotus).

ASSOCIATE: 30 g peanuts.

ASSISTANT: 30 g chestnuts.

SEASONING: white sugar.

STEPS:

(1) Boil chestnuts in enough water for ten minutes.

(2) Add Lian-zi (East Indian lotus) and peanuts and cook over low heat for about an hour. Add 1 teaspoonful of white sugar and bring to a boil again until the sugar has dissolved.

CONSUMPTION: have with meals.

INDICATIONS: heart fire syndrome of blood in urine.

ANALYSIS: Lian-zi can control bleeding through its constrictive effect; peanut is a common food to stop bleeding; chestnut can activate the blood and also stop bleeding; and white sugar improves the taste.

10.9 Diminished urination

1. **Hot Lung Syndrome**

SYMPTOMS AND SIGNS:

- Acute panting in a high-pitched sound and rapid expiration.
- Bitter taste in the mouth.
- Cough and vomit with pus and/or blood, accompanied by a foul odor.
- Coughing out yellowish, sticky sputum.
- Dry stools.
- Dripping of urine with difficult urination.
- Dry sensations in the mouth.
- Flaring nostrils.
- Hot sensations in the body.
- Light but periodic fever not unlike the tide.
- Nosebleed.
- Pain in the chest.
- Sore throat.
- Sore throat with dry sensations, and exhaling hot air from the nose.
- Paralysis.
- Presence of sputum that cannot be dislodged.
- Mental depression.
- Swollen, red throat.
- Urgent panting.

2. **Heart Fire Syndrome**

SYMPTOMS AND SIGNS:

- Bleeding from gums.
- Cold hands and feet.
- Difficult urination with reddish or very yellowish urine.
- Discharge of blood from the mouth.
- Dribbling after urination.
- Feeling depressed.
- Hot sensations in the center of palms.
- Mouth canker.
- Drowsy.
- Pain on urination.
- Palpitation.
- Ulcer on the tongue and canker in the mouth.
- Seminal emission.
- Insomnia.
- Abnormal thirst.

3. **Superficial Damp Heat Syndrome**

SYMPTOMS AND SIGNS:

- Burning sensation and itch in the genital area or burning sensation in the anus.
- Burning sensation on urination.
- Diarrhea with forceful discharge of stool.
- Discharge of yellowish red stool, turbid and with a foul odor.
- Edema.
- Excessive perspiration.
- Feeling depressed.
- Frequent itch and pain in the vulva.
- Low fever.
- Pain in the joints, with swelling and heaviness.
- Paralysis.
- Unusual perspiration in hands, feet, or in the face.
- Infrequent urination.
- Scanty, turbid urine.
- Short streams of reddish urine.
- Swollen tongue.
- Abnormal thirst.

4. **Energy Deficiency Syndrome**

SYMPTOMS AND SIGNS:

- Abdominal pain.
- Constipation with discharge of soft stools.
- Discharge of sticky, turbid stools or diarrhea.
- Dizziness.
- Fatigue following bowel movement.
- Headache (severe) that occurs after physical labor.
- Periodic headaches, headaches in the morning, or prolonged headaches.
- Inability to sit up from a reclining position without dizziness.
- Blurred vision.
- Numbness.
- Palpitation with anxiety.
- Perspiration in hands and feet.
- Ringing in ears that causes loss of hearing.
- Tremor in hands.
- Shortness of breath.
- Underweight with dry skin.
- Swallowing difficulty.
- Feeble voice.
- Slightly cold extremities.

5. **Excessive-Heat-in-the-Bladder Syndrome**

SYMPTOMS AND SIGNS:

- Discharge of urine containing pus and blood.
- Muddy urine.
- Obstructed, diminished urination.
- Pain (hot) inside the genitals on urination.
- Pain in lower abdomen with feeling of hardness and fullness.
- Yellowish red urine.

6. **Blood Coagulation Syndrome**

SYMPTOMS AND SIGNS:

- Abdominal pain.
- Bleeding from gums.
- Chest pain.
- Coughing with blood.
- Headache.
- Lumbago.
- Pain (acute) around umbilicus resisting massage, with palpable hard spots.
- Pain in region between navel and pubic hair with feeling of hardness.
- Pain in the hypochondrium.
- Pain in the loins as if being pierced with an awl.
- Pain in the ribs.
- Palpitation with anxiety.
- Partial suppression of lochia.
- Spasm.
- Stomachache.
- Swelling and congestion after eating.
- Vomiting of blood.

7. **Kidney Yang Deficiency Syndrome**

SYMPTOMS AND SIGNS:

- Chronic diarrhea.
- Coldness in the feet, legs, genital or lower hip area, or in the muscles.
- Cough and labored breathing.
- Diarrhea before dawn.
- Diarrhea with sticky, muddy stool.
- Discharge of watery-thin stool.
- Dizziness.
- Edema.

- Fatigue.
- Frequent urination at night.
- Cold extremities.
- Impotence.
- Infertility.
- Lack of appetite.
- Pain in the loins (lumbago).
- Palpitation.
- Panting.
- Perspiration in the forehead.
- Ringing in ears.
- Scanty urine.

INGREDIENTS FOR CREATING RECIPES

FOODS FOR EXCESS: watermelon, kidney bean, tofu, mung bean sprouts, wheat cucumber, carrot.

FOODS FOR DEFICIENCY: kidney bean, tofu, wheat, mutton, beef.

HERBS: Xiao-hui-xiang (fennel seed), Cong-bai (Welsh onion), Fu-ling (tuckahoe; Indian bread), Che-qian-zi (Asiatic plantain seed), Bai-zhu (white atractylodes), Hua-shi (talc), Qu-mai (rainbow pink), Sheng-di (dried glutinous rehmannia), Mu-tong (akebi), Dan-zhu-ye (light bamboo leaf).

Syndromes of disease and herbs to use:

1. **HOT LUNGS:** Hua-shi (talc), Qu-mai (rainbow pink), Sheng-di (dried glutinous rehmannia); cook with foods for excess.
2. **HEART FIRE:** Sheng-di (dried glutinous rehmannia), Mu-tong (akebi), Dan-zhu-ye (light bamboo leaf); cook with foods for excess.
3. **SUPERFICIAL DAMP HEAT:** Cong-bai (Welsh onion), Fu-ling (tuckahoe; Indian bread), Che-qian-zi (Asiatic plantain seed), Mu-tong (akebi); cook with foods for excess.
4. **ENERGY DEFICIENCY:** Fu-ling (tuckahoe; Indian bread), Bai-zhu (white atractylodes), Sheng-di (dried glutinous rehmannia); cook with foods for deficiency.
5. **EXCESSIVE-HEAT-IN-THE-BLADDER:** Fu-ling (tuckahoe; Indian bread), Che-qian-zi (Asiatic plantain seed), Hua-shi (talc), Qu-mai (rainbow pink), Sheng-di (dried glutinous rehmannia), Mu-tong (akebi); cook with foods for excess.
6. **BLOOD COAGULATION:** Xiao-hui-xiang (fennel seed), Fu-ling (tuckahoe; Indian bread); cook with foods for excess.
7. **KIDNEY YANG DEFICIENCY:** Xiao-hui-xiang (fennel seed), Bai-zhu (white atractylodes); cook with foods for deficiency.

RECIPE 69

MASTER: 15 g Sheng-di (dried glutinous rehmannia), 6 g Mu-tong (akebi), 9 g Dan-zhu-ye (light bamboo leaf).

ASSOCIATE: 50 g tofu.

ASSISTANT: 50 g wheat flour.

SEASONING: none.

STEPS:

(1) Decoct the three master ingredients; strain to obtain herbal soup.

(2) Boil tofu and wheat flour in water until cooked, then add the herbal soup.

CONSUMPTION: eat the tofu and drink the soup.

INDICATIONS: all syndromes of diminished urination and urination difficulty.

ANALYSIS: Sheng-di can clear heat and tone blood; Mu-tong can promote urination; Dan-zhu-ye can clear heat and promote urination; tofu can produce fluids and also promote urination; and wheat can clear heat and strengthen the kidneys. No seasoning is listed, since the recipe tastes quite good as is.

10.10 Enuresis (incontinent urination)

1. Spleen-Lung Energy Deficiency Syndrome

SYMPTOMS AND SIGNS:

- Abdominal swelling.
- Coughing with sputum and saliva.
- Decreased appetite.
- Diarrhea with sticky, muddy stool.
- Discharge of copious, clear, watery sputum.
- Eating little, accompanied by indigestion.
- Weak limbs.
- Fatigue.
- Frequent desire to urinate.
- Prolonged coughing.
- Rapid panting.
- Shortness of breath.
- Underweight.
- Dribbling of urine.

2. Kidney Energy Deficiency Syndrome

SYMPTOMS AND SIGNS:

- Hearing loss.
- Dizziness.
- Dribbling after urination.
- Fatigue.
- Frequent, scanty urination.
- Headache.
- Impotence.
- Lumbago.
- Prolonged dizziness.
- Ringing in ears.
- Seminal emission.

3. Looseness of Kidney Energy Syndrome

SYMPTOMS AND SIGNS:

- Bed-wetting.
- Clear, long streams of urine.
- Dizziness.
- Dribbling urination.
- Fatigue.
- Frequent urination, particularly at night.
- Incontinence of urine.
- Pain and softness in the loins and knees.
- Premature ejaculation.
- Ringing in ears.
- Seminal emission without erotic dreams.
- Abnormal vaginal discharge or between-menstruation bleeding.

INGREDIENTS FOR CREATING RECIPES

FOODS FOR DEFICIENCY: pork, beef, shiitake mushroom, shrimp.

HERBS: Fu-pen-zi (wild raspberry), Tian-hua-fen (Chinese trichosanthes), Bai-guo (ginkgo), Qian-shi (water lily), Lian-xu (lotus stamen).

Syndromes of disease and herbs to use:

1. **SPLEEN-LUNG ENERGY DEFICIENCY**: Tian-hua-fen (Chinese trichosanthes); cook with foods for deficiency.
2. **KIDNEY ENERGY DEFICIENCY:** Fu-pen-zi (wild raspberry); cook with foods for deficiency.
3. **LOOSENESS OF KIDNEY ENERGY:** Bai-guo (ginkgo), Qian-shi (water lily), Lian-xu (lotus stamen); cook with foods for deficiency.

RECIPE 70

MASTER: 100 g shiitake mushrooms.

ASSOCIATE: 100 g lean pork.

ASSISTANT: 5 g rice wine.

SEASONING: white sugar, sesame oil, soy sauce, salt, rice starch, corn oil.

STEPS:

(1) Wash shiitake mushroom and cut up the pork.

(2) Combine the sugar, sesame oil, soy sauce, salt, and rice starch (to taste) with enough water to make a seasoning juice.

(3) Put a little corn oil into a frying pan, add shiitake mushroom and pork and sauté over high heat for 15 minutes, adding the rice wine 10 to 20 seconds before removing from heat. Add seasoning juice.

CONSUMPTION: eat at mealtimes.

INDICATIONS: all syndromes of enuresis and incontinence of urination.

ANALYSIS: Shiitake mushroom can strengthen the kidneys and bone marrow to increase control over urination; lean pork is a yin tonic and acts on the kidneys; and rice wine speeds up the actions of the mushrooms and pork. Seasonings are designed to improve the taste.

CHAPTER 11

Blood, Endocrine, and Metabolism

11.1 Anemia

1. Heart-Spleen Deficiency Syndrome

SYMPTOMS AND SIGNS:

- Abdominal swelling.
- Bleeding symptoms.
- Watery-thin stools.
- Dizziness.
- Eating little.
- Fatigue.
- Forgetfulness.
- Impotence.
- Feeble voice.
- Nervousness.
- Night sweats.
- Palpitation.
- Poor appetite.
- Shortness of breath.
- Insomnia.
- Sallow, yellowish complexion.

2. Liver-Kidney Yin Deficiency Syndrome

SYMPTOMS AND SIGNS:

- Difficulty in both bowel movement and urination.
- Dizziness.
- Dry eyes or throat.
- Fatigue.
- Headache with pain in the bony ridge forming the eyebrow.
- Lumbago.
- Night-blindness.
- Night sweats.
- Pain in the hypochondrium.
- Hot hands and feet.
- Blood-shot eyes.
- Ringing in ears.
- Insomnia with forgetfulness.
- Withered complexion.
- Zygomatic regions on both sides appear tender and red.

3. Spleen-Kidney Yang Deficiency Syndrome

SYMPTOMS AND SIGNS:

- Cold hands and feet.
- Cold loins (lower back).
- Diarrhea before dawn.
- Diarrhea with sticky, muddy stool.
- Eating little.
- Edema that occurs all over the body.
- Fatigue.
- Aversion to cold.
- Weakness in the four limbs.
- Frequent, clear urination.
- Mental fatigue.
- Pale complexion.
- Palpitation.
- Poor appetite.
- Puffy face.
- Sputum rumbling with panting.

INGREDIENTS FOR CREATING RECIPES

FOODS FOR EXCESS: yellow soybean, litchi nut.

FOODS FOR DEFICIENCY: longan nut, glutinous rice, litchi nut, honey, pork liver, sheep or goat liver.

HERBS: Sang-shen (mulberry), Gou-qi-zi (matrimony vine fruit), Da-zao (red date), Ren-shen (Chinese ginseng), Dang-shen (root of pilose asiabell), Huang-qi (membranous milk vetch), Dang-gui (Chinese angelica), He-shou-wu (tuber of multiflower knotweed), E-jiao (donkey-hide gelatin).

Syndromes of disease and herbs to use:

1. **HEART-SPLEEN DEFICIENCY:** Sang-shen (mulberry), Gou-qi-zi (matrimony vine fruit), Da-zao (red date), Ren-shen (Chinese ginseng), Huang-qi (membranous milk vetch), Dang-shen (root of pilose asiabell); cook with foods for deficiency.
2. **LIVER-KIDNEY YIN DEFICIENCY:** Sang-shen (mulberry), Gou-qi-zi (matrimony vine fruits), Da-zao (red date), Dang-gui (Chinese angelica), He-shou-wu (tuber of multiflower knotweed); cook with foods for deficiency.
3. **SPLEEN-KIDNEY YANG DEFICIENCY:** Ren-shen (Chinese ginseng), Dang-shen (root of pilose asiabell), Huang-qi (membranous milk vetch), Dang-gui (Chinese angelica), He-shou-wu (tuber of multiflower knotweed); cook with foods for deficiency.

RECIPE 71

MASTER: 3 g Ren-shen (Chinese ginseng).

ASSOCIATE: 10 g Da-zao (red date).

ASSISTANT: none.

SEASONING: none.

STEPS:

Steam Da-zao (red date) until soft, remove seeds, then add Ren-shen (Chinese ginseng) to also steam until soft.

CONSUMPTION: eat at mealtimes.

INDICATIONS: all syndromes of anemia.

ANALYSIS: Both Ren-shen and Da-zao are energy tonics. They can cure anemia by increasing a person's energy; blood will be produced through the action of energy. This principle is called "yin comes from yang, yang comes from yin." Energy is yang, blood is yin.

RECIPE 72

MASTER: 10 g Gou-qi-zi (matrimony vine fruit).

ASSOCIATE: 10 g longan nut meat.

ASSISTANT: 30 g cherry.

SEASONING: white sugar.

STEPS:

(1) Boil Gou-qi-zi (matrimony vine fruit) and longan nut meat until they are plump. Add the cherries and boil again.

(2) Season with white sugar to taste.

INDICATIONS: all syndromes of anemia.

ANALYSIS: Gou-qi-zi is a yin tonic; longan nut is a blood tonic; cherry is an energy tonic, which supplements the blood tonic; and white sugar improves the taste.

11.2 Goiter

1. Liver Energy Congestion Syndrome

SYMPTOMS AND SIGNS:

- Abdominal obstruction.
- Abdominal pain.
- Bitter taste in the mouth.
- Convulsion.
- Dry tongue.
- Easily angered.
- Insomnia.
- Numbness.
- Pain in the hypochondrium.
- Poor appetite.
- Stomachache.
- Sensation of obstruction in the throat.
- Vomiting of blood.

2. Damp Phlegm Syndrome

SYMPTOMS AND SIGNS:

- Abdominal swelling with congested chest.
- Cough with excessive sputum.
- Dizziness with heavy sensations in the head.
- Nausea.
- Palpitation with anxiety.
- Poor appetite.

INGREDIENTS FOR CREATING RECIPES

FOODS FOR EXCESS: laver, seaweed, kelp, seagrass, saltwater clam, mussel.

HERBS: Xia-ku-cao (self heal), Xiang-fu (nutgrass flatsedge rhizome), Hai-piao-xiao (cuttlebone), Huang-yao-zi (Ceylon white yam), Mu-li (oyster shell).

Syndromes of disease and herbs to use:

1. **LIVER ENERGY CONGESTION:** Huang-yao-zi (Ceylon white yam), Xia-ku-cao (self heal), Hai-piao-xiao (cuttlebone), Xiang-fu (nutgrass flatsedge rhizome); cook with foods for excess.
2. **DAMP PHLEGM:** Huang-yao-zi (Ceylon white yam), Hai-piao-xiao (cuttlebone), Mu-li (oyster shell); cook with foods for excess.

RECIPE 73

MASTER: 10 g Huang-yao-zi (Ceylon white yam).

ASSOCIATE: 50 g jellyfish skin.

ASSISTANT: seaweed.

SEASONING: salt.

STEPS:

(1) Decoct Huang-yao-zi (Ceylon white yam) in water for 30 minutes; strain to obtain soup.

(2) Cut up jellyfish skin into small pieces and wash them in cold water.

(3) Boil seaweed for two minutes and drain.

(4) Mix jellyfish skin and seaweed into the herbal soup.

(3) Season with salt to taste.

CONSUMPTION: makes 2 servings to be consumed in one day.

INDICATION: both syndromes of goiter.

ANALYSIS: In the West, goiter is due to a lack of iodine in the diet, but Huang-yao-zi is an effective herb to treat goiter while containing no iodine. Jellyfish skin removes sputum, which is the cause of goiter; seaweed cures goiter because it can soften up hardness from the Chinese point of view; while salt also can soften up hardness.

11.3 Hyperthyroidism

1. Hot Stomach Syndrome

SYMPTOMS AND SIGNS:

- Bad breath.
- Bleeding from gums.
- Easily hungry.
- Swollen gums.
- Hiccups.
- Nosebleed.
- Pain in the gums with swelling.
- Sore throat.
- Perspiring in the head.
- Underweight.
- Stomachache.
- Thirst and craving for cold drinks.
- Vomiting with blood.
- Vomiting right after eating.

2. Liver Energy Congestion Syndrome

SYMPTOMS AND SIGNS:

- Abdominal obstruction.
- Abdominal pain.
- Convulsion.
- Insomnia.
- Numbness.
- Pain in the hypochondrium.
- Psychological tension.
- Stomachache.
- Subjective sensations of objects in the throat.
- Swollen tonsils.
- Vomiting of blood.
- Frequent anxiety.

3. Sputum Fire Syndrome

SYMPTOMS AND SIGNS:

- Aversion to heat.
- Big appetite.
- Easily frustrated or upset.
- Excessive perspiration.
- Hunger with little eating.
- Mental disturbances.
- Palpitation.
- Ringing in ears and hearing loss.
- Insomnia.
- Swollen tonsils.

4. Liver-Kidney Yin Deficiency Syndrome

SYMPTOMS AND SIGNS:

- Difficulty in both bowel movement and urination.
- Dizziness.
- Dry eyes or throat.
- Fatigue.
- Headache with pain in the bony ridge forming the eyebrow.
- Lumbago.
- Night-blindness.
- Night sweats.
- Pain in the hypochondrium.
- Hot hands and feet.
- Insomnia with forgetfulness.
- Withered complexion.

5. Deficiency Fire Syndrome

SYMPTOMS AND SIGNS:

- Easily angry.
- Coughing with blood.

- Dry cough without sputum.
- Coughing with sticky sputum.
- Dry sensations in the mouth.
- Dry or sore throat.
- Excessive perspiration.
- Feeling depressed.
- Forgetfulness.
- Hot sensations in body, center of hands, and feet, and warm skin and muscles.
- Light but periodic fever not unlike the tide.
- Night sweats.
- Red complexion.
- Ringing in ears.
- Seminal emission with dreams.
- Insomnia.
- Sputum with blood.

6. Deficiency of Energy and Yin Syndrome

SYMPTOMS AND SIGNS:

- Constipation.
- Dry cough.
- Dry stools.
- Excessive perspiration.
- Fatigue.
- Hot sensations in the palms of hands and soles of feet.
- Mild stomachache with swelling.
- Palpitation.
- Poor appetite.
- Ringing in ears.
- Scanty urine.
- Sore throat.
- Normal or abnormal thirst.
- Tidal fever in the afternoon.

INGREDIENTS FOR CREATING RECIPES

FOODS FOR EXCESS: radish, seaweed, kelp, seagrass.

FOODS FOR DEFICIENCY: oyster.

HERBS: Huang-yao-zi (Ceylon white yam), Dang-shen (root of pilose asiabell), Xia-ku-cao (self heal), Yuan-zhi (slender-leaved milkwort), Cong-bai (Welsh onion), Lian-zi (East Indian lotus), Ling-zhi, Zhi-mu (wind weed), Huang-bai (cork tree), Sheng-di (dried glutinous rehmannia), Ren-shen (Chinese ginseng), Mai-dong (lilyturf), Huang-jing (sealwort).

Syndromes of disease and herbs to use:

1. **HOT STOMACH:** Zhi-mu (wind weed), Huang-bai (cork tree), Sheng-di (dried glutinous rehmannia); cook with foods for excess.
2. **LIVER ENERGY CONGESTION:** Huang-yao-zi (Ceylon white yam), Xia-ku-cao (self heal); cook with foods for excess.
3. **SPUTUM FIRE:** Cong-bai (Welsh onion), Lian-zi (East Indian lotus), Ling-zhi; cook with foods for excess.
4. **LIVER-KIDNEY YIN DEFICIENCY:** Yuan-zhi (slender-leaved milkwort); cook with foods for excess.
5. **DEFICIENCY FIRE:** Zhi-mu (wind weed), Huang-bai (cork tree), Sheng-di (dried glutinous rehmannia); cook with foods for excess or deficiency.
6. **DEFICIENCY OF ENERGY AND YIN:** Dang-shen (root of pilose asiabell), Ren-shen (Chinese ginseng), Mai-dong (lilyturf), Huang-jing (sealwort); cook with foods for deficiency.

RECIPE 74

MASTER: 5 g Mai-dong (lilyturf), 12 g He-shou-wu (tuber of multiflower knotweed), 15 g Gou-qi-zi (matrimony vine fruit).

ASSOCIATE: 30 g seaweed.

ASSISTANT: 30 g radish.

SEASONING: rice wine, salt.

STEPS:

(1) Decoct the three master ingredients; strain to obtain herbal soup.

(2) Cook seaweed and radish in 3 cups water until cooked, then add to herbal soup.

(3) Season with rice wine and salt to taste.

CONSUMPTION: eat at mealtimes.

INDICATIONS: deficiency syndrome of hyperthyroidism.

ANALYSIS: Mai-dong and Gou-qi-zi are yin tonics, and He-shou-wu is a blood tonic. Tonics are good for deficiency. Seaweed and radish can sedate heat, which is beneficial to hyperthyroidism; rice wine can inject a degree of warmth into the recipe to prevent the recipe from getting too yin (called yin-yang balance), and salt can clear heat.

11.4 Hypothyroidism

1. Spleen-Kidney Yang Deficiency Syndrome

SYMPTOMS AND SIGNS:

- Physically weak and little inclination to talk.
- Cold hands and feet.
- Cold loins.
- Diarrhea before dawn.
- Diarrhea with sticky, muddy stool.
- Eating little.
- Edema that occurs all over the body.
- Fatigue.
- Aversion to cold.
- Weak limbs.
- Frequent clear urination.
- Impotence in men or irregular menstruation in women.
- Mental fatigue.
- Sputum rumbling with shortness of breath.

2. Heart-Kidney Yang Deficiency Syndrome

SYMPTOMS AND SIGNS:

- Chest pain.
- Cold limbs.
- Discharge of watery thin stool.
- Edema.
- Frequent urination.
- History of hydropericardium and cardiac troubles.
- Love of lying down.
- Palpitation.
- Nervousness.
- Sputum.

3. Deficiency of Kidney Yin and Kidney Yang Syndrome

SYMPTOMS AND SIGNS:

- Cough.
- Decreased sexual desire in men.
- Dry mouth.
- Edema.
- Fatigue.
- Gray hair and loss of hair.
- Impotence in men.
- Infertility in women.
- Lumbago.
- Mental fatigue.
- Labored breathing.
- Thirst.
- Weak legs.
- Yellowish urine.

INGREDIENTS FOR CREATING RECIPES

FOODS FOR EXCESS: sword bean, chili pepper.

FOODS FOR DEFICIENCY: chicken, lobster, walnut, chicken egg, duck.

HERBS: Gan-jiang (dried ginger), Rou-gui (Chinese cassia bark), Du-zhong (eucommia bark), Bu-gu-zhi (psoralea), Gui-zhi (cinnamon stick), Bai-zhu (white atractylodes), Gan-cao (licorice), Ren-shen (Chinese ginseng), Shan-yao (Chinese yam), Gou-qi-zi (matrimony vine fruit), Lu-jiao-jiao (deerhorn glue), Xiao-hui-xiang (fennel seed).

Syndromes of disease and herbs to use:

1. **SPLEEN-KIDNEY YANG DEFICIENCY:** Gan-jiang (dried ginger), Rou-gui (Chinese cassia bark), Du-zhong (eucommia bark), Bu-gu-zhi (psoralea), Gui-zhi (cinnamon stick), Bai-zhu (white atractylodes), Gan-cao (licorice); cook with foods for deficiency.
2. **HEART-KIDNEY YANG DEFICIENCY:** Gan-jiang (dried ginger), Rou-gui (Chinese cassia bark), Du-zhong (eucommia bark), Xiao-hui-xiang (fennel seed), Bu-gu-zhi (psoralea), Gui-zhi (cinnamon stick), Gan-cao (licorice); cook with foods for deficiency.
3. **DEFICIENCY OF KIDNEY YIN AND KIDNEY YANG:** Gan-jiang (dried ginger), Rou-gui (Chinese cassia bark), Du-zhong (eucommia bark), Bu-gu-zhi (psoralea), Gan-cao (licorice), Shan-yao (Chinese yam), Gou-qi-zi (matrimony vine fruit), Lu-jiao-jiao (deerhorn glue); cook with foods for deficiency.

RECIPE 75

MASTER: 5 g Gan-jiang (dried ginger), 5 g Bu-gu-zhi (psoralea), 5 g Gan-cao (licorice).

ASSOCIATE: 1 large lobster in its shell.

ASSISTANT: 20 g walnuts.

SEASONING: none.

STEPS:

(1) Decoct the three master ingredients; strain to obtain herbal soup.

(2) Put lobster and walnuts in a big bowl, add the soup and steam until cooked.

CONSUMPTION: eat the lobster and walnuts, drink the soup at mealtimes.

INDICATIONS: all syndromes of hypothyroidism.

ANALYSIS: Gan-jiang can warm the body; Bu-gu-zhi tones up kidney yang; Gan-cao is an energy tonic; and lobster and walnuts are yang tonics. This recipe makes use of yang tonics to warm the body as a way of curing hypothyroidism.

11.5 Diabetes mellitus

1. Lung Fire Syndrome

SYMPTOMS AND SIGNS:

- Dry nose and mouth.
- Frequent urination.
- Normal bowel movement.
- Sore throat, with redness and swelling.
- Extreme thirst with excessive intake of liquids.
- Vomiting of blood.

2. Stomach Fire Syndrome

SYMPTOMS AND SIGNS:

- Bitter taste in the mouth.
- Bleeding from gums with pain.
- Constipation with dry stool.
- Dry sensations in the mouth.
- Frequent hunger and eating.
- Headache.
- Hiccups.
- Underweight in spite of large intake of food.

- Morning sickness.
- Nosebleed.
- Pain in the gums with swelling.
- Red, swollen sore throat.
- Underweight.
- Toothache.
- Vomiting of blood.
- Vomiting right after eating.

3. Kidney Yin Deficiency Syndrome

SYMPTOMS AND SIGNS:

- Cough with sputum containing blood or coughing out fresh blood.
- Dry sensations in the mouth, particularly at night.
- Dry throat.
- Fatigue.
- Frequent urination.
- Hot sensations in any part of the body.
- Night sweats.
- Pain in the heel.
- Pain in the loins (lumbago).
- Retention of urine.
- Ringing in ears.
- Seminal emission with dreams.
- Insomnia.
- "Spots" in front of the eyes.
- Normal or unusual thirst.
- Toothache or loose teeth.
- Urine as thick as liquid fat.

INGREDIENTS FOR CREATING RECIPES

FOODS FOR EXCESS: corn, wheat bran, eggplant, Chinese wax gourd, pork skin, pear, freshwater clam.

FOODS FOR DEFICIENCY: pork pancreas, beef, milk, litchi nut, sesame seed, chicken egg, sea cucumber, pear.

HERBS: Mu-li (oyster shell), Shan-yao (Chinese yam), Shan-zhu-yu (fruit of medicinal cornel), Yu-mi-xu (corn silk), Yu-zhu (Solomon's seal), Dang-shen (root of pilose asiabell), Huang-qi (membranous milk vetch), Tian-hua-fen (Chinese trichosanthes), Sheng-di (dried glutinous rehmannia), Tian-dong (lucid asparagus), Lian-zi (East Indian lotus), Fu-ling (tuckahoe; Indian bread), Mai-dong (lilyturf), Wu-wei-zi (magnolia vine fruit), Gua-lou (snake gourd), Lu-gen (reed rhizome), Ren-shen (Chinese ginseng), Ge-gen (kudzu vine), Shu-di (processed glutinous rehmannia), Sang-shen (mulberry).

Syndromes of disease and herbs to use:

1. **LUNG FIRE:** Sheng-di (dried glutinous rehmannia), Yu-mi-xu (corn silk), Ge-gen (kudzu vine), Gua-lou (snake gourd), Lu-gen (reed rhizome); cook with foods for excess.
2. **STOMACH FIRE:** Sheng-di (dried glutinous rehmannia), Lu-gen (reed rhizome), Sheng-di (dried glutinous rehmannia), Tian-hua-fen (Chinese trichosanthes), Lian-zi (East Indian lotus); cook with foods for excess.
3. **KIDNEY YIN DEFICIENCY:** Sheng-di (dried glutinous rehmannia), Shan-yao (Chinese yam), Shan-zhu-yu (fruit of medicinal cornel), Yu-zhu (Solomon's seal), Dang-shen (root of pilose asiabell), Huang-qi (membranous milk vetch), Tian-hua-fen (Chinese trichosanthes), Tian-dong (lucid asparagus), Fu-ling (tuckahoe; Indian bread), Mai-dong (lilyturf), Wu-wei-zi (magnolia vine fruit), Ren-shen (Chinese ginseng), Shu-di (processed glutinous rehmannia), Sang-shen (mulberry); cook with foods for deficiency.

RECIPE 76

MASTER: 10 g Sheng-di (dried glutinous rehmannia).

ASSOCIATE: 200 g gold carp.

ASSISTANT: 2 chicken eggs.

SEASONING: salt and corn oil.

STEPS:

(1) Bake Sheng-di (dried glutinous rehmannia) and grind into powder.

(2) Break eggs and mix well with the herbal powder.

(3) Remove the internal organs and gills from the carp; leave the scales intact.

(4) Stuff the herb powder–egg mixture into the fish stomach and close with toothpicks.

(5) Season with salt and oil before steaming the fish until cooked, about 20 minutes.

CONSUMPTION: eat the fish and contents at mealtimes.

INDICATIONS: all syndromes of diabetes.

ANALYSIS: Sheng-di is a yin tonic and clears heat; gold carp is a spleen tonic; chicken egg is a yin tonic; salt can sedate heat; and corn oil can reduce cholesterol levels and lubricate the internal region.

11.6 Arthritis and rheumatoid arthritis

1. Wind Syndrome

SYMPTOMS AND SIGNS:

- Diarrhea with undigested food.
- Loose, watery stool.
- Aversion to wind.
- Headache accompanied by aversion to wind.
- Headache with heavy sensations in the head.
- Extremely itchy skin.
- Light cough.
- Nasal discharge.
- Numbness in facial skin.
- Pain in the joints all over the whole body that attacks suddenly.
- Pain in the joints that shifts from one joint to another.
- Body tremors.
- Sneezing.
- Muscle stiffness.
- Nasal congestion with heavy voice.
- Tickle in the throat.

2. Cold Syndrome

SYMPTOMS AND SIGNS:

- Abdominal pain.
- Absence of perspiration in hot weather.
- Absence of normal thirst.
- Excessive watering of eyes.
- Clear, long streams of urine.
- Cold chest or cold hands and feet.
- Cold sensations in the body.
- Muscle spasms.
- Coughing and vomiting with froth.
- Diarrhea with sticky, muddy stool.
- Aversion to cold.
- Hands and feet extremely cold.
- Headache with pain in back of neck.
- Preference for hot drinks.
- Pale complexion.
- Severe pain in the joints.

3. **Dampness Syndrome**

SYMPTOMS AND SIGNS:

- Abdominal pain with rumbling.
- Diarrhea.
- Diminished urination.
- Discharge of hard stool followed by sticky, turbid stool.
- Discharge of watery pus through openings of carbuncles.
- Discharge of yellowish sticky fluids from blisters that break open.
- Dizziness.
- Eczema.
- Edema on the dorsum of foot.
- Weak limbs.
- Headache as if the head were being wrapped up.
- Heavy sensation in any part of the body.
- Preference for hot drinks.
- Love of sleep and heavy sensations in the body.
- Pain always in the same joints and heavy sensations in the body.
- Pain in the loins as if sitting in water with heaviness in the body.
- Pain starting mostly from lower regions of the body.

4. **Heat Syndrome**

SYMPTOMS AND SIGNS:

- Acute onset of pain in the joints.
- Constipation.
- Diminished urination.
- Discharge of copious, yellowish sticky sputum.
- Dry lips.
- Escape of intestinal gas with noise.
- Light fever.
- Preference for cold drinks.
- Pain in the joints that shifts around.
- Pain in the joints with burning sensations.
- Severe pain with inability to extend or flex the joints.
- Red complexion, eyes, or urine.
- Scanty, short streams of urine.
- Stool with an extremely bad smell.
- Thirst with an incessant desire to drink.
- Swollen, red throat.
- Urine with an unusual odor.

INGREDIENTS FOR CREATING RECIPES

FOODS FOR EXCESS: watermelon, celery, cherry, wine, black soybean, carrot.

FOODS FOR DEFICIENCY: cherry, eel, mussel, polished rice, glutinous rice, mutton.

HERBS: Sang-zhi (mulberry twig), Huang-bai (cork tree), Sang-ji-sheng (mistletoe), Wei-ling-xian (Chinese clematis), Yi-yi-ren (Job's tears), Fang-feng (Chinese wind shelter), Mu-gua (Chinese flowering quince), Qin-jiao (large-leaved gentian), Du-huo (downy angelica), Chuan-xiong (hemlock parsley), Wu-jia-pi (slender acanthopanax root bark), Xu-duan (teazel), Niu-xi (two-toothed amaranthus), Zhi-mu (wind weed).

Syndromes of disease and herbs to use:

1. **WIND:** Sang-zhi (mulberry twig), Sang-ji-sheng (mistletoe), Wei-ling-xian (Chinese clematis), Fang-feng (Chinese wind shelter), Qin-jiao (large-leaved gentian), Du-huo (downy angelica), Chuan-xiong (hemlock parsley); cook with foods for excess, or cook with foods for deficiency in chronic cases.

2. **COLD:** Wu-jia-pi (slender acanthopanax root bark), Xu-duan (teazel), Niu-xi (two-toothed amaranthus); cook with foods for excess, or cook with foods for deficiency in chronic cases.

3. **DAMPNESS:** Sang-zhi (mulberry twig), Wei-ling-xian (Chinese clematis), Yi-yi-ren (Job's tears), Mu-gua (Chinese flowering quince), Qin-jiao (large-leaved gentian), Du-huo (downy angelica); cook with foods for excess, or cook with foods for deficiency in chronic cases.
4. **HEAT:** Huang-bai (cork tree), Zhi-mu (wind weed); cook with foods for excess, or cook with foods for deficiency in chronic cases.

RECIPE 77

MASTER: 10 g Yi-yi-ren (Job's tears).

ASSOCIATE: black soybeans, presoaked.

ASSISTANT: polished rice.

SEASONING: salt or sugar.

STEPS:

(1) Boil Yi-yi-ren (Job's tears), rice, and black soybeans together in water to make a congee.

(2) Season with either salt or sugar to taste, whichever is preferred.

CONSUMPTION: Eat at mealtimes.

INDICATIONS: dampness syndrome of rheumatism and arthritis.

ANALYSIS: Yi-yi-ren, a well-known herb for damp type of arthritis and rheumatism, helps to eliminate water from the body. Black soybean can also eliminate water from the body as well as promote blood circulation.

RECIPE 78

MASTER: 300 g Huang-jing (sealwort).

ASSOCIATE: 3,000 g (10 cups) rice wine.

ASSISTANT: 100 g white sugar.

SEASONING: none.

STEPS:

(1) Boil Huang-jing (sealwort) in water for two minutes, then remove from water to cool.

(2) Immerse the herb in rice wine.

(3) Add white sugar and seal it for three months.

CONSUMPTION: drink one cup before meals on an empty stomach, once daily.

INDICATIONS: all syndromes of arthritis and rheumatism except hot.

ANALYSIS: Huang-jing is a yin tonic and energy tonic, and rice wine can speed up the effects of Huang-jing and promote circulation; a combination of the two ingredients is commonly used to treat arthritis and rheumatism. White sugar is used to slow down the action of rice wine slightly used and also to tone the spleen.

11.7 Simple obesity

4. Spleen Dampness Syndrome

SYMPTOMS AND SIGNS:

- Chest discomfort without appetite.
- Diarrhea.
- Edema.
- Heavy sensations in head as if the head were covered with something.
- Heavy sensations in the body with discomfort.
- Preference for hot drinks.
- Nausea and vomiting.
- Poor appetite.
- Scanty urine.
- Stomach fullness and discomfort.
- Sweet and sticky taste in mouth.
- Little inclination to talk or move.

2. Spleen-Stomach Damp Heat Syndrome

SYMPTOMS AND SIGNS:

- Abdominal swelling.

- Bad breath.
- Bleeding from gums.
- Dizziness.
- Constipation.
- Easily hungry.
- Gums swelling.
- Hiccups.
- Bland taste in the mouth.
- Nosebleed.
- Sore throat.
- Perspiring in the head.
- Stomachache.
- Thirst and craving for cold drinks.
- Vomiting of blood.
- Vomiting right after eating.
- Vomiting with stomach discomfort as if hungry, empty, or hot.

3. Liver Energy Congestion Syndrome

SYMPTOMS AND SIGNS:

- Abdominal obstruction.
- Abdominal pain.
- Bitter taste in the mouth.
- Convulsion.
- Dry tongue.
- Easily angry.
- Numbness.
- Pain in the hypochondrium.
- Poor appetite.
- Stomachache.
- Feeling of throat obstruction.
- Vomiting of blood.

4. Energy Congestion and Blood Coagulation Syndrome

SYMPTOMS AND SIGNS:

- Abdominal swelling.
- Congested chest.
- Irregular menstruation with blood clots in women.
- Love of sighing.
- Lump in the abdomen that stays in the same region.
- Pain in the hypochondrium.
- Palpitation.
- Shortness of breath.

5. Internal Phlegm Syndrome

SYMPTOMS AND SIGNS:

- Abdominal swelling or rumbling.
- Congested chest.
- Dizziness.
- Headache.
- Heaviness in the body.
- Preference for hot drinks.
- Regular intake of sweet and/or greasy foods.
- Numbness.
- Pain in the chest or hypochondrium.
- Palpitation.
- Stomachache.
- Swollen tongue.
- Vomiting or cough with profuse watery sputum.

6. Spleen-Kidney Yang Deficiency Syndrome

SYMPTOMS AND SIGNS:

- Abdominal swelling.
- Cold extremities or loins.
- Diarrhea before dawn.
- Diarrhea with sticky, muddy stool.
- Eating little.
- Edema.
- Edema that occurs all over the body.
- Fatigue.
- Aversion to cold.
- Weak limbs.
- Frequent clear urination.
- Mental fatigue.
- Poor appetite.
- Scanty urine.
- Sputum rumbling with labored breathing.
- Watery stool.

INGREDIENTS FOR CREATING RECIPES

FOODS FOR EXCESS: common carp, kelp, Chinese wax gourd, seaweed, mung bean, bitter gourd, cucumber, azuki bean, corn.

FOODS FOR DEFICIENCY: polished rice, shiitake mushroom, liver, yam, beef kidney, chestnut.

HERBS: He-ye (lotus leaf), Shan-zha (Chinese hawthorn), Chi-xiao-dou (small red bean [similar to azuki]), Huang-qi (membranous milk vetch), Gui-zhi (cinnamon stick), Fu-ling (tuckahoe; Indian bread), Fang-feng (Chinese wind shelter), Jing-jie (Japanese ground-ivy), Ma-huang (Chinese ephedra), Chai-hu (hare's ear), Huang-qin (skullcap), Da-huang (rhubarb), Zhi-shi (China orange), Dang-gui (Chinese angelica), Shu-di (processed glutinous rehmannia), Tao-ren (peach kernel), Hong-hua (safflower), Ban-xia (half-summer pinellia), Chen-pi (dried tangerine peel), Bai-zhu (white atractylodes).

Syndromes of disease and herbs to use:

1. **SPLEEN DAMPNESS:** Chi-xiao-dou (small red bean), fang-ji, Huang-qi (membranous milk vetch), Gui-zhi (cinnamon stick), Fu-ling (tuckahoe; Indian bread); cook with foods for excess.
2. **SPLEEN-STOMACH DAMP HEAT:** Fang-feng (Chinese wind shelter), Jing-jie (Japanese ground-ivy), Ma-huang (Chinese ephedra); cook with foods for excess.
3. **LIVER ENERGY CONGESTION:** Chai-hu (hare's ear), Huang-qin (skullcap), Da-huang (rhubarb), Zhi-shi (China orange); cook with foods for excess.
4. **ENERGY CONGESTION AND BLOOD COAGULATION:** Shan-zha (Chinese hawthorn), Dang-gui (Chinese angelica), Shu-di (processed glutinous rehmannia), Tao-ren (peach kernel), Hong-hua (safflower); cook with foods for excess.
5. **INTERNAL PHLEGM:** Ban-xia (half-summer pinellia), Chen-pi (dried tangerine peel), Fu-ling (tuckahoe; Indian bread), Zhi-shi (China orange); cook with foods for excess.
6. **SPLEEN-KIDNEY YANG DEFICIENCY:** Huang-qi (membranous milk vetch), Bai-zhu (white atractylodes); cook with foods for deficiency.

RECIPE 79

MASTER: 9 g He-ye (lotus leaf).

ASSOCIATE: 9 g Shan-zha (Chinese hawthorn).

ASSISTANT: none.

SEASONING: none.

STEPS:

(1) Dry roast Shan-zha (Chinese hawthorn) until brownish, then grind into powder.

(2) Boil He-ye (lotus leaf) for 15 minutes in 3 cups water, then add the herbal powder.

(3) Remove the He-ye (lotus leaf) and discard.

CONSUMPTION: drink the soup at mealtimes.

INDICATIONS: simple obesity.

ANALYSIS: He-ye can clear heat and activates yang energy in the body to promote circulation. Shan-zha is a powerful digestive for fat, and it can also reduce high blood pressure and cholesterol. This is one of the few recipes with only two ingredients.

11.8 Osteoporosis

1. Blood Deficiency Syndrome

SYMPTOMS AND SIGNS:

- Abdominal pain.
- Constipation with discharge of hard stool.
- Difficult bowel movement.
- Dizziness.
- Dry, cracked lips and mouth.
- Fatigue.
- Fever.
- Feeling depressed.
- Headache in the afternoon or with dizziness.
- Pale lips.
- Reclining with an inability to sit up due to dizziness.
- Blurred vision.
- Muscle spasms.
- Night sweats.
- Palpitation with anxiety.
- Underweight with dry skin.
- Insomnia.
- Spasms of the four limbs.
- Pale complexion.

2. Blood Coagulation Syndrome

SYMPTOMS AND SIGNS:

- Abdominal pain.
- Bleeding from gums.
- Chest pain.
- Cough with blood.
- Headache.
- Lumbago.
- Pain (acute) around umbilicus, resisting massage, with hard spots felt by hands.
- Pain in region between navel and pubic hair with feeling of hardness.
- Pain in the hypochondrium.
- Pain in the loins as if being pierced with an awl.
- Pain in the ribs.
- Palpitation with anxiety.
- Partial suppression of lochia.
- Spasm.
- Stomachache.
- Swelling and congestion after eating.
- Vomiting of blood.

INGREDIENTS FOR CREATING RECIPES

FOODS FOR EXCESS: pork bone, cow bone, Chinese chive, tofu, black soybean, celery, eggplant, peach, spinach, garlic, kelp.

FOODS FOR DEFICIENCY: shiitake mushroom, tofu, shrimp, oyster, cantaloupe, chestnut, chicken egg, crab, glutinous rice, walnut, sword bean, honey.

HERBS: He-shou-wu (tuber of multiflower knotweed), Niu-xi (two-toothed amaranthus), Gu-sui-bu (rhizome of fortune's drynaria), Hai-piao-xiao (cuttlebone).

Syndromes of disease and herbs to use:

1. **BLOOD DEFICIENCY:** He-shou-wu (tuber of

multiflower knotweed), Gu-sui-bu (rhizome of fortune's drynaria); cook with foods for deficiency.

2. **BLOOD COAGULATION:** Niu-xi (two-toothed amaranthus), Hai-piao-xiao (cuttlebone); cook with foods for excess.

RECIPE 80

MASTER: 10 g He-shou-wu (tuber of multiflower knotweed).

ASSOCIATE: 100 g fresh oysters.

ASSISTANT: 50 g rice noodles.

SEASONING: salt, soy sauce, or miso.

STEPS:

(1) Decoct He-shou-wu (tuber of multiflower knotweed) in water; strain to obtain soup.

(2) Boil fresh oysters together with the noodles until cooked, then add the herbal soup.

(3) Season with salt, soy sauce, or miso to taste.

CONSUMPTION: eat at mealtimes.

INDICATIONS: blood deficiency syndrome of osteoporosis.

ANALYSIS: He-shou-wu acts on the kidneys and produces bone and marrow. Rice noodles are an energy tonic. Salt, soy sauce, or miso acts on the kidneys and also improves the taste.

11.9 Nosebleed

1. Hot Lungs Syndrome

SYMPTOMS AND SIGNS:

- Acute panting in a high-pitched sound and rapid expiration.
- Bitter taste in the mouth.
- Cough with subdued, feeble sounds.
- Coughing and vomiting of pus and blood with a foul odor.
- Coughing out yellowish, sticky sputum.
- Discharge of dry stool.
- Dry nasal passages, often accompanied by itch.
- Dry sensations in the mouth.
- Flickering of nostrils.
- Hot sensations in the body.
- Light but periodic fever not unlike the tide.
- Nosebleed with fresh-colored blood.
- Pain in the chest or in the throat.
- Sputum lodged in the throat.
- Mental depression.
- Urgent panting.

2. Hot Stomach Syndrome

SYMPTOMS AND SIGNS:

- Bad breath.
- Bleeding from gums.
- Dry nasal passages, often accompanied by itch.
- Nosebleed with red fresh-colored blood.
- Pain in the gums with swelling.
- Sore throat.
- Perspiring in the head.
- Stomachache.
- Thirst and craving for cold.
- Vomiting of blood.
- Vomiting right after eating.

3. Hot Liver Syndrome

SYMPTOMS AND SIGNS:

- Bitter taste in the mouth.
- Bloody urine.
- Hearing difficulties.

- Dry throat.
- Distended sensation in the head or headache.
- Profuse nosebleeding with red fresh-colored blood .
- Pain in the hypochondrium.
- Partial suppression of lochia.
- Pink eyes with swelling.
- Mental depression.
- Sour taste in the mouth.
- Spasms.
- Twitching.
- Vaginal discharge with a fishy, foul odor.

INGREDIENTS FOR CREATING RECIPES

FOODS FOR EXCESS: radish, fresh lotus rhizome, water chestnut, black fungus, pear, water spinach, peanut, litchi nut.

FOODS FOR DEFICIENCY: dried lotus rhizome, pear, chicken egg, chicken, longan nut, litchi nut.

HERBS: Sang-shen (mulberry), Gou-qi-zi (matrimony vine fruit), Da-zao (red date), Sheng-di (dried glutinous rehmannia), E-jiao (donkey-hide gelatin), Pu-huang (cattail pollen), Ce-bai-ye (oriental arbor vitae), He-ye (lotus leaf), Ai-ye (mugwort), Xiao-ji (cornfield thistle), Ma-bo (puff ball).

Syndromes of disease and herbs to use:

1. **HOT LUNGS:** Ce-bai-ye (oriental arbor vitae), Sang-shen (mulberry), Gou-qi-zi (matrimony vine fruit), Ai-ye (mugwort); cook with foods for excess.

2. **HOT STOMACH:** Ce-bai-ye (oriental arbor vitae), Sang-shen (mulberry), Gou-qi-zi (matrimony vine fruit), Da-zao (red date), He-ye (lotus leaf); cook with foods for excess.

3. **HOT LIVER:** Ce-bai-ye (oriental arbor vitae), Sang-shen (mulberry), Gou-qi-zi (matrimony vine fruit), Sheng-di (dried glutinous rehmannia), E-jiao (donkey-hide gelatin), He-ye (lotus leaf), Xiao-ji (cornfield thistle); cook with foods for excess.

RECIPE 81

MASTER: 30 g Sheng-di (dried glutinous rehmannia), 10 g E-jiao (donkey-hide gelatin), 15 g Pu-huang (cattail pollen).

ASSOCIATE: 30 g radish, sliced.

ASSISTANT: 30 black fungus, sliced.

SEASONING: salt or sugar.

STEPS:

(1) Decoct the three master ingredients; strain to obtain herbal soup.

(2) Boil the radish and black fungus until cooked. Add to the herbal soup.

CONSUMPTION: Eat at mealtimes.

INDICATIONS: all syndromes of nosebleed.

ANALYSIS: Sheng-di is a yin tonic and can clear heat as well. E-ji is a blood tonic, assisting in arresting bleeding, nosebleed in particular. Radish can cool the lungs and also stop nosebleed. Black fungus can also stop bleeding, including nosebleed, and salt or sugar improves the taste.

CHAPTER 12

Female Disorders

12.1 Premenstrual syndrome (PMS or premenstrual tension)

1. Energy Congestion and Blood Coagulation Syndrome

SYMPTOMS AND SIGNS:

- Abdominal bloating.
- Congested chest.
- Irregular menstruation with blood clots.
- Love of sighing.
- Hard spots in the abdomen that stay in the same region.
- Pain in the hypochondrium.
- Palpitation.
- Shortness of breath.

2. Cold Dampness Syndrome

SYMPTOMS AND SIGNS:

- Absence of perspiration.
- Thin, clear, blackish/dark-colored menstrual bleeding.
- Clear, watery vaginal discharge with a fishy smell.
- Cold limbs.
- Diarrhea with watery stools and abdominal pain.
- Aversion to cold.
- Heavy sensations in the body and head.
- Menstrual flow and vaginal discharge with a strong foul odor.
- Period pain.
- Poor appetite.

INGREDIENTS FOR CREATING RECIPES

FOODS FOR EXCESS: celery, rose, Chinese rose, yellow soybean, seaweed, day lily, mung bean, mung bean sprouts, corn, eggplant, cucumber.

FOODS FOR DEFICIENCY: chicken egg, wheat, polished rice, eel, walnut, honey, ham, grape, Irish potato, soy milk, pork, mutton.

HERBS: Bei-sha-shen (straight ladybell north), Yi-mu-cao (Siberian motherwort), Chuan-xiong (hemlock parsley), Mu-xiang (costus root), Dan-pi (peony), Mai-dong (lilyturf), Gou-qi-zi (matrimony vine fruit).

Syndromes of disease and herbs to use:

1. **ENERGY CONGESTION AND BLOOD COAGULATION:** Bei-sha-shen (straight ladybell north), Yi-mu-cao (Siberian motherwort), Chuan-xiong (hemlock parsley), Mu-xiang (costus root), Dan-pi (peony), Mai-dong (lilyturf), Gou-qi-zi (matrimony vine fruit); cook with foods for excess.

2. **COLD DAMPNESS:** Yi-mu-cao (Siberian motherwort), Chuan-xiong (hemlock parsley), Mu-xiang (costus root); cook with foods for excess or foods for deficiency.

RECIPE 82

MASTER: 6 g Chuan-xiong (hemlock parsley), 6 g Mu-xiang (costusroot).

ASSOCIATE: none.

ASSISTANT: none.

SEASONING: 1 teaspoon brown sugar.

STEPS:

(1) Decoct Chuan-xiong (hemlock parsley) and Mu-xiang (costus root) for thirty minutes; strain to obtain herbal soup.

(2) Add brown sugar.

CONSUMPTION: to drink anytime.

INDICATIONS: energy congestion and blood coagulation syndrome of premenstrual syndrome.

ANALYSIS: Chuan-xiong disperses the blood to correct blood coagulation; Mu-xiang promotes energy circulation to correct energy congestion; and brown sugar promotes blood circulation and improves the taste.

Note: Instead of using Chuan-xiong (hemlock parsley) and Mu-xiang (costus root), you can decoct 60 g roses and 100 g Dan-pi (peony) in the same way.

RECIPE 83

MASTER: 30 g Yi-mu-cao (Siberian motherwort).

ASSOCIATE: 250 g celery, chopped.

ASSISTANT: 1 chicken egg.

SEASONING: salt.

STEPS:

(1) Decoct Yi-mu-cao (Siberian motherwort) for thirty minutes; strain to obtain herbal soup.

(2) Boil celery in 2 1/2 cups of water, then mix in the egg before removing from heat. Add to herbal soup.

(3) Season with salt to taste.

CONSUMPTION: eat at mealtimes.

INDICATIONS: both syndromes of premenstrual syndrome.

ANALYSIS: Yi-mu-cao can disperse blood to correct blood coagulation; it is an important herb for regulating irregular menstruation. Celery can improve the condition of the liver to relieve anxiety and irritation; chicken egg is a blood tonic and lubricates dryness; and salt improves the taste.

12.2 Amenorrhea (absent period)

1. Wind Cold Syndrome

SYMPTOMS AND SIGNS:

- Absence of perspiration in hot weather.
- Normal breathing through the nose.
- Clear nasal discharge.
- Cough.
- Diarrhea.
- Aversion to cold.
- Dizziness.
- Headache with dizziness.
- Hoarseness at the beginning of illness.
- Itching in the throat.
- Light fever.
- Loss of voice.
- Nosebleed.

- Pain in the body shifting around with no fixed region.
- Pain in the joints.
- Nasal congestion.
- Vomiting.

2. **Damp Phlegm Syndrome**

SYMPTOMS AND SIGNS:

- Abdominal distention with congested chest.
- Coughing with excessive sputum.
- Dizziness with heavy sensations in the head.
- Headache.
- Hiccups.
- Nausea.
- Palpitation with nervousness.
- Frequent delayed periods.
- Poor appetite.
- Whitish vaginal discharge, especially if excessive.

3. **Internal Heat Syndrome**

SYMPTOMS AND SIGNS:

- Clenching teeth without grinding them.
- Cold fingertips.
- Cold hands and feet.
- Hot sensations in the center of palms and soles.

4. **Energy Stagnation Syndrome**

SYMPTOMS AND SIGNS:

- Abdominal pain that eases after releasing flatus.
- Belching or hiccups.
- Chest and rib tightness.
- Chest pain.
- Constipation with frequent false calls for a bowel movement.
- Irregular menstruation.
- Overdue menstruation.
- Pain in inner part of stomach with prickling sensation and bloating.
- Pain in the hypochondrium.
- Menstrual pain.
- Infrequent urination.
- Ringing in ears and hearing impairment.
- Stomachache.
- Subjective sensation of lump in the throat.
- Difficulty swallowing.
- Swelling and congestion after eating.

5. **Blood Deficiency Syndrome**

SYMPTOMS AND SIGNS:

- Abdominal pain.
- Constipation with discharge of hard stool.
- Difficult bowel movement.
- Dizziness.
- Dry, cracked lips and mouth.
- Excessive blood loss following childbirth.
- Fatigue.
- Fever.
- Depression.
- Headache in the afternoon or with dizziness.
- Colorless, pale lips.
- Dizziness upon standing or sitting from a reclining position.
- Menstrual flow with a light red color or like yellow water.
- Blurred vision.

- Involuntary muscle twitching.
- Night sweats.
- Palpitation with anxiety.
- Thin, with dry skin.
- Insomnia.
- Spasm in all four limbs.
- Pale complexion.

6. Blood Coagulation Syndrome

SYMPTOMS AND SIGNS:

- Abdominal pain.
- Bleeding from gums.
- Chest pain.
- Coughing with blood.
- Headache.
- Irregular periods at first, then overdue, and then no period.
- Lumbago.
- Pain (acute) around navel resisting massage, with hard spots felt by hands.
- Pain in region between navel and pubic hair with feeling of hardness.
- Pain in the hypochondrium.
- Pain in the loins as if being pierced with an awl.
- Pain in the ribs.
- Palpitation with anxiety.
- Partial suppression of lochia.
- Period pain.
- Spasm.
- Stomachache.
- Swelling and congestion after eating.
- Vomiting with blood.

7. Spleen Deficiency Syndrome

SYMPTOMS AND SIGNS:

- Abdominal pain relieved by massage.
- Belching.
- Clear, long streams of urine.
- Chronic diarrhea.
- Indigestion.
- Frequent whitish vaginal discharge.
- Poor appetite.
- Prolapse of any internal organ.
- Prolapse of rectum.
- Shortness of breath.
- Thin.
- Vaginal discharge with an odor.
- Vomiting of acid.

INGREDIENTS FOR CREATING RECIPES

FOODS FOR EXCESS: black fungus, fresh ling, fresh ginger, black soybean.

FOODS FOR DEFICIENCY: mutton, cuttlefish, chicken egg, pork trotter, pork liver, brown sugar.

HERBS: Ze-lan (water-horehound), Hong-hua (safflower), Tao-ren (peach kernel), Wang-bu-liu-xing (seed of cow-basil), Niu-xi (two-toothed amaranthus), Shan-zha (Chinese hawthorn), Yi-mu-cao (Siberian motherwort), xiang-fu (nutgrass flatsedge rhizome), San-leng (triangular rhizome), Ji-xing-zi (seed of garden balsam), Ren-shen (Chinese ginseng), Dang-gui (Chinese angelica), Chuan-xiong (hemlock parsley), Ban-xia (half-summer pinellia), Chen-pi (dried tangerine peel), Zhi-qiao (unripe citron), Shu-di (processed glutinous rehmannia), Huang-qin (skullcap), Huang-bai (cork tree), Bai-shao (white peony).

Syndromes of disease and herbs to use:

1. **WIND COLD:** Ren-shen (Chinese ginseng), Dang-gui (Chinese angelica), Chuan-xiong (hemlock parsley); cook with foods for excess.

2. **DAMP PHLEGM:** Ban-xia (half-summer pinellia), Chen-pi (dried tangerine peel), Zhi-qiao (unripe citron); cook with foods for excess.

3. **INTERNAL HEAT:** Shu-di (processed glutinous rehmannia), Huang-qin (skullcap), Huang-bai (cork tree); cook with foods for excess.

4. **ENERGY STAGNATION:** Ze-lan (water-horehound), Shan-zha (Chinese hawthorn), Xiang-fu (nutgrass flatsedge rhizome); cook with foods for excess.

5. **BLOOD DEFICIENCY:** Dang-gui (Chinese angelica), Shu-di (processed glutinous rehmannia), Bai-shao (white peony); cook with foods for deficiency.

6. **BLOOD COAGULATION:** Ze-lan (water-horehound), Hong-hua (safflower), Tao-ren (peach kernel), Wang-bu-liu-xing (seed of cow-basil), Niu-xi (two-toothed amaranthus), Yi-mu-cao (Siberian motherwort), San-leng (triangular rhizome), Ji-xing-zi (seed of garden balsam); cook with foods for excess.

7. **SPLEEN DEFICIENCY:** Ren-shen (Chinese ginseng), Dang-gui (Chinese angelica), Shu-di (processed glutinous rehmannia), Bai-shao (white peony); cook with foods for deficiency.

RECIPE 84

MASTER: 8 g Hong-hua (safflower).

ASSOCIATE: 30 g black soybeans, presoaked.

ASSISTANT: none.

SEASONING: brown sugar.

STEPS:

(1) Wrap Hong-hua (safflower) in a gauze bag.

(2) Boil soybeans in fresh water until almost cooked, then add the gauze bag to cook over low heat until soybeans are soft.

(3) Season with brown sugar to taste.

CONSUMPTION: eat at mealtimes.

INDICATIONS: blood coagulation syndrome of absent period.

ANALYSIS: all three ingredients in this recipe can activate the blood to correct blood coagulation. Brown sugar is also present to improve the taste.

RECIPE 85

MASTER: 15 g Dang-gui (Chinese angelica).

ASSOCIATE: 1 pork trotter.

ASSISTANT: none.

SEASONING: rice wine.

STEPS:

(1) Cut pork trotter into eight pieces and boil in water with Dang-gui (Chinese angelica) until cooked, about 1 hour.

(2) Remove Dang-gui (Chinese angelica) and discard.

(3) Season the broth with rice wine to taste.

CONSUMPTION: eat the pork trotter and drink the broth at mealtimes.

INDICATIONS: wind cold syndrome and deficiency syndromes of absent period.

ANALYSIS: Dang-gui is a blood tonic; it can warm the body. Pork trotter is also a blood tonic. Rice wine can speed up the actions of the other two ingredients, while also improving the taste.

12.3 Dysmenorrhea (period pain)

1. Wind Cold Syndrome

SYMPTOMS AND SIGNS:

- Absence of perspiration in hot weather.
- Normal breathing through the nose.
- Clear discharge from nose.
- Cough with a heavy sound and clear sputum.

- Diarrhea.
- Aversion to cold.
- Dizziness.
- Headache with dizziness.
- Hoarseness at the beginning of illness.
- Itchy sensation in the throat.
- Light fever.
- Loss of voice.
- Nosebleed.
- Shifting pain in the body.
- Pain in the joints.
- Nasal congestion.
- Vomiting.

2. Cold Dampness Syndrome

SYMPTOMS AND SIGNS:

- Absence of perspiration.
- Thin, clear, blackish/dark-colored menstrual flow.
- Clear and watery vaginal discharge with a fishy smell.
- Cold limbs.
- Diarrhea with discharge of watery stools and abdominal pain.
- Aversion to cold.
- Heavy sensations in the body and head.
- Menstrual flow and vaginal discharge with a strong smell.
- Period pain.
- Poor appetite.

3. Energy Stagnation Syndrome

SYMPTOMS AND SIGNS:

- Abdominal pain that eases after release of intestinal gas.
- Belching or hiccups.
- Chest and rib tightness.
- Chest pain.
- Constipation with frequent false calls for a bowel movement.
- Irregular menstruation.
- Overdue menstruation.
- Pain in inner part of stomach with prickling sensation and bloating.
- Pain in the hypochondrium.
- Period pain.
- Infrequent urination.
- Ringing in ears and difficulty hearing.
- Stomachache.
- Subjective sensation of lump in the throat.
- Difficulty swallowing.
- Bloating and congestion after eating.

4. Blood Deficiency Syndrome

SYMPTOMS AND SIGNS:

- Abdominal pain that occurs at onset of periods.
- Constipation with discharge of hard stool.
- Difficult bowel movement.
- Dizziness.
- Dry, cracked lips and mouth.
- Fatigue.
- Fever.
- Depression.
- Headache in the afternoon or with dizziness.
- Irregular menstruation.
- Pale lips.
- Reclining with an inability to sit up due to dizziness.
- Blurred vision.

- Muscle twitching that cannot be controlled.
- Night sweats.
- Overdue periods at first, followed by reduced flow, and finally stopping altogether.
- Palpitation accompanied by anxiety.
- Menstrual pain during period.
- Thin with dry skin.
- Insomnia.
- Spasms.
- Twitching of four limbs.
- Pale complexion.

5. Blood Coagulation Syndrome

SYMPTOMS AND SIGNS:

- Abdominal pain.
- Bleeding from gums.
- Chest pain.
- Coughing out blood.
- Headache.
- Irregular periods at first, then overdue, and then no period.
- Lumbago.
- Pain (acute) around umbilicus resisting massage, with hard spots felt by hands.
- Pain in region between the navel and pubic hair with feeling of hardness.
- Pain in the hypochondrium.
- Pain in the loins as if being pierced with an awl.
- Pain in the ribs.
- Palpitation accompanied by anxiety.
- Partial suppression of lochia.
- Period pain.
- Spasms.
- Stomachache.
- Swelling and congestion after eating.
- Vomiting of blood.

6. Kidney Deficiency Syndrome

SYMPTOMS AND SIGNS:

- Asthma.
- Chronic backache.
- Clear, watery vaginal discharge.
- Hearing difficulties.
- Diarrhea.
- Hair loss.
- Infertility.
- Frequent urination with no thirst or little liquid intake.
- Fatigue and sleepiness.
- No burning sensation on urination.
- Pain (falling) in the lower abdomen with fondness for massage.
- Menstrual pain.
- Chronic whitish vaginal discharge.
- Ringing in ears.
- Ringing in ears and hearing loss.
- Toothache.

INGREDIENTS FOR CREATING RECIPES

FOODS FOR EXCESS: fresh ginger, wine, sunflower, sunflower seed, celery, rose, tea, prickly ash, white pepper, chinese rose, Chinese chive, coriander (Chinese parsley).

FOODS FOR DEFICIENCY: brown sugar, mutton, shrimp, pork, chicken, polished rice.

HERBS: Yan-hu-suo (Chinese yanhusuo), Pu-huang (cattail pollen), Ai-ye (mugwort), Yi-mu-cao (Siberian motherwort), Chuan-xiong (hemlock parsley), Tao-ren (peach kernel), Hong-hua (safflower), Xiao-hui-xiang (fennel seed), Dan-shen (purple sage), Dang-gui

(Chinese angelica), Shu-di (processed glutinous rehmannia), Bai-shao (white peony), Bu-gu-zhi (psoralea).

Syndromes of disease and herbs to use:

1. **WIND COLD:** Ai-ye (mugwort), Xiao-hui-xiang (fennel seed), Dang-gui (Chinese angelica); cook with foods for excess.
2. **COLD DAMPNESS:** Ai-ye (mugwort), Xiao-hui-xiang (fennel seed), Dang-gui (Chinese angelica), Chuan-xiong (hemlock parsley); cook with foods for excess.
3. **ENERGY STAGNATION:** Yan-hu-suo (Chinese yanhusuo), Dan-shen (purple sage); cook with foods for excess.
4. **BLOOD DEFICIENCY:** Dang-gui (Chinese angelica), Shu-di (processed glutinous rehmannia), Bai-shao (white peony); cook with foods for deficiency.
5. **BLOOD COAGULATION:** Pu-huang (cattail pollen), Yi-mu-cao (Siberian motherwort), Chuan-xiong (hemlock parsley), Tao-ren (peach kernel), Hong-hua (safflower), Dan-shen (purple sage); cook with foods for excess.
6. **KIDNEY DEFICIENCY:** Bu-gu-zhi (psoralea), Bai-shao (white peony), Shu-di (processed glutinous rehmannia); cook with foods for deficiency.

RECIPE 86

MASTER: 20 g Yan-hu-suo (Chinese yanhusuo), 50 g Yi-mu-cao (Siberian motherwort).

ASSOCIATE: 2 chicken eggs.

ASSISTANT: none.

SEASONING: rock sugar.

STEPS:

(1) Boil the three ingredients in water until chicken eggs, with shells, are cooked.

(2) Peel the eggs and put them back in the water to boil for two minutes more.

CONSUMPTION: eat the eggs and drink the soup.

INDICATIONS: energy stagnation and blood coagulation syndrome of period pain.

ANALSIS: Yan-hu-suo disperses the blood and promotes energy circulation to correct blood coagulation and energy congestion simultaneously. Chicken egg is a blood tonic and also lubricates dryness. Rock sugar is an energy tonic and improves the taste of the recipe.

RECIPE 87

MASTER: 15 g Dang-gui (Chinese angelica).

ASSOCIATE: 250 g mutton.

ASSISTANT: 60 g fresh ginger, some peanut oil.

SEASONING: rice wine, green onion.

STEPS:

(1) Cut up mutton into small pieces and fry with peanut oil.

(2) Add water, Dang-gui, fresh ginger, and green onion to the mutton and boil until the mutton is cooked.

(3) Remove the Dang-gui.

CONSUMPTION: eat the mutton and drink the soup at mealtimes.

INDICATIONS: wind cold and cold dampness syndrome of period pain.

ANALYSIS: Dang-gui is a blood tonic; it can warm the body. Mutton, fresh ginger, rice wine, and green onion can all warm the internal region; and peanut oil lubricates dryness.

12.4 Leukorrhea (vaginal discharge)

1. Energy Deficiency Syndrome

SYMPTOMS AND SIGNS:

- Abdominal pain.
- Constipation with soft stools.
- Discharge of sticky, turbid stool or diarrhea.

- Dizziness.
- Fatigue following bowel movement.
- Headache (severe) that occurs with fatigue after labor.
- Recurring headaches, headache in the morning, or prolonged headache.
- Reclining with an inability to sit up due to dizziness.
- Blurred vision.
- Numbness.
- Palpitation accompanied by anxiety.
- Perspiration in hands and feet.
- Ringing in ears that impairs hearing.
- Trembling hands.
- Shortness of breath.
- Thin with dry skin.
- Difficulty swallowing.
- Feeble voice.
- Slightly cold fingertips and toes.

2. Sputum Syndrome

SYMPTOMS AND SIGNS:

- Abdominal bloating or rumbling.
- Congested chest.
- Diarrhea.
- Dizziness.
- Headache.
- Heavy sensation in the body.
- Craving for hot drinks.
- Love of sweet or greasy foods.
- Numbness.
- Pain in the chest or hypochondrium.
- Palpitation.
- Stomachache.
- Swollen tongue.
- Vomiting or coughing with excessive watery sputum.

INGREDIENTS FOR CREATING RECIPES

FOODS FOR EXCESS: sunflower stem, buckwheat, litchi nut, towel gourd, black pepper, broad bean, Chinese chive, eggplant, water spinach, tofu.

FOODS FOR DEFICIENCY: brown sugar, litchi nut, glutinous rice, chicken, mussel, tofu, polished rice, chicken egg, pork skin, pork trotter, rock sugar.

HERBS: Lian-xu (lotus stamen), Bai-bian-dou (hyacinth bean), Qian-shi (water lily), Shan-yao (Chinese yam), Che-qian-zi (Asiatic plantain seed), Bai-guo (ginkgo), Jin-ying-zi (Cherokee rose), Rou-gui (Chinese cassia bark), Fu-ling (tuckahoe; Indian bread), Lian-zi (East Indian lotus), Ai-ye (mugwort), Da-zao (red date), Qian-shi (water lily).

Syndromes of disease and herbs to use:

1. **ENERGY DEFICIENCY:** Shan-yao (Chinese yam), Rou-gui (Chinese cassia bark), Fu-ling (tuckahoe; Indian bread), Ai-ye (mugwort), Da-zao (red date), Qian-shi (water lily); cook with foods for deficiency.
2. **SPUTUM:** Lian-xu (lotus stamen), Bai-bian-dou (hyacinth bean), Qian-shi (water lily), Che-qian-zi (Asiatic plantain seed), Bai-guo (ginkgo), Jin-ying-zi (Cherokee rose), Lian-zi (East Indian lotus); cook with foods for excess.

RECIPE 88

MASTER: 10 g Shan-yao (Chinese yam).

ASSOCIATE: 1 block tofu.

ASSISTANT: 50 g glutinous rice.

SEASONING: rock sugar.

STEPS:

(1) Grind Shan-yao into powder and cut the tofu into cubes.

(2) Boil the rice in 3 cups of water. While the water is boiling, add the tofu and herbal

powder. Continue to boil for ten minutes.

(3) Remove from heat and season with rock sugar, stirring until it dissolves.

CONSUMPTION: have as a midday meal.

INDICATIONS: energy deficiency syndrome of vaginal discharge.

ANALYSIS: All the ingredients in this recipe are energy tonics, including rock sugar, which also improves the taste.

RECIPE 89

MASTER: 60 g Qian-shi (water lily).

ASSOCIATE: 60 g Lian-zi (East Indian lotus).

ASSISTANT: 30 g glutinous rice.

SEASONING: brown sugar.

STEPS:

(1) Boil the three ingredients in enough water to make a congee.

(2) Season with brown sugar to taste.

CONSUMPTION: eat at mealtimes.

INDICATIONS: both syndromes of vaginal discharge.

ANALYSIS: Qian-shi and Lian-zi are both constrictive, which can stop discharge; glutinous rice is an energy tonic; and brown sugar improves the taste.

12.5 Metrorrhagia (uterine bleeding)

1. Sputum Congestion Syndrome

SYMPTOMS AND SIGNS:

- Normal breathing through the nose.
- Cold limbs.
- Congested chest.
- Cough.
- Headache.
- Craving for hot drinks.
- Morning sickness.
- Palpitation with nervousness.
- Light-colored menstrual flow.
- Perspiration that stops quickly.
- Subjective sensation of lump in the throat.

2. Energy Deficiency Syndrome

SYMPTOMS AND SIGNS:

- Abdominal pain.
- Complete suppression of urine during pregnancy.
- Constipation with discharge of soft stools.
- Discharge of sticky, turbid stool or diarrhea.
- Dizziness.
- Fatigue following bowel movement.
- Severe headache that occurs with fatigue after labor.
- Recurring headaches, headache in the morning, or prolonged headache.
- Inability to sit up from a reclining position due to dizziness.
- Blurred vision.
- Numbness.
- Palpitation accompanied by anxiety.
- Perspiration in hands and feet.
- Prolonged headache.
- Ringing in ears that causes hearing impairment.
- Trembling of both hands.
- Shortness of breath.
- Thin with dry skin.
- Difficulty swallowing.
- Feeble voice.
- Slightly cold fingers and toes.

3. **Energy Stagnation Syndrome**

SYMPTOMS AND SIGNS:

- Abdominal pain that eases after release of intestinal gas.
- Belching or hiccups.
- Chest and rib discomfort.
- Chest pain.
- Constipation with frequent false calls for a bowel movement.
- Irregular menstruation.
- Overdue menstruation.
- Pain in inner part of stomach with prickling sensation and distention.
- Pain in the hypochondrium.
- Period pain.
- Infrequent urination.
- Ringing in ears and hearing difficulty.
- Stomachache.
- Subjective sensation of lump in the throat.
- Difficulty swallowing.
- Swelling and congestion after eating.

4. **Hot Blood Syndrome**

SYMPTOMS AND SIGNS:

- Abdominal pain.
- Bleeding of various kinds, including nosebleed.
- Deep-red or violet-colored menstrual flow.
- Menstrual flow with a foul odor.
- Premature periods.
- Skin ulcers.
- Vaginal bleeding other than menstrual.
- Urination difficulty.

5. **Blood Coagulation Syndrome**

SYMPTOMS AND SIGNS:

- Abdominal pain.
- Bleeding from gums.
- Chest pain.
- Coughing with blood.
- Headache.
- Irregular period at first, then overdue, and then no period.
- Lumbago.
- Pain (acute) around umbilicus resisting massage, with hard spots felt by hands.
- Pain in region between navel and pubic hair with feeling of hardness.
- Pain in the hypochondrium.
- Pain in the loins as if being pierced with an awl.
- Pain in the ribs.
- Palpitation accompanied by anxiety.
- Partial suppression of lochia.
- Painful period.
- Spasm.
- Stomachache.
- Swelling and congestion after eating.
- Vomiting of blood.

6. **Spleen Deficiency Syndrome**

SYMPTOMS AND SIGNS:

- Abdominal pain with a fondness for massage.
- Belching.
- Clear, long streams of urine.
- Chronic diarrhea.
- Indigestion.

- Prefer to be reclining.
- Excessive whitish vaginal discharge.
- Poor appetite.
- Prolapse of any internal organ.
- Prolapse of rectum.
- Shortness of breath.
- Underweight.
- Vaginal discharge with a slight foul odor.
- Vomiting of acid.

7. Kidney Deficiency Syndrome

SYMPTOMS AND SIGNS:

- Asthma.
- Chronic backache.
- Clear, watery, whitish vaginal discharge.
- Hearing difficulty.
- Diarrhea.
- Falling hair.
- Infertility.
- Large quantities of urine with no thirst or drink.
- Preference for reclining and sleeping.
- No burning sensation on urination.
- Pain (falling) in the lower abdomen with fondness for massage.
- Period pain.
- Ringing in ears.
- Ringing in ears and hearing impairment.
- Toothache.
- Whitish vaginal discharge, especially prolonged.

INGREDIENTS FOR CREATING RECIPES

FOODS FOR EXCESS: vinegar, litchi nut, water chestnut, buckwheat, broad bean, black fungus, sunflower, pork skin, shepherd's purse.

FOODS FOR DEFICIENCY: mussel, longan nut, white fungus, pork.

HERBS: Sha-ren (grains of paradise), E-jiao (donkey-hide gelatin), Pu-huang (cattail pollen), Hai-piao-xiao (cuttlebone), Ai-ye (mugwort), Ce-bai-ye (oriental arbor vitae), Xian-he-cao (agrimony), Huang-yao-zi (Ceylon white yam), Da-zao (red date), Yu-mi-xu (corn silk), Sheng-di (dried glutinous rehmannia), Yi-mu-cao (Siberian motherwort), Bu-gu-zhi (psoralea), Gan-cao (licorice).

Syndromes of disease and herbs to use:

1. **SPUTUM CONGESTION:** Hai-piao-xiao (cuttlebone), Ce-bai-ye (oriental arbor vitae), Xian-he-cao (agrimony); cook with foods for excess.
2. **ENERGY DEFICIENCY:** E-jiao (donkey-hide gelatin), Hai-piao-xiao (cuttlebone), Ce-bai-ye (oriental arbor vitae), Xian-he-cao (agrimony), Da-zao (red date), Gan-cao (licorice); cook with foods for deficiency.
3. **ENERGY STAGNATION:** Sha-ren (grains of paradise), Hai-piao-xiao (cuttlebone), Ai-ye (mugwort), Xian-he-cao (agrimony), Ce-bai-ye (oriental arbor vitae); cook with foods for excess.
4. **HOT BLOOD:** Hai-piao-xiao (cuttlebone), Ce-bai-ye (oriental arbor vitae), Xian-he-cao (agrimony), Huang-yao-zi (Ceylon white yam), Yu-mi-xu (corn silk), Sheng-di (dried glutinous rehmannia); cook with foods for excess.
5. **BLOOD COAGULATION:** Pu-huang (cattail pollen), Hai-piao-xiao (cuttlebone), Ai-ye (mugwort), Ce-bai-ye (oriental arbor vitae), Xian-he-cao (agrimony), Yi-mu-cao (Siberian motherwort); cook with foods for excess.
6. **SPLEEN DEFICIENCY:** E-jiao (donkey-hide gelatin), Hai-piao-xiao (cuttlebone), Ce-bai-ye (oriental arbor vitae), Xian-he-cao (agrimony), Da-zao (red date), Gan-cao (licorice); cook with foods for deficiency.
7. **KIDNEY DEFICIENCY:** E-jiao (donkey-hide

gelatin), Hai-piao-xiao (cuttlebone), Ce-bai-ye (oriental arbor vitae), Xian-he-cao (agrimony), Da-zao (red date), Bu-gu-zhi (psoralea), Gan-cao (licorice); cook with foods for deficiency.

RECIPE 90

MASTER: 60 g longan nuts.

ASSOCIATE: 30 g litchi nuts.

ASSISTANT: 15 g peanut oil.

SEASONING: none.

STEPS:

(1) Shell the longan and litchi nuts.

(2) Pour peanut oil into the frying pan and heat until hot. Add the longan and litchi nut meat and fry for a few seconds.

CONSUMPTION: Have twice each day.

INDICATIONS: energy and kidney deficiency syndromes of metrorrhagia.

ANALYSIS: longan nut is a blood tonic, frequently used to treat bleeding from the uterus; litchi nut is a yin tonic and disperses the blood to correct blood coagulation; and peanut oil is yin tonic and lubricates dryness.

RECIPE 91

MASTER: 30 g Hai-piao-xiao (cuttlebone).

ASSOCIATE: 90 g pork.

ASSISTANT: none.

SEASONING: salt.

STEPS:

(1) Cut up the pork into large pieces and wash clean; crush cuttlebone.

(2) Place pork, cuttlebone, salt, and an adequate amount of water in a steamer and steam until the ingredients are cooked.

CONSUMPTION: eat the pork.

INDICATIONS: all syndromes of metrorrhagia.

ANALYSIS: Hai-piao-xiao is constrictive, helping to control bleeding; pork is a yin tonic, lubricating internal dryness; and salt improves the taste.

RECIPE 92

MASTER: 30 g shepherd's purse.

ASSOCIATE: 60 g fresh lotus root.

ASSISTANT: 3 g Sheng-di (dried glutinous rehmannia), 15 g peanut oil.

SEASONING: salt or miso.

STEPS:

(1) Wash shepherd's purse and lotus root.

(2) Over high heat, pour peanut oil into an earthenware pot; add the three ingredients and fry.

(3) Season with salt or miso to taste. Discard Sheng-di.

CONSUMPTION: eat the shepherd's purse and lotus root.

INDICATIONS: hot blood syndrome of metrorrhagia.

ANALYSIS: Shepherd's purse and fresh lotus root are commonly used to stop bleeding. Sheng-di is a yin tonic, helping to clear heat. Peanut oil is a yin tonic and lubricates drynesss. Salt or miso can clear heat and improve the taste.

12.6 Menorrhagia (excessive menstrual bleeding)

1. Damp Phlegm Syndrome

SYMPTOMS AND SIGNS:

- Abdominal distention with congested chest.
- Coughing with excessive sputum.
- Dizziness with heavy sensations in the head.
- Headache.
- Hiccups.
- Nausea.
- Palpitation with nervousness.
- Late periods.

- Poor appetite.
- Whitish vaginal discharge, especially excessive.

2. **Energy Deficiency Syndrome**

SYMPTOMS AND SIGNS:

- Abdominal pain.
- Constipation with discharge of soft stools.
- Discharge of sticky, turbid stool or diarrhea.
- Dizziness.
- Fatigue following bowel movement.
- Severe headache that occured with fatigue after previous labor.
- Recurring headaches, headache in the morning, or prolonged headache.
- Inability to sit up from a reclining position due to dizziness.
- Blurred vision.
- Numbness.
- Palpitation accompanied by anxiety.
- Perspiration in hands and feet.
- Prolonged headache.
- Ringing in ears that causes hearing impairment.
- Trembling of both hands.
- Shortness of breath.
- Thin with dry skin.
- Difficulty swallowing.
- Feeble voice.
- Slightly cold fingers and toes.

3. **Hot Blood Syndrome**

SYMPTOMS AND SIGNS:

- Abdominal pain.
- Bleeding of various kinds.
- Deep-red or violet-colored menstrual flow.
- Menstrual flow with a foul odor.
- Premature periods.
- Skin ulcers.
- Urination difficulty.

INGREDIENTS FOR CREATING RECIPES

FOODS FOR EXCESS: fresh ginger, black fungus.

FOODS FOR DEFICIENCY: chicken egg, mussel.

HERBS: Wu-mei (black plum), Jin-ying-zi (Cherokee rose), Tian-dong (lucid asparagus), Shu-di (processed glutinous rehmannia), E-jiao (donkey-hide gelatin), Sheng-di (dried glutinous rehmannia), Bai-ji (amethyst orchid).

Syndromes of disease and herbs to use:

1. **DAMP PHLEGM:** Wu-mei (black plum), Jin-ying-zi (Cherokee rose), Bai-ji (amethyst orchid); cook with foods for excess.

2. **ENERGY DEFICIENCY:** Wu-mei (black plum), Jin-ying-zi (Cherokee rose), Tian-dong (lucid asparagus), Shu-di (processed glutinous rehmannia), E-jiao (donkey-hide gelatin); cook with foods for deficiency.

3. **HOT BLOOD:** Wu-mei (black plum), Jin-ying-zi (Cherokee rose), Sheng-di (dried glutinous rehmannia); cook with foods for excess.

RECIPE 93

MASTER: 5 g E-jiao (donkey-hide gelatin).

ASSOCIATE: 30 g brown sugar.

ASSISTANT: none.

SEASONING: none.

STEPS:

(1) Boil E-jiao (donkey-hide gelatin) in 2 cups of water until water is reduced to 1 cup.

(2) Add brown sugar and boil for a few minutes longer.

CONSUMPTION: drink the soup hot, once daily.

INDICATIONS: energy deficiency syndrome of metrorrhagia.

ANALYSIS: E-jiao, a blood tonic which is sticky in nature, can stop bleeding particularly in the deficiency syndrome of bleeding. Brown sugar, an energy tonic, is often used in a recipe to stop bleeding.

12.7 Oligomenorrhea (scanty or infrequent menstrual flow)

1. Blood Deficiency Syndrome

SYMPTOMS AND SIGNS:

- Abdominal pain that occurs at onset of periods.
- Constipation with discharge of hard stool.
- Difficult bowel movement.
- Dizziness.
- Dry, cracked lips and mouth.
- Fatigue.
- Fever.
- Feeling depressed.
- Headache in the afternoon or with dizziness.
- Irregular menstruation.
- Pale lips.
- Inability to sit up from a reclining position due to dizziness.
- Blurred vision.
- Muscles spasms.
- Night sweats.
- Overdue periods at first, then reduced, and then stopping.
- Palpitation accompanied by anxiety.
- Period pain.
- Thin with dry skin.
- Insomnia.
- Twitching in the four limbs.
- Pale complexion.

2. Damp Phlegm Syndrome

SYMPTOMS AND SIGNS:

- Abdominal swelling with congested chest.
- Coughing out excessive sputum.
- Dizziness with heavy sensations in the head.
- Frequent coughs during previous pregnancy that prolonged or caused fetal motion.
- Headache.
- Hiccups.
- Nausea.
- Palpitation with nervousness.
- Frequent overdue periods.
- Poor appetite.
- Whitish vaginal discharge, especially excessive.

3. Spleen Dampness Syndrome

SYMPTOMS AND SIGNS:

- Chest discomfort without appetite.
- Diarrhea.
- Edema.
- Heavy sensations in head as if the head were covered with something.
- Heavy sensations in the body with discomfort.
- Craving for hot drinks.
- Nausea and vomiting.
- Poor appetite.
- Scanty urine.
- Stomach fullness and discomfort.

- Sweet-sticky taste in mouth.
- Too lazy to talk or move.
- Vaginal discharge with a fishy, foul odor.
- Whitish or bloody vaginal discharge.

4. **Cold Blood Syndrome**

SYMPTOMS AND SIGNS:

- Abdominal pain.
- Cold and stabbing pain in lower abdomen before periods.
- Irregular menstruation.
- Menstrual flow not unlike juice of black beans.
- Overdue period.
- Period pain.

5. **Blood Deficiency Syndrome**

SYMPTOMS AND SIGNS:

- Abdominal pain.
- Constipation with discharge of hard stool.
- Difficult bowel movement.
- Dizziness.
- Dry, cracked lips and mouth.
- Fatigue.
- Fever.
- Feeling depressed.
- Headache in the afternoon or with dizziness.
- Irregular menstruation.
- Pale lips.
- Low energy and feeble voice.
- Inability to sit up from a reclining position due to dizziness.
- Blurred vision.
- Muscle spasms.
- Night sweats.
- Pale complexion, lips, and nails.
- Palpitation accompanied by anxiety.
- Thin with dry skin.
- Insomnia.
- Twitching in the four limbs.
- Pale complexion.

6. **Deficiency of Energy and Blood Syndrome**

SYMPTOMS AND SIGNS:

- Bleeding of various kinds with light-colored blood, often seen in consumptive diseases.
- Dizziness.
- Fatigue.
- "Flying objects" in front of the eyes.
- Insomnia.
- Low energy.
- Feeble voice.
- No burning sensation on urination.
- Numbness of limbs.
- Pale complexion and lips.
- Pale nails.
- Palpitation.

7. **Blood Coagulation Syndrome**

SYMPTOMS AND SIGNS:

- Abdominal pain.
- Bleeding from gums.
- Chest pain.
- Coughing with blood.
- Headache.
- Irregular periods at first, then overdue, and then no period.
- Lumbago.

- Pain (acute) around umbilicus resisting massage, with hard spots felt by hands.
- Pain in region between navel and pubic hair with feeling of hardness.
- Pain in the hypochondrium.
- Pain in the loins as if being pierced with an awl.
- Pain in the ribs.
- Palpitation accompanied by anxiety.
- Partial suppression of lochia.
- Period pain.
- Spasms.
- Stomachache.
- Swelling and congestion after eating.
- Vomiting of blood.

8. Kidney Deficiency Syndrome

SYMPTOMS AND SIGNS:

- Asthma.
- Chronic backache.
- Clear, watery, white vaginal discharge.
- Hearing loss.
- Diarrhea.
- Falling hair.
- Infertility.
- Large quantities of urine with no thirst or drink.
- Prefer to recline and sleep.
- No burning sensation on urination.
- Pain (falling) in the lower abdomen with fondness for massage.
- Period pain.
- Ringing in ears.
- Ringing in ears and hearing loss.
- Toothache.
- Whitish vaginal discharge, especially prolonged.

INGREDIENTS FOR CREATING RECIPES

FOODS FOR EXCESS: fresh ginger, celery, black soybean.

FOODS FOR DEFICIENCY: chicken, chicken liver, duck, pork trotter, chicken egg, brown sugar, mutton.

HERBS: Ai-ye (mugwort), Bai-zi-ren (oriental arborvitae kernel), Niu-xi (two-toothed amaranthus), Shan-zha (Chinese hawthorn), Dang-gui (Chinese angelica), Dang-shen (root of pilose asiabell), Shan-yao (Chinese yam), Huang-qi (membranous milk vetch), Fu-ling (tuckahoe; Indian bread), Cang-zhu (gray atractylodes), Ban-xia (half-summer pinellia), Chen-pi (tangerine peel), Chi-xiao-dou (small red bean [like azuki bean]), Huang-qi (membranous milk vetch), Gui-zhi (cinnamon stick), Bai-shao (white peony), Ren-shen (Chinese ginseng), Bai-zhu (white atractylodes), Tao-ren (peach kernel), Hong-hua (safflower), Chuan-xiong (hemlock parsley), E-jiao (donkey-hide gelatin), Hai-piao-xiao (cuttlebone), Ce-bai-ye (oriental arborvitae), Xian-he-cao (agrimony), Da-zao (red date), Bu-gu-zhi (psoralea), Gan-cao (licorice).

Syndromes of disease and herbs to use:

1. **BLOOD DEFICIENCY:** Dang-gui (Chinese angelica), Dang-shen (root of pilose asiabell), Shan-yao (Chinese yam), Huang-qi (membranous milk vetch); cook with foods for deficiency.
2. **DAMP PHLEGM:** Fu-ling (tuckahoe; Indian bread), Cang-zhu (gray atractylodes), Ban-xia (half-summer pinellia), Chen-pi (dried tangerine peel); cook with foods for excess.
3. **SPLEEN DAMPNESS;** Chi-xiao-dou (small red bean), Huang-qi (membranous milk vetch), Gui-zhi (cinnamon stick), Fu-ling (tuckahoe; Indian bread); cook with foods for excess.
4. **COLD BLOOD:** Dang-gui (Chinese angelica), Huang-qi (membranous milk vetch), Gui-

zhi (cinnamon stick); cook with foods for excess.

5. **BLOOD DEFICIENCY:** Dang-gui (Chinese angelica), Huang-qi (membranous milk vetch), Bai-shao (white peony); cook with foods for deficiency.

6. **DEFICIENCY OF ENERGY AND BLOOD:** Dang-gui (Chinese angelica), Dang-shen (root of pilose asiabell), Ren-shen (Chinese ginseng), Bai-zhu (white atractylodes); cook with foods for deficiency.

7. **BLOOD COAGULATION:** Tao-ren (peach kernel), Hong-hua (safflower), Dang-gui (Chinese angelica), Chuan-xiong (hemlock parsley); cook with foods for excess.

8. **KIDNEY DEFICIENCY:** E-jiao (donkey-hide gelatin), Hai-piao-xiao (cuttlebone), Ce-bai-ye (oriental arborvitae), Xian-he-cao (agrimony), Da-zao (red date), Bu-gu-zhi (psoralea), Gan-cao (licorice); cook with foods for deficiency.

RECIPE 94

MASTER: 10 g Dang-gui (Chinese angelica), 25 g Huang-qi (membranous milk vetch).

ASSOCIATE: 500 g mutton.

ASSISTANT: 60 g fresh ginger.

SEASONING: black pepper.

STEPS:

(1) Put Dang-gui (Chinese angelica) and Huang-qi (membranous milk vetch) in a gauze bag.

(2) Cut the mutton into small pieces. Peel and slice the fresh ginger.

(3) Put the gauze bag, mutton, and ginger in water and boil over low heat until mutton is cooked, about 20 minutes.

(4) Remove the gauze bag and add black pepper to taste before consuming.

CONSUMPTION: eat the mutton and drink the soup twice daily, at mealtimes.

INDICATIONS: deficiency syndromes of oligomenorrhea.

ANALYSIS: Dang-gui is a blood tonic; Huang-qi is an energy tonic; mutton and fresh ginger can warm up the body; and black pepper reinforces the warming effect of this recipe while also improving the taste.

12.8 Menopause

1. Kidney Yang Deficiency Syndrome

SYMPTOMS AND SIGNS:

- Chronic diarrhea.
- Cold feet, cold loins and legs, or cold sensations in the vaginal area or in the muscles.
- Coughing and panting after light exertion.
- Diarrhea before dawn.
- Diarrhea that consists of sticky, muddy stool.
- Discharge of watery thin stool.
- Dizziness.
- Edema.
- Fatigue.
- Frequent urination at night.
- Cool or cold hands and feet.
- Infertility.
- Lack of appetite.
- Pain in the loins (lumbago).
- Palpitation.
- Panting.
- Period pain which eases with menstrual flow.
- Perspiration in the forehead.
- Pre-period pain in the abdomen with hard, full sensation in the lower abdomen.
- Ringing in ears.

- Scanty periods of a dark, violet color.
- Scanty urine.

2. Liver Kidney Yin Deficiency Syndrome

SYMPTOMS AND SIGNS:

- Difficulty in both bowel movement and urination.
- Dizziness.
- Dry eyes or throat.
- Fatigue.
- Headache with pain in the bony ridge forming the eyebrow.
- Lumbago.
- Night-blindness.
- Night sweats.
- Pain in the hypochondrium.
- Hot palms of hands and soles of feet.
- Insomnia with forgetfulness.
- Dry, withered complexion.

INGREDIENTS FOR CREATING RECIPES

FOODS FOR EXCESS: pork skin.

FOODS FOR DEFICIENCY: chestnut, mutton, glutinous rice, white sugar, wheat, chicken, pork, longan nuts.

HERBS: Da-zao (red date), Gan-cao (licorice), Ling-zhi (lucid ganoderma), Shan-yao (Chinese yam), Bai-he (lily), Bai-shao (white peony), Ce-bai-ye (oriental arborvitae), Suan-zao-ren (jujube), Fu-shen (poria with hostwood), Gou-qi-zi (matrimony vine fruit).

Syndromes of disease and herbs to use:

1. **KIDNEY YANG DEFICIENCY**: Ling-zhi (lucid ganoderma), Shan-yao (Chinese yam), Ce-bai-ye (oriental arborvitae); cook with foods for deficiency.

2. **LIVER KIDNEY YIN DEFICIENCY:** Da-zao (red date), Gan-cao (licorice), Ling-zhi (lucid ganoderma), Shan-yao (Chinese yam), Bai-he (lily), Bai-shao (white peony), Ce-bai-ye (oriental arborvitae), Suan-zao-ren (jujube), Fu-shen (poria with hostwood); cook with foods for deficiency.

RECIPE 95

MASTER: 50 g Ling-zhi (lucid ganoderma).

ASSOCIATE: 50 g glutinous rice.

ASSISTANT: 50 g wheat flour.

SEASONING: white sugar.

STEPS:

(1) Boil the Ling-zhi (lucid ganoderma), glutinous rice, and wheat flour in enough water to make a congee.

(2) Season with white sugar to taste.

CONSUMPTION: have at mealtimes.

INDICATIONS: both syndromes of menopause.

ANALYSIS: Ling-zhi, a general tonic, can improve the spirits and complexion; glutinous rice is an energy tonic; wheat flour can calm the spirits; and white sugar improves the taste.

RECIPE 96

MASTER: 15 g Shan-yao (Chinese yam).

ASSOCIATE: 25 g longan nut meat, 100 g glutinous rice.

ASSISTANT: 10 g Da-zao (red date).

SEASONING: honey.

STEPS:

(1) Cut Shan-yao (Chinese yam) into small pieces.

(2) Boil the Shan-yao, longan nut meat, glutinous rice, and Da-zao (red date) in water to make a congee.

(3) Season with honey to taste.

CONSUMPTION: eat as a side dish at mealtimes.

INDICATIONS: both syndromes of menopause.

ANALYSIS: Shan-yao is an energy tonic; longan nut is a blood tonic; glutinous rice and Da-zao are also energy tonics; and honey lubricates internal dryness while also improving the taste.

12.9 Frigidity (absence of sexual desire and orgasm)

1. **Liver Energy Congestion Syndrome**

SYMPTOMS AND SIGNS:

- Abdominal pain.
- Muscle spasms.
- Irregular periods.
- Menstrual pain.
- Morning sickness.
- Numbness.
- Pain in the hypochondrium.
- Early or late periods.
- Shortage of milk secretion after childbirth.
- Stomachache.
- Subjective sensations of objects in the throat.
- Vomiting of blood.
- Whitish vaginal discharge.

2. **Kidney Yang Deficiency Syndrome**

SYMPTOMS AND SIGNS:

- Chronic diarrhea.
- Cold feet, cold loins and legs, or cold sensations in the vaginal area or in the muscles.
- Coughing and panting after light exertion.
- Diarrhea before dawn.
- Diarrhea that consits of sticky, muddy stool.
- Discharge of watery thin stool.
- Dizziness.
- Edema.
- Fatigue.
- Frequent urination at night.
- Cool or cold hands.
- Infertility.
- Lack of appetite.
- Pain in the loins (lumbago).
- Palpitation.
- Shortness of breath.
- Period pain eases with menstrual flow.
- Perspiration in the forehead.
- Pre-period pain in the abdomen with hard, full sensation in the lower abdomen.
- Ringing in ears.
- Scanty periods with a dark, violet color.
- Scanty urine.
- Suppression of menses.

3. **Kidney Yin Deficiency Syndrome**

SYMPTOMS AND SIGNS:

- Cough with sputum containing blood or coughing out fresh blood.
- Dry sensations in the mouth particularly at night.
- Dry throat.
- Fatigue.
- Frequent urination.
- Hot sensations in any part of the body.
- Night sweats.
- Pain in the heel.
- Pain in the loins (lumbago).
- Retention of urine.
- Ringing in ears.
- Insomnia.

- "Spots" in front of the eyes.
- Unusual thirst.
- Toothache or loose teeth.
- Urine as thick as liquid fat.

INGREDIENTS FOR CREATING RECIPES

FOODS FOR EXCESS: common carp, crab, pea, squash seed, orange leaf, sword bean, peanut, tofu, sorghum, common button mushroom.

FOODS FOR DEFICIENCY: honey, sparrow, lobster, Chinese chive, walnut, sparrow egg, mussel, shrimp, oyster, loach, pork, mutton, sea cucumber.

HERBS: Huang-jing (sealwort), Gou-qi-zi (matrimony vine fruit), Fu-pen-zi (wild raspberry), Ai-ye (mugwort), Dang-gui (Chinese angelica), Ba-ji-tian (morinda root), Yin-yang-huo (longspur epimendium), Jiu-cai-zi (Chinese chive seed), She-chuang-zi (snake bed seed), Chai-hu (hare's ear), Zhi-shi (China orange), Sheng-ma (skunk bugbane).

Syndromes of disease and herbs to use:

1. **LIVER ENERGY CONGESTION:** Chai-hu (hare's ear), Zhi-shi (China orange), Sheng-ma (skunk bugbane); cook with foods for excess.
2. **KIDNEY YANG DEFICIENCY:** Ai-ye (mugwort), Ba-ji-tian (morinda root), Yin-yang-huo (longspur epimendium), Jiu-cai-zi (Chinese chive seed), She-chuang-zi (snake bed seed); cook with foods for deficiency.
3. **KIDNEY YIN DEFICIENCY**: Huang-jing (sealwort), Gou-qi-zi (matrimony vine fruit), Fu-pen-zi (wild raspberry); cook with foods for deficiency.

RECIPE 97

MASTER: 8 g Huang-jing (sealwort), 15 g Gou-qi-zi (matrimony vine fruit).

ASSOCIATE: 1 lobster.

ASSISTANT: 50 g shrimp.

SEASONING: salt.

STEPS:

(1) Decoct Huang-jing (sealwort) and Gou-qi-zi (matrimony vine fruit) for thirty minutes; strain to obtain herbal soup.

(2) Boil lobster and shrimp, with shells, in ample water until cooked.

(3) Remove lobster and shrimp from water and add to the herbal soup.

(4) Season with salt to taste.

CONSUMPTION: eat at mealtimes.

INDICATIONS: deficiency syndromes of frigidity in women.

ANALYSIS: Huang-jing is a yin tonic, Gou-qi-zi is a blood tonic, and lobster and shrimp are yang tonics. Salt acts on the kidneys and also improves the taste.

RECIPE 98

MASTER: 9 g each, Yin-yang-huo (longspur epimendium), Jiu-cai-zi (Chinese chive seed), She-chuang-zi (snake bed seed).

ASSOCIATE: 1 whole chicken.

ASSISTANT: 3 teaspoonfuls of rice wine.

SEASONING: salt.

STEPS:

(1) Put the three master ingredients in a gauze bag.

(2) Boil the chicken in ample water with the rice wine and gauze bag until cooked, about 25 to 35 minutes.

(3) Remove the bag and discard, and season with salt to taste.

CONSUMPTION: eat at mealtimes.

INDICATIONS: deficiency syndromes of frigidity in women.

ANALYSIS: The three master ingredients are all yang tonics; chicken is an energy tonic; rice wine can speed up the effects of the other ingredients, and salt acts on the kidneys and improves the taste.

12.10 Shortage of milk in nursing mothers

1. **Blood Deficiency Syndrome**

SYMPTOMS AND SIGNS:

- Abdominal pain.
- Constipation with discharge of hard stool.
- Difficult bowel movement.
- Dizziness.
- Dry, cracked lips and mouth.
- Fatigue.
- Fever.
- Feeling depressed.
- Headache in the afternoon or with dizziness.
- Irregular menstruation.
- Pale, lightly colored lips .
- Low energy and feeble voice.
- Inability to sit up from a reclining position due to dizziness.
- Blurred vision.
- Muscle spasms.
- Night sweats.
- Pale complexion, lips, and nails.
- Palpitation accompanied by anxiety.
- Thin with dry skin.
- Insomnia.
- Twitching in the four limbs.
- Pale complexion.

2. **Liver Energy Congestion Syndrome**

SYMPTOMS AND SIGNS:

- Abdominal obstruction.
- Abdominal pain.
- Bitter taste in the mouth.
- Muscle spasms.
- Dry tongue.
- Easily angry.
- Numbness.
- Pain in the hypochondrium.
- Early periods.
- Poor appetite.
- Stomachache.
- Subjective sensations of objects in the throat.
- Vomiting of blood.
- Whitish vaginal discharge.

INGREDIENTS FOR CREATING RECIPES

FOODS FOR EXCESS: common carp, crab, pea, squash seed, orange leaf, sword bean, peanut, tofu, towel gourd, sorghum, common button mushroom.

FOODS FOR DEFICIENCY: sesame seed, pork, pork liver, pork trotter, chicken, wheat, tofu, shiitake mushroom, mutton, white sugar, shrimp.

HERBS: Da-zao (red date), Cong-bai (Welsh onion), Wang-bu-liu-xing (seed of cow-basil), Lou-lu (rhaponticum root), Chi-xiao-dou (small red bean [like azuki bean]), Zi-su-ye (purple perilla leaf), Chen-pi (dried tangerine peel), Gao-liang-jiang (lesser galangal), Dang-gui (Chinese angelica), Huang-qi (membranous milk vetch), Chai-hu (hare's ear), Qing-pi (green tangerine peel), Xiang-fu (nutgrass flatsedge rhizome), Mu-tong (akebi).

Syndromes of disease and herbs to use:

1. **BLOOD DEFICIENCY:** Da-zao (red date), Cong-bai (Welsh onion), Lou-lu (rhaponticum root), Wang-bu-liu-xing (seed of cow-basil), Mu-tong (akebi), Gao-liang-jiang (lesser galangal); cook with foods for deficiency.
2. **LIVER ENERGY CONGESTION:** Wang-bu-liu-xing (seed of cow-basil), Chi-xiao-dou (small red bean), Chai-hu (hare's ear),

Qing-pi (green orange peel), Xiang-fu (nutgrass flatsedge rhizome); cook with foods for excess.

RECIPE 99

MASTER: 1 pork trotter.

ASSOCIATE: 15 g Cong-bai (Welsh onion or white heads of green onion).

ASSISTANT: 90 g tofu, 50 ml rice wine.

SEASONING: soy sauce.

STEPS:

(1) Wash and clean the pork trotter and cut into 8 pieces. Place in an earthenware pot along with Cong-bai (Welsh onion) and tofu.

(2) Add 1 to 2 glasses of water and boil over low heat.

(3) Add rice wine and soy sauce before removing from heat.

CONSUMPTION: eat at mealtimes; in general, 5 to 7 times should be sufficient.

INDICATIONS: blood deficiency syndrome of shortage of milk secretion.

ANALYSIS: Pork trotter, a blood tonic, is commonly used to promote milk secretion. Cong-bai promotes energy circulation; tofu is an energy tonic; rice wine speeds up the effects of the other ingredients; and soy sauce improves the taste.

RECIPE 100

MASTER: 100 g shrimp.

ASSOCIATE: 1 pork trotter.

ASSISTANT: 60 ml rice wine.

SEASONING: none.

STEPS:

(1) Clean the shrimp as you would in normal cooking.

(2) Cut the pork trotter in 2 slices, then further cut each slice into 3 or 4 pieces.

(3) Put water in an earthenware pot and steam the two ingredients over high heat.

(4) When they are cooked, add the rice wine.

CONSUMPTION: eat the contents and drink the soup. In general, 5 to 7 times should be sufficient.

INDICATIONS: blood deficiency syndrome of shortage of milk secretion.

ANALYSIS: Shrimp is a yang tonic; pork trotter is a blood tonic. Both are commonly used to promote milk secretion. Rice wine speeds up the effects of the other ingredients.

NOTE: No herbs are used in this recipe; food cures may be effective without the use of herbs, as in this case.

RECIPE 101

MASTER: 5 g Mu-tong (akebi).

ASSOCIATE: 150 g octopus.

ASSISTANT: 1 pork trotter.

SEASONING: salt.

STEPS:

(1) Wash the octopus and cut it up into 3 1.5-cm pieces.

(2) Slice the pork trotter in two, and then cut each slice further into 3–4 pieces.

(3) Place octopus, pork trotter, and Mu-tong (akebi) in an earthenware pot and add enough water to boil over high heat until cooked.

(4) Remove Mu-tong (akebi) from the pot and discard.

CONSUMPTION: eat the contents and drink the soup. In general, 5 to 7 times should be sufficient.

INDICATIONS: blood deficiency syndrome of shortage of milk secretion.

ANALYSIS: Mu-tong is commonly used to promote milk secretion; octopus is an energy and blood tonic; pork trotter is also a blood tonic, commonly used to promote milk secretion; and salt improves the taste.

RECIPE 102

MASTER: 15 g Chi-xiao-dou (small red beans).

ASSOCIATE: 100 g gold carp.

ASSISTANT: 1 pork trotter.

SEASONING: salt.

STEPS:

(1) Cut away the scales and remove internal organs of the carp, and wash clean.

(2) Cut the pork trotter in two slices, then cut each slice further into 4 pieces.

(3) Place the three ingredients in an earthenware pot and boil in water over high heat until cooked.

(4) Season with salt to taste.

CONSUMPTION: eat the carp, pork trotter, and Chi-xiao-dou and drink the soup.

INDICATIONS: liver energy congestion syndrome of shortage of milk secretion.

ANALYSIS: Chi-xiao-dou is a leading food to promote milk secretion; gold carp is a spleen tonic; and pork trotter is a blood tonic also commonly used to promote milk secretion. Salt improves the taste.

12.11 Morning sickness

1. Sputum Congestion Syndrome

SYMPTOMS AND SIGNS:

- Breathing through the nose.
- Cold limbs.
- Congested chest.
- Cough.
- Headache.
- Palpitation with nervousness.
- Perspiration that stops quickly.
- Subjective sensation of lump in the throat.

2. Spleen-Stomach Yang Deficiency Syndrome

SYMPTOMS AND SIGNS:

- Belching.
- Copious phlegm in the throat.
- Diarrhea.
- Eating in the morning and vomiting in the evening.
- Slightly cold hands and feet.
- Hiccups.
- Craving for hot drinks.
- Preference for massage with heat.
- Stomachache.
- Vomiting of clear saliva.

3. Hot Stomach Syndrome

SYMPTOMS AND SIGNS:

- Bad breath.
- Bleeding from gums.
- Dry nose.
- Nosebleed of a bright red color.
- Pain in the gums with swelling.
- Sore throat.
- Perspiring in the head.
- Stomachache.
- Thirst and craving for cold drinks.
- Vomiting of blood.
- Vomiting right after eating.
- Vomiting with stomach discomfort.

4. Hot Liver Syndrome

SYMPTOMS AND SIGNS:

- Bitter taste in the mouth.
- Bloody urine.
- Hearing impairment.

- Dry throat.
- Head swelling sensation or headache.
- Nosebleed of a bright red color.
- Pain in the hypochondrium.
- Partial suppression of lochia.
- Pink eyes with swelling.
- Mental depression.
- Sour taste in the mouth.
- Spasms.
- Twitching.
- Vaginal discharge with a fishy, foul odor.

5. Spleen-Stomach Energy Deficiency Syndrome

SYMPTOMS AND SIGNS:

- Abdominal swelling.
- Belching.
- Diarrhea often triggered by eating cold or greasy foods.
- Diarrhea that consists of watery stools.
- Fatigue.
- Indigestion with poor appetite.
- Prolapse of the uterus.
- Ringing in ears and hearing loss.
- Withered yellowish complexion.
- Sallow complexion.

INGREDIENTS FOR CREATING RECIPES

FOODS FOR EXCESS: orange leaf, grapevine leaf, common carp, fresh lotus root, grapefruit, watermelon, mung bean, fresh ginger, Chinese chive, coriander (Chinese parsley).

FOODS FOR DEFICIENCY: glutinous rice, dried lotus root, sugar cane, mutton, grape.

HERBS: Zi-su-ye (purple perilla leaf), Huang-lian (goldthread), Zhu-ru (bamboo shavings), Bai-bian-dou (hyacinth bean), Shi-di (Japanese persimmon), Sha-ren (grains of paradise), Mu-xiang (costus root), Ban-xia (half-summer pinellia), Chen-pi (dried tangerine peel), Sang-shen (mulberry), Gou-qi-zi (matrimony vine fruit), Da-zao (red date), E-jiao (donkey-hide gelatin), Bai-zhu (white atractylodes), Shan-yao (Chinese yam), Huang-qi (membranous milk vetch), Lu-gen (reed rhizome).

Syndromes of disease and herbs to use:

1. **SPUTUM CONGESTION:** Zi-su-ye (purple perilla leaf), Sha-ren (grains of paradise), Mu-xiang (costus root), Ban-xia (half-summer pinellia), Chen-pi (dried tangerine peel); cook with foods for excess.
2. **SPLEEN-STOMACH YANG DEFICIENCY:** Zhu-ru (bamboo shavings), Sha-ren (grains of paradise), Mu-xiang (costus root); cook with foods for excess.
3. **HOT STOMACH:** Sang-shen (mulberry), Gou-qi-zi (matrimony vine fruit), Da-zao (red date), Bai-bian-dou (hyacinth bean), Shi-di (Japanese persimmon); cook with foods for excess.
4. **HOT LIVER:** Sang-shen (mulberry), Gou-qi-zi (matrimony vine fruit), Sheng-di (dried glutinous rehmannia), E-jiao (donkey-hide gelatin): cook with foods for excess.
5. **SPLEEN-STOMACH ENERGY DEFICIENCY:** Bai-zhu (white atractylodes), Shan-yao (Chinese yam), Huang-qi (membranous milk vetch); cook with foods for deficiency.

RECIPE 103

MASTER: 10 g Shan-yao (Chinese yam).

ASSOCIATE: 30 g grapes.

ASSISTANT: 20 g mung beans.

SEASONING: salt.

STEPS:

(1) Place the three ingredients in an earthenware pot. Add water and bring to a boil. Simmer until all ingredients are cooked and soft.

CONSUMPTION: eat the contents and drink the soup.

INDICATION: spleen-stomach energy deficiency syndrome of morning sickness.

ANALYSIS: Shan-yao is an energy tonic; grape is a yin and blood tonic; mung bean cools the stomach; and salt improves taste.

12.12 Infertility

1. Deficiency of Energy and Blood Syndrome

SYMPTOMS AND SIGNS:

- Bleeding of various kinds with light-colored blood, often seen in consumptive diseases.
- Dizziness.
- Fatigue.
- "Flying objects" in front of the eyes.
- Insomnia.
- Irregular menstruation.
- Low energy.
- Feeble voice.
- Menstrual flow in light-red color.
- Mentally depressed.
- Regular menstruation, but with very scanty flow, lasting for one or two days only.
- Numbness of limbs.
- Pale complexion and lips.
- Pale nails.
- Palpitation.

2. Yin Deficiency Syndrome

SYMPTOMS AND SIGNS:

- Bleeding from gums.
- Constipation.
- Dizziness.
- Dry, scanty stool; dry sensations in the mouth; dry throat.
- Fatigue.
- Headache in the afternoon.
- Low fever in the afternoon.
- Menstrual flow in a dark color.
- Night sweats.
- Nosebleed.
- Red, swollen sore throat.
- Hot palms of hands and soles of feet.
- Palpitation accompanied by anxiety.
- Regular menstruation with scanty flow, lasting for one day or half a day.
- Short streams of red urine.
- Underweight.
- Insomnia.
- Difficulty swallowing.
- Toothache.
- Vomiting of blood or nosebleed during periods.

3. Deficiency Cold

SYMPTOMS AND SIGNS:

- Cold pain or cold sensations in the lower abdomen or cold sensations in the vaginal area.
- Dark, blackish-red menstrual flow.
- Failure of the fetus to grow during previous pregnancy.
- Frequent miscarriage.
- Functional disturbances of the ovary.
- Pale complexion.
- Poor appetite.
- Thin, watery menstrual flow in light color.

4. Hot Blood Syndrome

SYMPTOMS AND SIGNS:

- Abdominal pain that occurs at onset of periods.
- Anal bleeding before periods.
- Fever after previous childbirth.
- Irregular periods.
- Heavy menstrual flow.
- Menstrual flow with an unusual odor.
- Nosebleed.
- Periods ten days early or two periods within one month.
- Dark red or violet-colored menstrual flow.
- Skin ulcers.
- Abnormal vaginal bleeding.
- Vomiting of blood during periods.

5. Liver Energy Congestion Syndrome

SYMPTOMS AND SIGNS:

- Abdominal pain.
- Muscle spasms.
- Irregular periods.
- Menstrual pain.
- Morning sickness.
- Numbness.
- Pain in the hypochondrium.
- Early or overdue periods.
- Shortage of milk secretion after previous childbirth.
- Stomachache.
- Subjective sensations of objects in the throat.
- Vomiting of blood.
- Whitish vaginal discharge.

6. Damp Phlegm Syndrome

SYMPTOMS AND SIGNS:

- Discharge of sputum that can be coughed out easily or discharge of white, watery sputum.
- Dizziness, especially prolonged.
- Frequent coughs during previous pregnancy that prolonged or caused fetal motion.
- Headache.
- Hiccups.
- Light red menstrual flow.
- Turbid, sticky menstrual flow.
- Pain in the chest.
- Abnormal panting.
- Frequent overdue periods.
- Excessive menstrual flow.
- Excessive sleep or insomnia.
- Suppression of menses.
- Vomiting.
- Whitish vaginal discharge, especially excessive.
- Frequent morning sickness during previous pregnancy.

INGREDIENTS FOR CREATING RECIPES

FOODS FOR EXCESS: fresh ginger, Chinese chive.

FOODS FOR DEFICIENCY: mutton, lobster, chicken, chicken egg, pork kidney, polished rice.

HERBS: Cong-bai (Welsh onion), Lu-jiao-jiao (deerhorn glue), Bai-shao (white peony), Dang-gui (Chinese angelica), Yi-mu-cao (Siberian motherwort), Shu-di (processed glutinous rehmannia), Shan-zhu-yu (fruit of medicinal cornel), Ai-ye (mugwort), Chuan-xiong (hemlock parsley), Wu-zhu-yu (evodia), Di-gu-pi (root bark of Chinese wolfberry), Huang-bai (cork tree), Chai-hu (hare's ear), Ban-xia (half-summer pinellia), Chen-pi (dried tangerine peel), Fu-ling (tuckahoe; Indian bread), Xiang-fu (nutgrass flatsedge rhizome).

Syndromes of disease and herbs to use:

1. **DEFICIENCY OF ENERGY AND BLOOD:** Bai-shao (white peony), Dang-gui (Chinese angelica), Yi-mu-cao (Siberian motherwort), Shu-di (processed glutinous rehmannia), Lu-jiao-jiao (deerhorn glue); cook with foods for deficiency.

2. **YIN DEFICIENCY:** Bai-shao (white peony), Shan-zhu-yu (fruit of medicinal cornel), Shu-di (processed glutinous rehmannia), Lu-jiao-jiao (deerhorn glue); cook with foods for deficiency.

3. **DEFICIENCY COLD:** Cong-bai (Welsh onion), Ai-ye (mugwort), Bai-shao (white peony), Chuan-xiong (hemlock parsley), Dang-gui (Chinese angelica), Shu-di (processed glutinous rehmannia), Wu-zhu-yu (evodia); cook with foods for deficiency.

4. **HOT BLOOD:** Bai-shao (white peony), Di-gu-pi (root bark of Chinese wolfberry), Shu-di (processed glutinous rehmannia), Huang-bai (cork tree); cook with foods for excess.

5. **LIVER ENERGY CONGESTION:** Bai-shao (white peony), Chai-hu (hare's ear), Dang-gui (Chinese angelica); cook with foods for excess.

6. **DAMP PHLEGM:** Ban-xia (half-summer pinellia), Chen-pi (dried tangerine peel), Fu-ling (tuckahoe; Indian bread), Chuan-xiong (hemlock parsley), Xiang-fu (nutgrass flatsedge rhizome); cook with foods for excess.

RECIPE 104

MASTER: 5 g Bai-shao (white peony).

ASSOCIATE: 5 g Dang-gui (Chinese angelica).

ASSISTANT: 100 g polished rice.

SEASONING: salt.

STEPS:

(1) Decoct Bai-shao (white peony) and Dang-gui (Chinese angelica) in enough water for thirty minutes; strain to obtain herbal soup.

(2) Boil rice in water to make a very thick congree.

(3) Combine the herbal soup with the concentrated congee.

(4) Season with salt to taste.

CONSUMPTION: eat on an empty stomach.

INDICATIONS: deficiency of energy and blood syndrome of infertility in women.

ANALYSIS: Bai-shao is a blood and yin tonic and Dang-gui is a blood tonic. The two herbs are often used together to correct irregular menstruation and infertility. Polished rice is an energy tonic. Salt improves the taste of this recipe.

PART IV

BUILDING UP THE IMMUNE SYSTEM

CHAPTER 13 The Immune System and Chinese Medicine

If I were asked, "In what way can traditional Chinese medicine benefit human health the most?" I would reply without hesitation that its most outstanding feature is to bolster the immune system for the maintenance of good health and prevention of disease. A Chinese medical classic published in the third century B.C. pointed this out quite clearly: "A good doctor will prevent disease rather than cure it, for the same reason that a good ruler will prevent a revolt rather than wait for it to start and then suppress it. To treat a disease, or to put down a revolt, for that matter, is like digging a well after one feels thirsty or making weapons after the war breaks out—a belated attempt to restore human health or social order."

People do not share the same immune system

The Chinese have long observed that not all people have the same immune system. On the contrary, each individual has a unique immune system. This can be demonstrated by observing people in everyday life. Some people may have cold limbs and get sick more often in winter, while others may feel hot and get sick more often in summer; still others may feel neither cold nor hot, but allergic to some foods or dust. A famous Chinese doctor in the seventeenth century by the name of Wu You Ke tried to make a point about the fact that people have different immune systems. He revealed a keen observation when he said, "When people get intoxicated, normally their pulses will be stronger and faster, they will feel more high-spirited and warmer than usual, and their faces and eyes will look red. This is only a general assumption which is not true on closer examination. If we observe people more carefully, we will notice that their reactions to alcohol are rather different. Some people talk illogically and act irrationally once they are intoxicated, and after they sober up, they don't remember a thing; some remain rational when they are drunk; some look pale though they have a red complexion as a rule; others feel more energetic rather than weaker; still others shiver with cold. Moreover, there are people who get drunk easily and sober up quickly; there are others who don't get drunk easily, but take a long time to sober up; then there are people who yawn and sneeze when they are intoxicated, and those who become dizzy, have blurred vision, and develop headaches. This is because individuals have differenty quantities of energy and blood in them. They have inherited differently shaped internal organs, which is why they have different reactions to intoxication."

The fact that each individual has a unique immune system is also borne out by the use of immunosuppressant drugs, used to suppress a patient's immune system after transplant surgery in order to prevent the rejection of foreign tissues. One would think that it is vital to boost a patient's immune system at all times, and particularly after surgery to fight infection, but contrary to this common belief a doctor will try to reduce immunity, increasing the risk of infection and the development of certain cancers. Isn't this a medical paradox? Paradoxical as it may seem, this practice in transplant surgery bears out traditional Chinese beliefs that each individual has a unique immune system; one individual's body will not accept another individual's tissues if their immune systems are incompatible.

Where does one's immunity come from? There is innate immunity, which is passed on to each individual from the parents. There is also acquired immunity, which is developed through correct nourishment in life.

In what way do people's immune systems differ from each other? An individual's immune system may be stronger in one respect, but weaker in another respect. To bolster an individual's immune system, it is necessary to know what aspect of his or her immune system is strong and what aspect is weak, so that the weak aspect can be strengthened while maintaining the strong aspect. If a person's immune system as a whole is weak, as in the elderly, it is necessary to bolster the entire system.

Protective immunity

In Chinese medicine, there are three basic strategies to bolster the immune system: enhance protective immunity, organic immunity, and adaptive immunity.

Protective immunity is the protection of the body against invading bacteria, viruses, and fungi. It also counteracts development of cancer cells, allergy, and hypersensitivity. Protective immunity is in jeopardy when the body is in a state of energy, blood, yin, or yang deficiency. Deficiency means a shortage of something, and each type of deficiency is reflected by a set of symptoms. In the case of energy deficiency, a person may constantly feel tired for no apparent reason, speak in a feeble voice, have a poor appetite for a lengthy period, discharge watery stools, and perspire excessively. If you have a few of these symptoms, chances are that you may have energy deficiency. Energy deficiency may lead to leukocytopenia (low leukocytes or white blood corpuscles), bronchial asthma, myasthenia gravis (weakness of muscles), and common cold or skin infection.

What are the symptoms that point to blood deficiency? A person may constantly feel dizzy with blurred vision, experience palpitation and nervousness fairly often, look pale or have a very dry complexion, and have pale nails and tongue. If you have a few of these symptoms, chances are you may have a blood deficiency. Blood deficiency may lead to hemolytic anemia, such hemorrhagic states as thrombocytopenic purpura and anaphylactoid purpura, and hives.

What are the symptoms that point to yin deficiency? Yin refers to bodily fluids and seminal fluid in men. A person may constantly feel thirsty and dry in the mouth, feel hot sensations in the body, have dry skin, perspire at night (night sweats), cough out a small quantity of mucus or blood, have constipation often and discharge short streams of urine, and have red lips and cheeks. If you have a few of these symptoms, chances are you may have a yin deficiency. Yin deficiency may lead to anaphylactoid purpura, lupus erythematosus (a systemic disease), rheumatism, rheumatic arthritis, radiation damage, pulmonary tuberculosis, and chronic hepatitis.

What are the symptoms that point to yang deficiency? Yang refers to yang energy in the body in general and yang energy in the kidneys in particular. A person may feel tired with cold sensations in the limbs, have lower back pain and shortness of breath, discharge long streams of urine, and have a pale complexion and tongue. If you have a few of these symptoms, chances are you may have a yang deficiency. Yang deficiency may lead to bronchial asthma, asthmatic tracheitis, allergic rhinitis, myasthenia gravis, scleroderma (a skin disease), rheumatism, rheumatoid arthritis, chronic nephritis, leukocytopenia, vitiligo, psoriasis, and bone tuberculosis.

Organic immunity

Organic immunity refers to the ability of internal organs to maintain their proper functions and stay free from the invasion of pathogens, which may have penetrated the body, posing a threat to the internal organs.

Modern Chinese research has indicated that the immune system has a great deal to do with internal organs, notably the lungs, spleen, and kidneys. It is common knowledge that the skin provides an effective barrier to the vast majority of disease-causing agents. The lungs take charge by building up a protective barrier in the skin to prevent disease-causing agents from entering the body through it. However, most disease-causing agents are able to gain entry into the body through the respiratory tract, that is, the nose and the throat, which are also controlled by the lungs. Thus, the Chinese credit the lungs with providing the first line of immune defense. A weakening of this line of defense may lead to skin or respiratory infection, pneumonia, or allergy-related diseases, such as allergic rhinitis, bronchial asthma, and hives.

The spleen is an important organ to bolster acquired immunity, because it is in charge of digestion and absorption of nutrients, and thus responsible for delivering them to various parts of the body. When the spleen is deficient, the immune system will become weaker, which may lead to intestinal infection and infection of the soft tissues in the skin.

The kidneys are important organs to bolster innate immunity. The Chinese believe that the kidneys are the roots of life, containing great power to resist the attack of pathogens. When the kidneys are short of yin energy, it is called kidney yin deficiency.

Deficiency may give rise to such symptoms as blurred vision, dizziness, dry mouth and throat, night sweats, thirst, urinary disorders eventually leading to diabetes, hypertension, prostatitis, tonsillitis, and tuberculosis of the bone and joints. When the kidneys are short of yang energy, it is called kidney yang deficiency. This may give rise to chronic diarrhea, edema, aversion to cold, frequent urination at night, shortness of breath, seminal emission in men, and eventually lead to bronchial asthma, diabetes, hypothyroidism, lumbago, neurasthenia, and otogenic vertigo. Many Chinese researchers have pointed to the importance of the lungs, spleen, and kidneys to the immune system.

When the body is under the attack of an invading organism or tumor cell, called an antigen, the body's immune system must respond to the invasion: an immune response. There are two types of immune responses: humoral responses in humoral immunity and cellular responses in cellular immunity.

Humoral responses center on the activities of antibodies (immunoglobulins). There are five classes of antibodies, IgM, IgG, IgA, IgD, and IgE. Among them IgG (immunoglobulin G) comprises about 75 percent of the antibodies of the normal person. In addition, white blood cells called phagocytes (commonly known as devouring cells) play an important role in humoral immunity, because they can destroy invading microorganisms by devouring them.

Cellular responses center on the activities of T-cells (T-Lymphocytes) in response to the invasion. T-cells do not produce antibodies; they travel to and attach to the abnormal cells and destroy them.

Immunity is most closely related to the lungs, then to the spleen, and then to the kidneys, regarding T-cells. Lung deficiency has the greatest impact on the immune system, indicating that when lungs are in distress, T-cells increase to launch an attack.

Adaptive immunity

Adaptive immunity is the capacity of the body to react to a vast range of different invading organisms, allergy-causing substances, tumor cells, and other disease-causing factors. Adaptive immunity is different from protective immunity or organic immunity in that it refers to the body's *positive response* to invading elements, whereas protective immunity and organic immunity simply protect the body from the attack. Adaptive immunity must produce phagocytes that target specific disease-causing organisms in order to devour them. Some Chinese herbs have a cold energy and a bitter taste, which have been found to increase the number of phagocytes and their devouring power. These herbs have been used as immunostimulants to increase the efficiency of the body's immune system.

There are two ways to build up adaptive immunity: first, by using foods and herbs to detoxify, effective in the treatment of carbuncles, sore throat, diarrhea and dysentery, for prevention of leukopenia, and also useful for cancer patients undergoing chemotherapy and radiation; second, by using foods and herbs to cool, such as by reducing fever in chronic consumptive diseases and in inflammatory diseases.

CHAPTER 14

Recipes to Build Up Protective Immunity

In each recipe, one to five herbs has been selected for cooking. A cooking recipe to promote health is like an herbal formula in Chinese medicine, except that an herbal formula may contain anywhere from one to twelve or more herbs, while a cooking recipe may contain one to five. Rock sugar may be replaced by honey when not available.

ENERGY TONICS

FOODS: beef, bird's nest, broomcorn, cherry, chicken, coconut meat, date, eel, grape, Irish potato, kidney bean, mushroom, sweet potato, rice, rock sugar, shark's fin, shiitake mushroom, squash, sturgeon, tofu, white string bean.

HERBS: Huang-qi (membranous milk vetch), Ren-shen (Chinese ginseng), Bai-zhu (white atractylodes), Gan-cao (licorice), Shan-yao (Chinese yam).

RECIPE 105

MASTER: 30 g Ren-shen (Chinese ginseng), 200 g chicken.

ASSOCIATE: 20 g He-shou-wu (multiflower knotweed tuber), 15 g Shan-yao (Chinese yam), 15 g Gou-qi-zi (matrimony vine fruit).

ASSISTANT: 20 shiitake mushrooms, 1 egg white.

SEASONING: 15 g yellow wine, salt to taste, teaspoon of starch.

STEPS:

(1) Dry roast Ren-shen (Chinese ginseng) and He-shou-wu (multiflower knotweed tuber) and grind into powder; set aside for later use.

(2) Grind Shan-yao (Chinese yam) into powder; set aside for later use.

(3) Mince chicken and combine with the wine and salt, then add the ginseng and multiflower knotweed tuber powders. Finally add the egg white and Chinese yam powder to make a thick paste.

(4) Divide this paste into 10 equal portions. Place a portion between two shiitake mushrooms to make a "shiitake sandwich."

(5) Steam the shiitake sandwiches in a steamer for 20 minutes.

(6) In a pot, add yellow wine, salt, Gou-qi-zi (matrimony vine fruit), and one cup of water and bring to a boil. Finally, add starch to make a thick sauce. Pour on top of the shiitake sandwiches.

CONSUMPTION: have the sandwiches three times a week.

INDICATIONS: premature aging, facial wrinkles, poor complexion.

ANALYSIS: This recipe is primarily an energy tonic and secondarily a blood tonic. He-shou-wu is for the blood, while Gou-gi-zi is a yin tonic. Chinese women often use this recipe to stay youthful.

BLOOD TONICS

FOODS: beef liver, chicken egg, grape, ham, litchi nut, longan, mandarin fish, oyster, pork liver, sea cucumber, spinach, white fungus, raisin.

HERBS: Dang-gui (Chinese angelica root), He-shou-wu (multiflower knotweed tuber), Huang-jing (sealwort), Gou-qi-zi (matrimony vine fruit), E-jiao (donkey-hide gelatin).

RECIPE 106

MASTER: 30 g Gou-qi-zi (matrimony vine fruit).

ASSOCIATE: 40 g white fungus.

ASSISTANT: 200 g rock sugar.

SEASONING: none.

STEPS:

(1) Soak Gou-qi-zi (matrimony vine fruit) and white fungus in warm water for two minutes. Rinse and set aside.

(2) Boil rock sugar in 700 ml of water to dissolve, then strain to obtain a sweet syrup.

(3) Place Gou-qi-zi, white fungus, and the syrup in a bowl or container, then place it in a pot filled with water. Cover the pot, bring to a boil for 5 minutes, then reduce to low heat. Continue to simmer for two hours. Make sure that there is sufficient water, or add water as necessary so that you don't burn the pot.

(4) Remove from heat and serve warm.

CONSUMPTION: serve as a soup at mealtimes, twice a week on a regular basis.

INDICATIONS: dry skin, blurred vision, lumbago, impotence, seminal emission.

ANALYSIS: Gou-qi-zi (matrimony vine fruit) is a blood tonic as well as a kidney tonic. White fungus and rock sugar are used to reinforce the toning effect of this herb.

RECIPE 107

MASTER: 10 pieces of Da-zao (red date).

ASSOCIATE: 15 g Dang-shen (purple sage), 15 g Huang-qi (membranous milk vetch).

ASSISTANT: 80 g longan nuts.

SEASONING: 40 g raisins.

STEPS:

(1) Decoct Dang-shen (purple sage) and Huang-qi (membranous milk vetch); strain to obtain herbal soup.

(2) Remove shells and seeds from longan nuts.

(3) In a pot, add the herbal soup and 900 ml water, longan nuts, and raisins and cook for 20 minutes over medium heat.

CONSUMPTION: serve as a soup at mealtimes, twice a week on a regular basis.

INDICATIONS: palpitation, insomnia, neurasthenia, nervousness, poor appetite, seminal emission.

ANALYSIS: Da-zao is a mild blood tonic, which may be consumed on a regular basis. Huang-qi and Dang-shen are both energy tonics. Longan nuts and raisins, also blood tonics, reinforce the effects of Da-zao.

YIN TONICS

FOODS: abalone, air bladder of shark (also called "swim bladder"), apple, asparagus, bird's nest, brown sugar, cantaloupe, cheese, chicken egg, clam, coconut milk, crab, cuttlefish, date, duck, duck egg, honey, kidney bean, kumquat, lard, lemon, maltose, mandarin orange, mango, mussel, oyster, pea, pear, pineapple, pork, rice, royal jelly, sea cucumber, shrimp, string bean, tofu, tomato, walnut, watermelon, white sugar.

HERBS: Shu-di (processed glutinous rehmannia), Wu-wei-zi (magnolia vine fruit), Shan-zhu-yu (medicinal cornel fruit), Nu-zhen-zi (wax tree), Mai-dong (lilyturf), Tian-dong (lucid asparagus).

RECIPE 108

MASTER: 200 g pork.

ASSOCIATE: 250 g fresh watermelon peel.

ASSISTANT: 1 egg white.

SEASONING: 2 teaspoons each salt, wine, peanut oil, starch, and sesame oil.

STEPS:

(1) Rinse watermelon peel and slice thin. Sprinkle a little salt and put aside for 15 minutes.

(2) Slice pork into thin pieces, then mix with the egg white, salt, wine, and starch.

(3) In a frying pan over medium heat, add peanut oil. When the oil is hot, add the pork. As soon as it changes color, remove the pork from the frying pan and discard the oil.

(4) Return the slices of pork to the frying pan and add the watermelon slices. Saute for 30 seconds, then remove from the frying pan and sprinkle with sesame oil.

CONSUMPTION: eat at mealtimes, three times per week for two months.

INDICATIONS: fatigue and thirst during recuperation from an illness, constipation, or sunstroke.

ANALYSIS: Pork is a yin tonic, watermelon can clear heat, peanut oil and sesame oil can lubricate. Thus, this recipe has a triple effect: to tone yin energy, clear heat, and lubricate the internal region. The Chinese take this as a moderate yin tonic to facilitate recovery from an illness.

RECIPE 109

MASTER: 12 g Shan-zhu-yu (medicinal cornel fruit), 12 g Wu-wei-zi (magnolia vine fruit).

ASSOCIATE: 300 g Irish potatoes

ASSISTANT: 500 g tofu, 20 g starch, 2 egg whites, 50 g peanuts.

SEASONING: 100 g flour, 50 g black sesame seeds, 20 g soy sauce, 20 g rice wine, 1 kg peanut oil.

STEPS:

(1) Decoct Shan-zhu-yu (medicinal cornel fruit) and Wu-wei-zi (magnolia vine fruit) together; strain to obtain herbal soup.

(2) Peel potatoes and steam until soft. Coat the potatoes with the flour and mashed tofu.

(3) Stir fry peanuts until toasted, then remove outer skins. Dry roast sesame seeds.

(4) Crush peanuts and sesame seeds and mix with egg whites and starch to make a paste. Make a hole in each potato ball and squeeze paste into it. Heat about 1 cup of the peanut oil and deep fry the potato balls until lightly browned.

(5) Mix herbal soup, soy sauce, and rice wine with the remaining oil (10 g) to make a concentrated seasoning sauce. Serve the sauce with the potato balls.

CONSUMPTION: have the entire portion as a main dish for the evening meal. Cook once a week for one month.

INDICATIONS: frequent urination, seminal emission, lumbago, low energy.

ANALYSIS: Both Shan-zhu-yu and Wu-wei-zi can tone the kidneys, increasing the yin of this organ. The other ingredients lubricate the internal region and warm the kidneys.

YANG TONICS

FOODS: air bladder of shark, beef kidney, chestnut, clove, clove oil, fennel seed, lobster, pistachio nut, raspberry, shrimp, star anise, strawberry, sword bean (jack bean), beef, pork kidney, shiitake mushroom, bamboo shoot, celery, water chestnut, soy sauce, starch.

HERBS: Yin-yang-huo (longspur epimedium), Bu-gu-zhi (psoralea), Wu-jia-pi (acanthopanax root bark), Du-zhong (eucommia bark), Rou-gui (Chinese cassia bark).

RECIPE 110

MASTER: 10 g Rou-gui (Chinese cassia bark)

ASSOCIATE: 6 g Gan-cao (licorice).

ASSISTANT: 300 g beef.

SEASONING: sliced green onion, peeled and sliced fresh ginger, white sugar, sesame oil, soy sauce, salt.

STEPS:

(1) Cut beef into large chunks and boil in water over high heat for 8 minutes or until 30% cooked. Cool, then cut into smaller pieces.

(2) Heat sesame oil in a frying pan, add the pieces of beef and sauté for 1 minute. Add the soy sauce and salt and stir fry for another 2 minutes. Add 2 cups of water, Rou-gui, Gan-cao, green onion, and ginger and simmer over low heat for 2 hours. Add white sugar and continue to simmer until all the water is gone.

(3) Stir fry the contents in the same frying pan over medium-high heat until the oil makes a crackling noise. Discard the ginger, cassia bark, and licorice.

CONSUMPTION: serve as a side dish, once every other day for two weeks.

INDICATIONS: bronchial asthma and asthmatic tracheitis with aversion to cold, edema, lumbago, leucocytopenia, rheumatism, rheumatoid arthritis.

ANALYSIS: Rou-gui, a yang tonic, can warm the body; Gan-cao and beef, energy tonics, can strengthen body energy. This recipe is primarily to build up yang energy in the body and secondarily to increase body energy.

RECIPE 111

MASTER: 15 g Du-zhong (eucommia bark).

ASSOCIATE: 10 g Bu-gu-zhi (psoralea).

ASSISTANT: 250 g pork kidneys.

SEASONING: 3 stalks green onion; 10 slices peeled fresh ginger; 1 teaspoon each soy sauce, vinegar, wine, salt, and sesame oil.

STEPS:

(1) Decoct Du-zhong (eucommia bark) and Bu-gu-zhi (psoralea); strain to obtain herbal soup. Slice the green onion and ginger.

(2) Quarter each pork kidney to look like a flower, called "kidney flower" in Chinese.

(3) Heat sesame oil in a frying pan until it begins to smoke, then add kidney flowers. Stir fry until their color changes, then add sliced green onions, ginger, soy sauce, vinegar, and wine. After stir frying a minute or two, add the herbal soup to simmer for 5 minutes.

CONSUMPTION: serve as a side dish, once a week for a month.

INDICATIONS: headache, vertigo, ringing in the ears, hearing problems, lumbago.

ANALYSIS: Du-zhong, Bu-gu-zhi (psoralia), and pork kidney are kidney tonics. This recipe is ideal for kidney yang deficiency, manifested as cold lower limbs, cold feet in particular.

RECIPE 112

MASTER: 30 g Wu-jia-pi (acanthopanax root bark).

ASSOCIATE: 600 g tofu.

ASSISTANT: 30 g shiitake mushrooms, 30 g bamboo shoots, 25 g celery, 25 g water chestnuts, 10 g starch, 12 g soy sauce.

SEASONING: 20 g rice wine, 8 g white sugar, 10 g green onion, 2 g salt, 800 g peanut oil.

STEPS:

(1) Prepare a herbal decoction: put Wu-jia-pi in 200 ml water and bring to a boil, then lower heat and simmer until water is reduced by half. Strain and set aside.

(2) Drain excess water from tofu and cut into large cubes; set aside for later use.

(3) In a frying pan over high heat, cook peanut oil until it is reduced by 15%. Add the cubes of tofu and fry until golden.

(4) When cubes become firm, remove and leave to cool on paper towels.

(5) Slice mushrooms, bamboo shoots, water chestnuts, and celery into bite-size pieces and mix together. Mix in salt and starch to make a stuffing.

(6) Make a hole in each cube of tofu, and squeeze some stuffing into it.

(7) Place cubes of tofu in a steamer for twenty minutes.

(8) Chop the green onion and celery.

(9) Make the sauce: place a frying pan over high heat with 20 g peanut oil. Add soy sauce, herbal soup, white sugar, rice wine, and green onion and bring to a boil, then remove from heat.

(10) Pour sauce over the tofu.

CONSUMPTION: serve as a side dish at mealtimes, once every two days.

INDICATIONS: leukopenia, rheumatic arthritis, rheumatoid arthritis, chronic tracheitis, prevention of acute altitude stress.

ANALYSIS: Research indicates Wu-jia-pi can increase the production of blood by the bone marrow, drastically increase the number of macrophages in the spleen, and counteract infection and inflammation; fried tofu can increase yang energy and warm the body.

NOTE: This is a vegetarian dish, but if meat is desired, lamb or pork may be used along with other stuffing ingredients in the recipe.

CHAPTER 15

Recipes to Build Up Organic Immunity

Foods and herbs listed to enhance organic immunity are divided according to the organs involved. For example, foods and herbs listed to enhance organic immunity of the lungs act on the lungs. Each organ has immunity; when immunity is deficient in the organ, that organ will be vulnerable to the attack of disease.

The Chinese believe that when a given internal organ is weak, it is beneficial to consume the corresponding animal organ. Thus, pork kidney or beef kidney, for example, is beneficial to the human kidney.

LUNG TONICS

FOODS: air bladder of shark, cheese, garlic, milk, rice, walnut, whitebait, duck, pears.

HERBS: Chuan-bei (tendril-leaved fritillary bulb), Huang-qi (membranous milk vetch), Ren-shen (Chinese ginseng), Dong-chong-xia-cao (Chinese caterpillar fungus).

RECIPE 113

MASTER: 10 g Dong-chong-xia-cao (Chinese caterpillar fungus).

ASSOCIATE: 1 duck.

ASSISTANT: 10 g Cong-bai (Welsh onion).

SEASONING: 15 g wine, 5 g peeled fresh ginger, 3 g black pepper, 3 g salt.

STEPS:

(1) Cut open the duck and remove organs. Soak the duck in hot water for 1 minute, then remove and set aside.

(2) Rinse Dong-chong-xia-cao (Chinese caterpillar fungus) in warm water. Chop the Cong-bai (Welsh onion) and ginger.

(3) Stuff the Dong-chong-xia-cao, onion, and ginger into the duck stomach. Add two tablespoons of water, salt, and pepper, and close the stomach with toothpicks.

(4) Steam the duck in a steamer for 1.5 hours, remove from the steamer, and discard the onion and ginger from the stomach.

CONSUMPTION: serve as a side dish at mealtimes, twice a week.

INDICATIONS: cough, asthma, excessive perspiration, impotence, seminal emission.

ANALYSIS: Dong-chong-xia-cao (Chinese caterpillar fungus) is a lung and kidney tonic, consumed with other food among the Chinese people. Duck is also a lung and kidney tonic. The two ingredients work together to build up the organic immunity of the lungs and kidneys.

NOTE: This recipe was written by a Chinese physician in 1765.

RECIPE 114

MASTER: 12 g Chuan-bei (tendril-leaved fritillary bulb).

ASSOCIATE: 8 pears.

ASSISTANT: 100 g glutinous rice, 100 g wax gourd or cucumber.

SEASONING: 180 g rock sugar.

STEPS:

(1) Decoct Chuan-bei and strain to obtain herbal soup. Set the soup aside. Cook the glutinous rice in the usual way.

(2) Mince wax gourd (or cucumber) into the size of soybeans.

(3) With a small knife, peel the pears, cut away the base, and remove seeds. Soak the pears (and their bases) in boiling water for 20 seconds, transfer to cold water, then remove to dry.

(4) Mix rice, wax gourd (or cucumber) and half of the rock sugar. Stuff the mixture into the pears, then cover with the bases. Put them on a plate to steam in a steamer for 40 minutes.

(5) Boil 200 ml of water, add herbal soup and the remaining rock sugar, and dissolve to make a syrup for topping the pears.

CONSUMPTION: have as a snack, 2 pears at a time, twice daily. Store the rest in the refrigerator.

INDICATIONS: dry cough, discharge of blood from the mouth, asthma.

ANALYSIS: Both Chuan-bei and pears can lubricate the lungs, good for a dry cough. Glutinous rice is a lung tonic.

SPLEEN TONICS

FOODS: apple, cucumber, beef, bird's nest, caraway seed, carrot, chestnut, ham, horse bean (broad bean/fava bean) pistachio nut, date, rice, glutinous rice, royal jelly, string bean.

HERBS: Dang-shen (root of pilose asiabell), Bai-zhu (white atractylodes), Yi-yi-ren (Job's tears), Fu-ling (Indian bread), Da-zao (red date), Huang-qi (membranous milk vetch), Chen-pi (tangerine peel), Bai-bian-dou (hyacinth bean).

RECIPE 115

MASTER: 10 g Dang-shen (root of pilose asiabell).

ASSOCIATE: 20 g Da-zao (red date).

ASSISTANT: 250 g glutinous rice.

SEASONING: 50 g white sugar.

STEPS:

(1) Decoct Dang-shen and Da-zao; strain to obtain herbal soup. Set aside the herbs for later use.

(2) Add sugar to the soup and boil over low heat.

(3) Cook the glutinous rice in the usual way.

(4) Spoon cooked rice onto a plate, place the two herbs on top of the rice, then pour the herbal sauce over all.

CONSUMPTION: serve as a side dish at breakfast, three times a week for two months.

INDICATIONS: chronic fatigue, palpitation, insomnia, poor appetite, chronic diarrhea.

ANALYSIS: The two herbs used are both spleen tonics, strengthening the spleen's ability to digest and absorb nutrients. Glutinous rice and white sugar are both pleasing to the spleen.

NOTE: This is a time-honored recipe written centuries ago.

RECIPE 116

MASTER: 15 g Huang-qi (membranous milk vetch).

ASSOCIATE: 20 g Chen-pi (tangerine peel).

ASSISTANT: one medium-sized whole chicken.

SEASONING: 2 stalks Cong-bai (Welsh onion), 5 slices peeled fresh ginger, 15 g "yellow wine" (see Note), 2 teaspoons sesame oil.

STEPS:

(1) Decoct Huang-qi for 40 minutes over low heat. Make sure there is a sufficient amount of water to cook the chicken in it. Strain to obtain herbal soup.

(2) Add the chicken, Cong-bai, ginger, and yellow wine together in the herbal soup and bring to a boil. Reduce heat and simmer for 40 minutes, then remove the chicken from the soup.

(3) Heat sesame oil in a frying pan to fry Chen-pi until aromatic—called "Chen-pi oil."

(4) Chop the chicken, and pour Chen-pi oil over it—called "oily chicken."

CONSUMPTION: serve as a side dish at mealtimes, once a week.

INDICATIONS: fatigue, chronic cough, asthma.

ANALYSIS: Huang-qi can tonify spleen energy, Chen-pi can promote energy circulation; both are essential for the spleen. Again, chicken is also a spleen tonic, and ginger and yellow wine can promote energy circulation. Thus this recipe has a double function, to bolster spleen energy and promote energy circulation.

NOTE: The Chinese call rice wine "yellow wine." It contains 10 to 20 percent alcohol, suitable for drinking with the meal.

RECIPE 117

MASTER: 1.5 kg Shan-yao (Chinese yam) powder.

ASSOCIATE: 3 kg wheat flour.

ASSISTANT: 10 chicken eggs.

SEASONING: 5 g peeled fresh ginger, salt, lard, black pepper, green onion slices.

STEPS:

(1) In a bowl, combine the flour, Shan-yao powder, eggs and salt. Add enough water to make a dough. Work the dough until you have a large, flat, thin pancake. Cut the pancake into strips to make noodles.

(2) Boil water in a pot and add a desired quantity of lard, green onion, and fresh ginger. Add a desired quantity of noodle strips and cook. When the noodles are ready (about 6 to 8 minutes), add salt to taste. Keep the remaining noodles in a refrigerator for use next time.

CONSUMPTION: serve as a main dish at mealtimes, for regular consumption.

INDICATIONS: chronic diarrhea, dysentery, seminal emission in men and vaginal discharge in women, frequent urination.

ANALYSIS: Shan-yao (Chinese yam) is an excellent spleen tonic, and can check diarrhea and reduce blood sugar levels as well. Chicken egg is a spleen and stomach tonic. Thus, the two ingredients work together to build up the organic immunity of the spleen.

KIDNEY TONICS

FOODS: beef kidney, chestnut, chicken liver, fennel, millet, mussel, pork kidney, sea cucumber, string bean, walnut, wheat, wild cabbage.

HERBS: Tu-si-zi (dodder seed), Ba-ji-tian (morinda root), Shan-zhu-yu (medicinal cornel fruit), Wu-wei-zi (magnolia vine fruit), Du-zhong (eucommia bark).

RECIPE 118

MASTER: 2 pork kidneys.

ASSOCIATE: 50 g polished rice.

ASSISTANT: 3 stalks Cong-bai (Welsh onion).

SEASONING: five-spice powder (prickly ash, star anise, cinnamon, clove, and fennel ground into powder in equal quantities), peeled fresh ginger, salt.

STEPS:

(1) Cut Cong-bai and fresh ginger into large slices.

(2) Rinse pork kidneys and cut into small pieces.

(3) Boil the kidneys and rice in water to make a congee (the quantity of water can be adjusted to your preference).

(4) When the congee is ready, add the Cong-bai, fresh ginger, salt, and five-spice powder to taste.

CONSUMPTION: serve at breakfast, once a week on a regular basis.

INDICATIONS: lumbago, walking difficulty, deafness, particularly waning strength in the elderly.

ANALYSIS: Pork kidney is good for the kidneys; polished rice is an energy tonic; Cong-bai, fresh ginger, and five-spice powder can warm the kidneys.

NOTE: This recipe was written by a Chinese physician in 1578.

RECIPE 119

MASTER: 15 g Du-zhong (eucommia bark).

ASSOCIATE: 2 pork kidneys.

ASSISTANT: 30 g walnuts.

SEASONING: 1 g salt.

STEPS:

(1) Rinse kidneys and cut them in half.

(2) Bring 3 cups of water to a boil; add the kidneys, Du-zhong (eucommia bark) and walnuts and cook for 3 minutes, then reduce heat and simmer for 20 minutes.

(3) Remove the kidneys from the water and season with salt. Discard the remainder.

CONSUMPTION: serve as a side dish at mealtimes, once a week on a regular basis.

INDICATIONS: lumbago, cold feet, frequent urination, impotence, blurred vision.

ANALYSIS: Du-zhong (eucommia bark) is a strong kidney tonic; pork kidney is good for the kidneys; walnuts warm the kidneys; and salt tones the kidneys when used in small quantities. All the ingredients in this recipe are for the kidneys, helping to strengthen and maintain their organic immunity.

CHAPTER 16

Recipes to Build Up Adaptive Immunity

In adaptive immunity, detoxifying foods and herbs function to assist the body in developing specific immunities against individual invading agents such as bacteria, viruses, toxins, and foreign tissues from other animals. One detoxifying food and herb may be able to specifically destroy one virus, while another detoxifying food and herb may be able to destroy another virus.

Unlike detoxifying foods and herbs, cooling foods and herbs regulate the body to create a condition under which the invading agents cannot survive inside the body. We all know that plants will blossom and migratory birds will return every year when the climate is warm. Many bacteria and viruses will thrive in a relatively warm or hot internal condition of the body. Heat-clearing foods and herbs can adjust the internal condition to a cooler state so that bacteria and viruses cannot survive in that condition.

DETOXIFYING FOODS AND HERBS

FOODS: azuki bean, aloe vera, asparagus, bamboo shoot, banana, bitter gourd, burdock, chicken egg white, crab, fig, mung bean, Irish potato, preserved duck egg, romaine lettuce, salt, miso, squash, tofu, water spinach, wheat, mushroom, water chestnut.

HERBS: Huang-qin (skullcap), Huang-lian (goldthread), Ku-shen (bitter sophora), Xia-ku-cao (self-heal), Ye-ju-hua (wild chrysanthemum), Pu-gong-ying (Asian dandelion), Zhi-zi (gardenia), Bai-hua-she-she-cao (herb of spreading hedyotis).

RECIPE 120

MASTER: 40 g Bai-hua-she-she-cao (herb of spreading hedyotis).

ASSOCIATE: 250 g fresh mushroom.

ASSISTANT: 150 g water chestnut.

SEASONING: garlic, fresh ginger, salt, peanut oil, sesame oil to taste.

STEPS:

(1) Decoct Bai-hua-she-she-cao (herb of spreading hedyotis) in water; strain to obtain herbal soup.

(2) Rinse mushrooms and water chestnuts,

and peel the garlic and ginger. Chop all ingredients into small pieces.

(3) Heat peanut oil in a frying pan until the oil begins to smoke, add the garlic and ginger and stir fry until aromatic. Next add the water chestnuts and mushrooms and stir fry for 2 minutes, then add the herbal soup and salt. Season with sesame oil before eating.

CONSUMPTION: have as a side dish, once a day on a regular basis.

INDICATIONS: various cancers, frequent sore throat.

ANALYSIS: Bai-hua-she-she-cao has been found to be effective in the treatment of many kinds of cancer, hepatitis, nephritis, psoriasis, laryngitis, and mouth cankers.

RECIPE 121

MASTER: 5 g Huang-lian (goldthread), 5 g Huang-qin (skullcap).

ASSOCIATE: 250 g fresh celery leaves.

ASSISTANT: 100 g tofu.

SEASONING: white sugar, sesame oil, soy sauce to taste.

STEPS:

(1) Decoct Huang-lian (goldthread) and Huang-qin (skullcap); strain to obtain herbal soup. Bring the soup to a boil again and blanch the celery leaves and tofu for 20 seconds in the soup before removing. Chop tofu into oblong pieces.

(2) Mix celery leaves and tofu together on a plate, and season with sugar, sesame oil, and soy sauce to taste.

CONSUMPTION: eat at mealtimes, twice a week.

INDICATIONS: hypertension, headache, canker sores in the mouth, constipation.

ANALYSIS: In this recipe, two herbs are used to clear heat and detoxify; both taste very bitter, but since they are decocted only for blanching celery leaves and tofu, their flavor should be minimal. Celery is a good vegetable to reduce high blood pressure even when eaten by itself. Tofu can assist the two herbs to clear heat. This recipe is particularly effective for those with high blood pressure and headache at the same time.

COOLING FOODS AND HERBS

FOODS: bamboo shoot, barley, cabbage, cantaloupe, crab, cucumber, eggplant, clam, jellyfish, kidney bean, kiwi fruit, laver, millet, mung bean, pear, rice, seaweed, tomato, watercress, watermelon, wheat, wheat bran.

HERBS: Chai-hu (hare's ear), Di-gu-pi (Chinese wolfberry root bark).

RECIPE 122

MASTER: 25 g Di-gu-pi (Chinese wolfberry root bark).

ASSOCIATE: 300 g tomato

ASSISTANT: 250 g tofu, 70 g shiitake mushrooms, 100 g day lily, 50 g water chestnuts.

SEASONING: 4 g salt, 10 g fresh coriander, 10 g sesame oil, 60 g peanut oil, 12 g starch, 8 g Cong-bai (Welsh onion), 2 g black pepper.

STEPS:

(1) Place Di-gu-pi in 500 ml water, bring to a boil, then simmer until water is reduced to 250 ml; strain to obtain herbal soup.

(2) Quarter each tomato, halve the shiitake mushrooms and water chestnuts, and separate coriander stems from the leaves.

(3) Over high heat, boil day lily in 2 cups of water until the water is reduced by half; strain to obtain clear soup.

(4) Pour peanut oil into a hot frying pan, add the Cong-bai (Welsh onion), day lily broth, herbal soup, salt, tofu, shiitake mushrooms, and water chestnuts, and boil for 5 minutes. Add coriander stems, tomato, and starch, and cook until you have a thick tomato stew.

(5) Remove from heat and add sesame oil, black pepper, and coriander leaves before eating.

CONSUMPTION: have as a side dish at mealtimes, twice a week for two months.

INDICATIONS: allergy, pneumonia, tracheitis, low fever in chronic and consumptive diseases such as pulmonary tuberculosis and pneumonia.

ANALYSIS: Di-gu-pi, an anti-inflammatory and anti-allergy herb, has been found to be effective in the treatment of chronic urticaria (hives), drug allergy, allergic purpura, contact dermatitis, lymphatic tuberculosis, and pneumonia. One research study reports that among the 150 cases of malaria treated by this herb, 145 cases were quickly brought under control. In addition, this herb is also effective for hypertension and diabetes. Tomato is a vegetable and also a fruit; it can clear heat and produce fluids, and is good for thirst, as in diabetes.

Conversion Table
(Approximate Equivalents)

Gram	Ounce	Milliliter	Cup	Teaspoon	Tablespoon
1	0.03	1		1/4	
2	0.07	2			
3	0.11	3			
4	0.14	4			
5	0.18	5		1	
6	0.21	6			
7	0.25	7			
8	0.28	8			
9	0.32	9			
10	0.35	10		2	1/2
11	0.39	11			
12	0.42	12		3	
13	0.45	13			
14	0.49	14		4	1
15	0.53	15			
25	0.88			7	2
35	1.23				
45	1.59				3
55	1.94		1/4		4
65	2.29				
75	2.64				
85	3.00				
95	3.35				
100	3.53				
115	4.06		1/2		
125	4.41	130			
150	5.30				
175	6.18				
200	7.05				
225	8		1		16
250	8.82				
300	10.58				
350	12.34				
400	14.11				
450	15.87				
453.6	16.00		2		
500	17.64				
600	21.16				
700	24.69				
800	28.22				
900	30.75				
1000	35.27	1040			